HOME HEALTH CARE FOR GERIATRICS

About the Authors

Dr. Ramandeep Bawa is working as Assistant Professor (Guest Faculty) in University Institute of Fashion Technology, Panjab University, Chandigarh. She is Ph.D., Post Doctoral fellow (fellowship grant received from Indian Council of Social Science Research) in the Centre for Advanced Studies in Anthropology at Panjab University, Chandigarh, India. She is M.Sc. in Clothing and Textiles and MBA in Marketing. She has over 8 years of experience in Research and Teaching and over 3 years of industrial experience as a Senior Merchandiser.

She has authored one book and has a total of 25 research articles published in National and International journals and has presented over 15 research papers in various National and International seminars/conferences/symposium. She was also working as a Group head with 'Hauz Health Care Services', a franchise of LIFE CIRCLE SENIOR SERVICES in partnership with 'GROUPE SOS FRANCE'.

Dr. A.K. Sinha is currently working as an ICSSR Senior Fellow. He was Professor in Social Anthropology, Panjab University, Chandigarh. To his credit are more than one hundred and ninety publications. He has authored 8 books, co-authored five books and edited five volumes. He has been teaching Social Anthropology since 1987. His major interests include Tribal studies, Anthropology of food, Panchayati Raj Institutions, Gender Studies and Medical Anthropology.

HOME HEALTH CARE FOR GERIATRICS

Challenges, Experiences and Wellness

Ramandeep Bawa
A.K. Sinha

CONCEPT PUBLISHING COMPANY PVT. LTD.
NEW DELHI - 110 059

ISBN: 978-93-6344-977-0

First Published 2025

Published and Printed by

Concept
Since 1974

Concept Publishing Company Pvt. Ltd.
A/15-16, Commercial Block, Mohan Garden
New Delhi-110059 (India)
T: +91-11-41101460
E: publishing@conceptpub.com, *W*: www.conceptpub.com

Cataloging in Publication--Courtesy: D.K. Agencies (P) Ltd. <docinfo@dkagencies.com>

Bawa, Ramandeep, author.
Home health care for geriatrics : challenges, experiences and wellness / Ramandeep Bawa, A.K. Sinha.
pages cm
Study conducted in Chandigarh, Panchkula in Haryana and Mohali in Punjab of India.
Includes bibliographical references and index.
ISBN 9789363449770

1. Older people--Home care--India--Chandīgarh. 2. Older people--Home care-India --Panchkula. 3. Older people--Home care--India--Mohali. 4. Older people--Medical care--India--Chandīgarh. 5. Older people--Medical care--India--Panchkula. 6. Older people --Medical care--India--Mohali. 7. Caregivers--India--Chandīgarh. 8. Caregivers--India--Panchkula. 9. Caregivers--India--Mohali. I. Sinha, Anil Kishore, author. II. Title.

LCC HV1484.I4B39 2025 | DDC 362.60954 23

Preface

Within the world of healthcare, there exists a field often overshadowed by the bustling corridors of hospitals and clinics—a world where care goes beyond the confines of institutional walls and finds its true essence in the comfort of one's own home. This is the world of home care, where caregivers, also known by other titles such as personal care assistants or general duty assistants, and nursing staffs play a key role in nurturing the health and well-being of individuals in need.

In the pages that follow, we research into the heart of home care, delving into the multifaceted nature of this service. From the meticulous tasks of hygiene maintenance to the support provided to patients and families, caregivers, nurses and doctors uphold the spirit of compassion and dedication that defines the field.

Amidst the exploration, the profound impact of the COVID-19 pandemic on the healthcare landscape cannot be ignored. As we evaluated the pandemic's effects on the healthcare system in India, we witnessed health care facilities facing a dual challenge: addressing the needs of COVID-19 patients while ensuring timely care for non-COVID patients, especially those with chronic conditions. To tackle the situation, many home care providers, hospitals, and agencies levelled up their operations, extending home health care services to vulnerable patients. This shift not only reduced strain on hospital resources but also provided patients with opportunity for high-quality care at lower prices.

Indeed, home care services have emerged as an essential component of patient care. An integrated approach, accompanied with tele-consultations and diagnostic modalities at home, promises a bright future for home health care services. To ensure successful and long term care for the elderly, the agencies should understand the demand and value for trained manpower.

Through the lens of caregiver narratives, patient perspectives, and the evolving landscape of healthcare. The authors aims to shed light on the transformative power of home care and support these unsung heroes who embody the essence of care, compassion, and humanity in its purest form. The authors endeavours' to built a model that focus on the experiences of home care workers, the emotional stress they face at their work place, the conditions under which they perform their duty and the support they require from the clients, their family members and agencies.

The lack of health care for the elderly is a matter of grave concern. The state of the elderly in the country is such that they are without any social or health safety nets in the sunset years of their lives. Among this section, the most deprived are the ones which are bedbound or in need of home care round the clock.

With these perspectives in sight, the book is an attempt to help the readers understand the state of the home health care sector highlighting the role, responsibilities, experiences and burden of patients, family caregivers, nurses and personal care assistants in home care.

Happy Reading

Ramandeep Bawa
A.K. Sinha

Acknowledgements

Dedicated to three handsome guys in my life, my soul-mate Rameet and adorable sons, Anshveer and Ayaansh.

My sincere thanks to my Parents and all Family members.

Special thanks to the lovely children in my family – Sehaj, Mehak, Mehar, Riva, Pragunn and Gurshabad.

Ramandeep Bawa

Contents

List of Plates, Tables, Figures and Maps

PLATES

TABLES

FIGURES

Maps

1

Home Health Care for the Elderly Population

We make a living by what we get, but we make a life by what we give.

–Winston Churchill.

1.1 Elderly Health

A dramatic demographic transition has been observed in the past 50 years in India (the world's second most populous country), showing the tripling of the older population over the age of 60 years (Government of India, 2011). This pattern of increase in the elderly population is poised to continue. It is also estimated that the proportion of Indians aged 60 and older will rise from 7.5 per cent in 2010 to 11.1 per cent in 2025 (United Nations Department of Economic and Social Affairs [UNDESA], 2008).However, this percentage that seems too small in absolute terms is indeed a remarkable figure. According to a report by Price Waterhouse Coopers, an estimated 189 million people in the country will be more than 60 years of age by 2025 needing higher health care services.[1,2] According to UN by 2050 the population of 60 and older in India would likely go up to 20 per cent.[3] India's demographic structure is expected to shift dramatically from a young to an aging population resulting in 316 million elderly persons by 2050.[4]

This high at-risk elderly population is afflicted with multiple chronic diseases like anaemia, chest pain, chronic bronchitis, diabetes, digestive disorders, high blood pressure, kidney problems, vision problems, rheumatism, and depression (Angra *et al.*, 1997; Kumari and Sarasa, 2001; Raju, 2000; Roy, 1994; Shah and Prabhakar, 1997). However, cardiovascular diseases are the major cause of death among the elderly (Jha *et al.*, 2006).

As the conceptual model of elderly health in India is being developed, we have begun with a perusal of the larger health scenario in India while finding that "health care, far from helping people rise out of poverty, has become an important cause of household impoverishment and debt, the average national health indicators, though showing improvements in the recent decade, hide vast regional and social disparities." Although, in this scenario, some privileged individuals enjoy excellent health outcomes, while others have experienced "the worst imaginable conditions" (Patel *et al.*, 2011).

Among the elderly population, several barriers to good health are observed. These range from pathological progression (Lynch *et al.*, 2009) to nuclearization of family, dependency (Gupta and Sankar, 2002; Rajan and Prasad, 2008), and reductions in earning potential (Selvaraj *et al.*, 2010). Although, there is a trend of feminization of the elderly population; according to the 2001 Census reports the gender ratio among the Indian elderly aged 60 years and older is 1,028 females for 1,000 males (Rajan and Aiyar, 2008). It is, however, expected that by 2016, 51 per cent of the elderly Indian population will be women (Kumari and Sarasa, 2001; Rao, 2006). It is also an observed fact that most women report poor health status as compared to males, however, a greater proportion of men are hospitalized as compared to females (87 *versus* 67 per 1,000 aged persons) (Rajan and Sreerupa, 2008).

Unmet health needs are a cause of concern as was witnessed among the 33.1 per cent of the elderly population in India who in 2001reported to have lost their spouses (Rajan and Aiyar, 2008), of whom a larger proportion of the population were females. It was also noticed that 50 per cent of the female elderly were widows *versus* only 15 per cent of elderly males were widowers. Many studies have reflected that widows are disproportionately vulnerable to disability, illness, and poor health care utilization (Sreerupa, 2006) due to a variety of mobility, employment, property, and financial constraints (Dreze, 1990).

Along with the stigma of aging, this elderly population also faces other social and health conditions such as depression, dementia, depression, incontinence lack of voluntary control over urination, or widowhood, as social barriers to health, which are manifested in Indian society in different and unique ways (World Health Organization [WHO], 2002).

Now-a-days the concept of "living apart but together" is a common prevalence. This implies that living in joint families has been discontinued, which has a negative implication on the health of the elderly as in times of health crisis, it is the family one seeks and strong social support should be immediately available (Sokolovsky, 2001). However, even this provision, if available would somewhere lead to "disclosure of neglect", where the needs and problems of the elderly are invisible to those who offer them support in terms of their acute health crises (Sokolovsky, 2001). It is also indicated through research in our country that it is not the number of family ties that matters but it is the quality of particularities that is related to health. Moreover, in some cases, having strong ties with a neighbour or a child may have a more health-protective impact than having many weaker ties with community members and the host of the family (Sudha *et al.*, 2006).

1.2 Concept of Home Health Care

Home-based health care goes far back in time. It has been present since the existence of the nursing and medical professions. Health care was always available to people in the form of house calls and this was the standard practice adopted by health care professionals long before the development of hospitals and office-based medical care (Landers *et al.*, 2016).

Home-based primary care is a model that makes use of home care physicians and nurse practitioners, in connection with an interdisciplinary team of professionals, including skilled home health professionals. "Home-based primary care" and "hospital-at-home" are models of care provided at home to serve patients with health conditions that are sometimes acute, or severe depending upon the health problem. The skills needed to provide these services increase accordingly. The hospital-at-home models serves hospital home admissions for those patients who need hospital-level care in the home. Those receiving this kind of highest acuity level of home-based care in the homes have experienced 19 per cent lower costs, and much higher satisfaction, and while compared with similar in-patients who are admitted to hospitals, home-care patients have shown much better care outcomes (Cryer, 2012).

"Medicare skilled home health care" or "home health care" refers to services offered by medicare-certified home health agencies under the medicare home health benefit. By contrast, "home-based care" refers to a wide array of different types of care provided in the home by a wide range of parties/agencies. Home-based care includes both formal caregiving and informal personal care services, Medicare skilled home health care (skilled nursing and therapy), physician house calls, and even "hospital-at-home" services (Landers *et al.*, 2016).

1.3 History and Origin of Home Health Care

In the early 19th century, taking care of the sick (who are chronically ill, or are dying) and giving birth were all considered part of domestic life, while hospitals were meant for those patients (for their last resort)who did not have any families. Families with good finances tend to hire doctors, nurses, or midwives to serve the patient's in their homes.

Home care was started by "The Charleston Ladies Benevolent Society" in 1813. Benevolent ladies (serving a charitable rather than profit-making purpose) across the United States started organizations for helping the sick and poor people and provided medical care, and other types of charitable help, to the "worthy" poor. These organizations trained nurses and provided care to the sick and poor people thus preventing the spread of any contagious diseases.

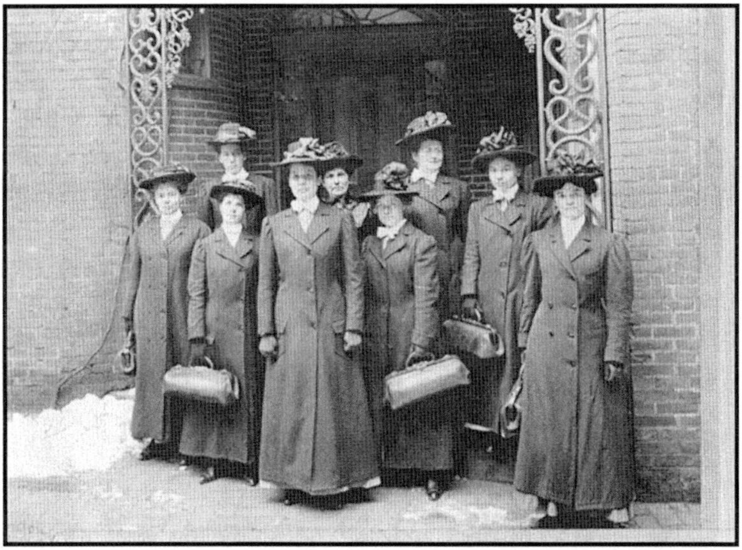

Plate 1.1: Nurses outside their office ready to serve the chronically ill patients ready for the day's work. Visiting Nurse Society of Philadelphia, c.1909.

Source: https://www.nursing.upenn.edu/live/image/gid/97/width/650/src_region/0,0,634,450/3931_visiting_nurses_outside_their_offices.jpg

From the very beginning, the realization of serving chronic patients was the sole responsibility of these organizations. However, still, these organizations were vexed with questions like which of the chronically ill patients requires immediate care, how long the patient be taken care of and what type of care should be provided. Along with the handling of these three critical questions, The Ladies

Benevolent Society struggled with the family circumstances and chronic illness of the patients. The chronically ill challenged the economic finances of the organization and discharging the needy chronically ill patients violated the basic norms of duty of this benevolent society. It was a tough task for society to distinguish who deserved care among the chronically ill.

As this society's mission was to serve patients in acute distress, they limited their care to the patients who were provided with the certificate of medical necessity. The nursing ladies later concluded that some problems could not be taken care of at home. The mid-century saw the launch of Charleston's hospital which offered alternatives to various care continuums which cannot be cared of at home. Charleston's continuous efforts to deliver home care, especially to the poor and needy remained an excellent protocol on the landscape of the United States. By the end of the 19th century, Industrialization, Urbanization, Immigration of population, and the continuous rise of infectious diseases turned the aura of larger cities into unhealthy places to live (Wilkerson, 2001; 2007).

1.3.1 *The Visiting Nurse Arrives as a Legacy of Home Care*

Guided by the English precedent and inspired by Florence Nightingale, the introduction of the words 'visiting nurse' was a precedent step towards social and religious obligation dominating the activities of earlier generations like the ladies of Charleston. The image of nurse climbing a tenement (Plate 1.2) (a large building divided into apartments, usually in poor areas of a city)and protect society from dangerous infectious diseases appealed to numerous century reformers.

By 1909, over 600 organizations were sponsoring the work of visiting nurses. Visiting nurses appealed to the emerging society striving for leadership and recognition. Their work for the societal uplift enhanced the status of the nurse who was working, in the homes of the poor, nurses at this time occupied the centre stage and attained a distinct position within society. Wealthy ladies managed and supervised the care provided by their nurses to the patients.

Nurses were expected to be eminent practitioners in their work – showing patience, humour, good judgment, and the required scientific knowledge for the care of the sick. But as the work grew, these organizations could not survive under few volunteers who were donating time for a good cause. Lady managers reluctantly recognized that their organizations required revamping and redefinition of authority. Nurse Superintendent was the new name for the management of any organization providing care for the sick. These nursing superintendents were well-educated and belong to good families. They have a sympathetic attitude and a clear vision of the future. As the nurses began to dominate home care, the lady managers finally receded in the background (Wilkerson, 2001; 2007).

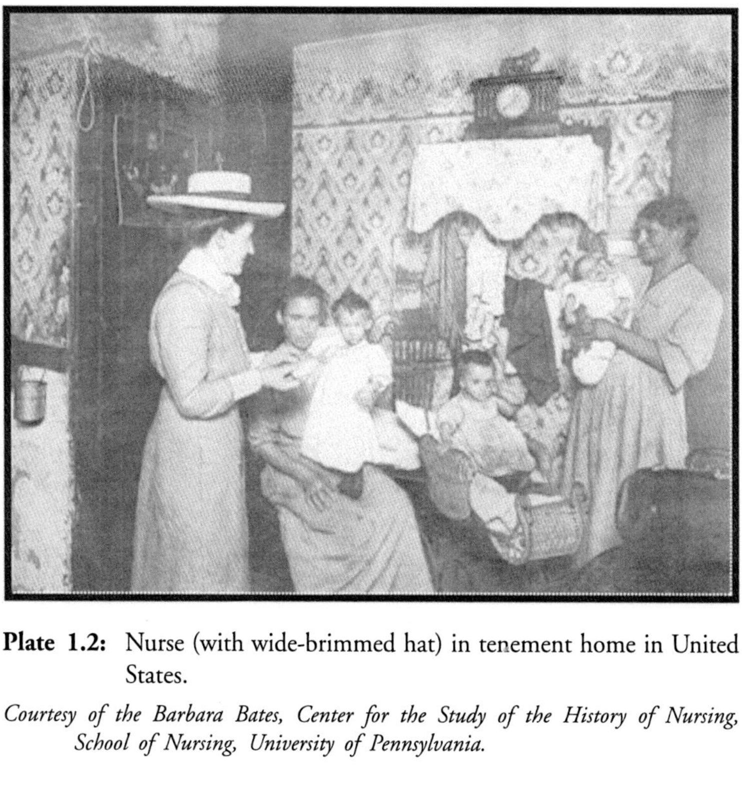

Plate 1.2: Nurse (with wide-brimmed hat) in tenement home in United States.

Courtesy of the Barbara Bates, Center for the Study of the History of Nursing, School of Nursing, University of Pennsylvania.

1.3.2 Nurses at Home

Nurses who found patients alone at home simply took charge and exercised considerable authority over the patient. On daily rounds, visiting nurses attended to the patient's medical needs, and environment, and took care of their nourishment. They helped patients in emergencies, gave necessary treatments, bought the latest portable medical equipment, provided health education to all age groups, and welcomed visitors. Their patients were mostly women, children, men, mothers, newborns, workers, elderly, and the injured.

In addition to general care, these nurses also contributed clothes, food, child care, housekeeping services, and assistance to exhausted families from caregiving responsibilities.

1.3.3 Lillian Wald and Professionalization of Visiting Nurses

Lillian Wald demonstrated a new concept for patient care at home, she invented the term public health nurse to describe a nursing practice that considered sickness within its social and economic context. She considered that the duties of the nurse were not only to provide bedside care to the sick but they should also be able to identify the underlying cause of misery and illness. Wald was truly credited with the professionalization of visiting nurses.

She possessed a charismatic ability to analyze overwhelming problems that resulted in innovative remedies. Like her colleagues, she discovered that to care for the sick, much more is required than medicines. As a public health nurse, she secured reforms in industry, health, education, recreation, and housing.

1.3.4 Introducing Home Care Insurance Coverage

Among Wald's most innovative and remarkable works, the highlight was the establishment of insurance cover for home care. Wald convinced the Metropolitan Life Insurance (MLI) Company to regulate the cost-effectiveness of its policies. For a moderate amount, MLI included the benefit of a visiting nurse (Plate 1.3) and in the long term, reducing the number of death benefits. This experiment was a huge success.

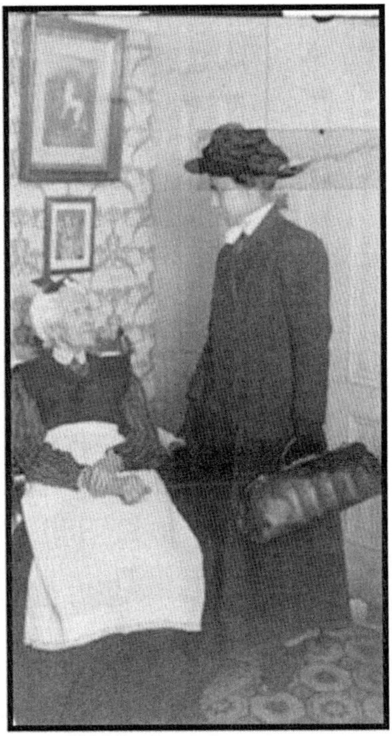

Plate 1.3: Visiting nurse with the patient in the home, Visiting Nurse Society of Philadelphia, c.1910.

As of 1913, this insurance company supported 20 to 30 per cent of the annual budget of many visiting nurse associations. Although in 1916, the visiting nurse service was available to maximum policy holders, it was estimated that about 221,566 policyholders received care of over one million visits made by the nursing staff. While the visiting nurse associations were satisfied and contented with MLI's financial support, they were less interested in conducting their work and were much oriented towards making a business out of it. Ultimately, visiting nurse associations found the transition from benevolent factor to the most cost-effective care in conflict with their mission and values. MLI publically claimed that their nursing service saved lives and money while privately; they were more concerned about the business part of the visiting nurse association. Furthermore, nurses always placed the care of the sick over cost containment, which proved uncontrollable in the view of MLI. By 1920, MLI denied payment to nurses, this figure was as high as 24 per cent. Naturally, the care of the chronically sick was a problem from a business perspective.

By 1920, there was a change in the health care system, hospitals became an indispensable institution and an accepted part of medical care. Policy holders now increasingly sought hospital care when they were seriously ill and lived longer (Wilkerson, 2001; 2007).

1.3.5 A New Home Care Movement—Federal Policy for Home Care

By the 1930s and 1940s, the locus of care for the chronically ill was compromised in the hospitals, and home care was preferred, this was considered a less expensive alternative to hospital care. Initially, it was concluded that only in the case of seriously sick patients where the coverage was limited, home care would a better option to be included in the insurance programmes. In the 1960s, finally, home care was included in medicare, medicaid, and the older American Act. It was through home care the hospital beds could be emptied that added to its inclusion in the medicare programme. This resulted in the arrival of a vast array of narrowly defined community-based services for the elderly. However, the outcome of services for the patients was very confusing with a wide assortment of programmes with different eligibility criteria, payment issues, the system of reimbursement, and also coverage limitations created a wide gap in the services people received when they had to stay at home because of their illness.

Over the years, the ambiguity over the interpretation of benefits had created the opportunity for home care providers to recast their medicare regulations and cater to a broader set of patient needs. On 1st October, 1997, the Balanced Budget Act of 1997 transformed the medicare home care benefit which had been enacted in 1965.

The outcome was over 3,000 agencies closed, the number of visits per patient was reduced and the public funding for the home care was dramatically reduced. Moreover, financial issues lead to fewer visits and a rapid transfer of care to the family members.

The professional home care staff (nurses and caregivers) provides a spectrum of services including professional caregiving, activities of daily living such as bathing, grooming, and dressing to technical services provided by nursing staff to serve, support, and empower patients and their families with their care. However, yet the burden of family caregiving yet remains a multifaceted issue (Wilkerson, 2001).

1.4 Delivering Health Care at Home—Role of Nurses and Caregivers

Home health care environment differs from hospitals and other institutional environments where nurses work. To begin with, home health care nurses work alone in the field with support resources available from a central office and spend more time on paperwork than hospital nurses, they also have to spend more time dealing with reimbursement issues (National Association for Home Health Care & Hospice, 2006; Anthony and Milone, 2005).

Caregivers fall into 2 broad categories: caregivers working on a payroll who are part of the formal health care sector (e.g., home care workers) and unpaid "informal" caregivers (usually family members) (Townsend *et al.*, 1990, Browne *et al.*, 1994, Addington-Hall *et al.*, 1992) who are motivated by a deeper commitment to the patient. Sergi-Swinehart (1985) has called this tradition of family caregiving fundamental to our society.

In the system of home health care, clinicians recognize that the care setting, i.e. the home is the inviolable domain of the patient. Therefore, compared to the hospitalized patient, home health care patient often has a greater role in determining how and even if certain interventions will be implemented. Professional clinicians have no authority over these caregivers. Further, the home environment and the intermittent nature of professional home health care services may limit the clinician's ability to observe the quality of care that informal caregivers deliver—unlike in the hospital, where care given by support staff may more easily be observed and evaluated.

When patients are discharged from the hospital and return home with the need for home nursing care, they move from highly supportive medical environments equipped with potentially many doctors, nurses, general duty assistants, and other professionals, to non-medical environments of the home with formal and informal caregiver support which is also supplemented by visits from home care nurses. It is also observed that both patients and caregivers mostly struggle to absorb the contradictory and confusing information imparted by multiple clinicians in the hospitals before discharge and by the home care nurses at home (Romagnoli, 2013).

The vast array of services provided at home are generally monitored and taken care of by the family caregivers, sometimes referred to as "informal services" (Johnson *et al.*, 2007). This phrase grossly underestimates the critical role family caregivers play in the care of patients at home. It is examined that among patients with multiple limitations on ADLs (activities of daily living), caregiving is crucial. Without caregivers at home, health care at home is rather impossible for those with functional limitations AARP (American Association of Retired Persons) investigated that 34.2 million adults alone served as caregivers in the year 2014 (AARP, 2015).

According to the Urban Institute's "The Retirement Project," in 2000, approximately about 2.2 million individuals received "formal personal care services," also defined as personal care services that are paid for by various means. This percentage has risen to 2.5 million in 2010 and was projected to increase to a mark of 2.9 million in 2020 (Johnson *et al.*, 2007).

1.5 Terminology

Nurse Officer: Based on the initial assessment of the elderly patient's requirements, a nurse officer prepares a patient care plan that includes a meditation plan, meals plan, exercise, massage, recreation, and daily routine. The nurse officer takes the patient's vitals on his/her visits to ensure the well-being of the patient. She/he also addresses the issues of the family regarding the home care attendants or nursing staff conduct. She/he is also responsible for placing a perfect nursing staff/caretaker as per the needs and requirements of the patient.

Nurse: A nurse is a licensed health care professional who practices independently or is supervised by a physician or surgeon, trained to look after sick or injured people.[5] The roles and responsibilities of nurses are further elaborated in Table 1.1.

Caregiver: A caregiver is a person who has received professional training or has prior experience in providing caregiving services to bedridden or chronically ill patients. The roles and responsibilities of caregivers are further elaborated in Table 1.1.

Patient: A person who receives treatment and diagnosis for a particular disease from health care professionals and the same is continued at home under the supervision of trained nurses and general duty assistants.

Client/Family Members: An individual who agrees to avail home health care services via a caregiver/nurse for himself/herself for their near ones.

Table 1.1: Roles and Responsibilities of Nurses and Caregivers Providing Home Care Services

Professional Caregiving Services	Home Nursing Services
Minimum qualification or experience required: Can be provided by GDA(General Duty assistant), Bed Side assistant, or Individuals who have adequate work experience.	**Minimum qualification or experience required:** Can be provided by ANM (Auxiliary Nurse Midwifery), GNM (General Nursing and Midwifery), or B.Sc. Nursing
Hygiene – Bed bath, hair grooming, denture care, eye, ear, and nose care, fingernail and toe nail care, perineal care for males and females	I.V cannula care and drug administration
Changing the patient's clothes	Blood sampling
Diaper changing	Tracheotomy care and Suctioning

(*Contd.*)

Professional Caregiving Services	Home Nursing Services
Assisting with commode, bedpan, and urinal	Urinary catheterization and catheter care
Repositioning bed-bound patients to help prevent bed sores	Oxygen administrator/concentrator/ CPAP/Portable ventilator at home
Mobility aids assistance	Medication administration
Assisting with oral medications	Checking vital parameters—Temperature, pulse, respiratory rate, blood pressure, blood oxygen level, and blood sugar (Insulin administration)
Assist in physiotherapy/daily exercises	Home Naso-gastric tube feeding
Basic food preparation for the patient (Dalia, khichdi, tea, milk, bread, boiled eggs, etc.) and recreational activities	Wound dressing
Home Naso-gastric tube feeding	Assist in physiotherapy/daily exercises
Checking vital parameters-Temperature, pulse, respiratory rate, blood pressure, blood oxygen level, and blood sugar (Insulin administration)	

Source: Life Circle Senior Services.

1.6 Role and Responsibilities of Caregivers

A caregiver is also known as the personal care assistant or general duty assistant who cares for the health and well-being of the individuals/patients who require help for the performance of daily tasks and activities. Depending on the level of support required, the responsibilities and duties of caregivers include maintenance of hygiene of the patient (Bed bath, Hair grooming, Denture care, Eye, Ear, and Nose care, fingernail and Toenail care, Perineal care for males and females), dressing, changing diapers, assisting with commode, bedpan, and urinal, repositioning bed-bound patients to help prevent bed sores, walking assistance and fall prevention. Additionally, caregiver activities also include assisting with oral medication, physiotherapy/daily exercises, Basic food preparation for the patient and recreational activities, checking vital parameters, and feeding through the nasogastric tube.

1.6.1 Hygiene of the Patient

Hygiene of the patient involves cleansing the skin, mouth, teeth, hair, nails, eyes, ears, nose, perineal area, and feet. All activities of daily living are performed by caregivers depending upon the underlying condition of the patients.

Purpose

- To reduce the risk of infection.
- To provide comfort.

Bed Bath

- Clean head to toe, front to back, distal to proximal.
- Secure I.V. lines for moving and turning patient.
- Use different sponge clothes for different areas.
- Change the water if cold or spoiled or very soapy.
- Change linen as needed.
- Do range of motion as needed.
- Do oral care, hair care, nail care.
- Leave bed in a low position, side rails up, and call bell in place.
- Report and document findings.

Hair Grooming/Care

- Ask the individual if he or she has a preference for his or her hairstyle that day.
- Teach and assist with drying wet hair with a towel/dryer.
- If the hairs are long, divide them into sections before combing or brushing.

Denture/Oral Care

- Depending on the condition of the patient's mouth, clean the dentures.

- Unconscious patients have no gag reflex, and position on their side for care.
- Assess whether the patient needs assistance with oral care.
- Assess for abnormalities, loose or missing teeth, swelling, and bleeding of gums.
- Check for unusual mouth odour.
- Provide mouth care by mouth care solutions as per recommended percentage and rinse with clean water.

Care of Eyes

- Clean eyes with a wet and warm cotton ball or clean cloth.
- Contact lenses are usually to be removed and stored in saline liquid.

Ear and Nose

- Wash external ear with wash clothed-covered finger.
- Clean nose by asking the patient to blow and remove crusted secretions in and around nose.

Fingernail and Toenail Care

Clean and trimmed fingernails and toenails are important for overall health. Germs often collect underneath the nails, frequent and thorough hand washing and foot care is a good way to prevent germs or fungus build-up. Toenails and fingernails should be kept clean, neatly trimmed, and smooth to prevent skin injury.

- Cleaning and trimming nails.
- Individuals with diabetes require professional assistance with nail care.
- Encourage individuals to do as much as they can for themselves.

Perineal Care for Males

- Explain to the individual to hold his penis and wash and rinse the tip.

- Always wash from the small opening (urethra) where that urine flows, outward or towards the end of the penis.
- Use a different cloth to wipe the urethral opening and dry thoroughly.
- Teach the individual to wash, rinse and dry the shaft of the penis.
- Moisture between skin folds may cause cracking of the skin and skin breakdown.

Perineal Care for Females

- Put on disposable gloves.
- Separate the folds of skin in her genitals, called the labia, and using the washcloth, wash with one down stroke the sides of the labia.
- Using a different side of the washcloth, wash down the middle of the labia. Rinse from front to back.
- Always wash from the pubic area (front of the genitals) to the anal area to prevent contaminating the urethral opening (where the urine comes out) with germs or bacteria from the anal area.
- Teach the individual to wash and rinse the anal area, moving front to back.
- Use a different part of the washcloth for each wipe.

1.6.2 Changing Patient Clothes

After cleansing all the areas of skin, mouth, teeth, hair, nails, eyes, ears, nose, perineal area, and feet, the next step involves dressing the patient.

Important Caregiver Tips

- While dressing a patient, it is important to make them feel comfortable.
- Always encourage the patients to dress/undress unless and until the interference is required if they face any difficulty in changing.

- Patient's generally do not prefer wearing shoes all the time, it is advisable to use slip-resistant slippers and putting a pair of gripper socks while going to sleep as they will benefit during nighttime going to the washroom.
- Adaptations to their clothing such as snap buttons or magnets instead of buttons and zippers can eliminate the struggle of dressing and make them more independent.

1.6.3 Changing Diapers

Changing diapers is important as it prevents the perineal area from rashes and pressure sores.

Procedure for Changing an Adult Diaper

- Wash hands thoroughly with soap and warm water.
- Put on a pair of medical gloves.
- Raise the bed to a height following the comfort of the patient.
- Ease the patient onto their sides, and gently bend their knees towards the chest.
- Unfasten the diapers and roll the diapers inwards, tuck any mess inside when rolling.
- Once the diaper is removed, throw it in the trash bag.
- Use moistened wipes for cleaning the area from front to back and make sure that all the skin folds are clean and dry.
- Apply skin creams to the buttock area, and carefully visualize the skin for any bedsores.
- Position the diaper, tucking it a little under the hips, and close the diaper using the tabs.
- Removing gloves, and dispose them.

1.6.4 Assisting with Commode, Bedpan and Urinal

The patient who are bedridden are assisted by the caregiver with the commode, bedpan and urinal at home.

Assisting with the Commode (Procedure to be followed)

- Be careful while shifting the patient from bed or chair onto the commode.
- Make sure the wheels on the commode are locked.
- One should be careful, that they don't lose balance while sitting down on the commode.
- For cleaning, wet wipes are better than toilet paper. Be sure to clean the area from front to back.
- In case the caregiver have used gloves, remove them and throw it in the trash bag.
- Help the patient stand up off the commode.
- Empty the commode bucket into the toilet.
- Rinse and wash the commode bucket using a disinfectant diluted with water.
- Wash and dry your hands.

Bedpan (Procedure to be followed)

- Washing of hands and putting on gloves.
- Covering the patient with a sheet or blanket while taking off their pants/lowers and underwear.
- Sprinkle a small amount of talcum powder on the bed pan so that it can easily slide under the buttocks.
- Make sure to hold the bedpan (Plate 1.4) in place and ensure use of moistened wipes to clean the patient.
- Empty the bedpan in the toilet.
- Rinse and wash the bedpan with a disinfected diluted with water.

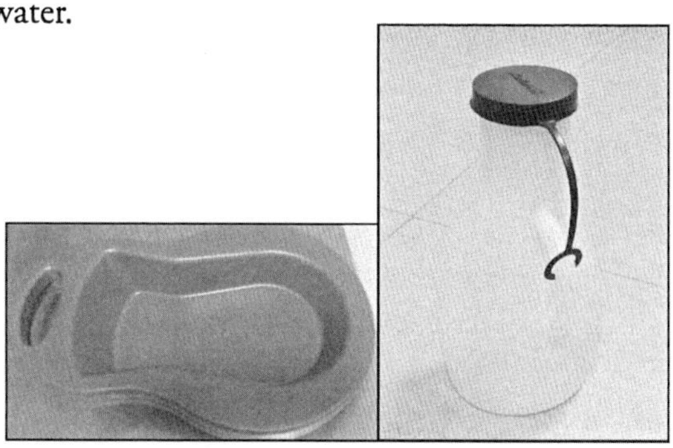

Plate 1.4: Bedpan and Urinal.

Urinals

In case of putting urinals (Plate 1.4), between their legs, spread the legs. If the patient needs help, one should hold the urinal while they urinate.

1.6.5 Repositioning Bed-Bound Patients to Help Prevent Bed Sores

Repositioning is defined as the movement of patients from one position to another in an effort to prevent pressure on any part of the body.

Guidelines for Repositioning the Patients

- Repositioning a bedridden patient is followed by the "Rule of 30".
- The Rule of 30 means that the head of the bed is elevated at not more than 30 degrees angle from the horizontal position and the body is placed in 30 degrees.
- The patient's hips and shoulders should be tilted at 30 degrees from the supine.
- Make use of pillows to reduce pressure over the hips or buttocks. Also, ensure that the patient's ankles, knees and elbows are not resting on each other.

1.6.6 Mobility Aids Assistance

Mobility aids are devices to help people who have disabilities or injuries and elderly adults who are at risk of falling. Common types of mobility aids include canes, crutches, walkers and wheel chairs.

Important Steps to be Taken

- Exercises for balance and strength.
- Regular vision check-up.
- Keeping the floor clutter free.
- Remove small rugs from the floor to prevent slipping.
- Add side rails or bars near the bathing area or next to the toilet area for additional support.

1.6.7 Oral Medications

Oral administration of medications is defined as preparing, administering and duration of medications.

Important Things to Remember

- Explain about drug, duration, action and side effects to the patient.
- Hand hygiene to be followed.
- Make sure that the patient is in an upright position, never give pills or liquids in lying down position.
- Take tablets or capsules into medication cup. Tablets or capsules are not to be taken in hand.
- Offer fluids before administering tablets or capsules to facilitate administration and prevent them from sticking to the sides of the patient's mouth.
- Patients who wear dentures may not be aware of the presence of medication in the mouth. Inspect the mouth to ensure all medications have been swallowed.
- Give one pill at a time.
- If the food interferes with the absorption of the drugs, administer between meals or an empty stomach.
- Stay with the patient to make sure that all medications are being taken and swallowed.

1.6.8 Assist in Physiotherapy/Daily Exercises

Physical therapy exercises are designed to help patients maintain and restore their physical health. The elderly population who had an accident, or undergone surgery or stroke are required to receive physiotherapy exercises for strengthening their muscles, improvement in motion, and reduce pain (Plate 1.6). For example, if the patients have undergone any hip or knee replacement surgery, they need to put heat pads or sometimes ice packs to relieve the pain. In (Plate 1.5), Ultrasound therapy is used for pain management, inflammation, and swelling.

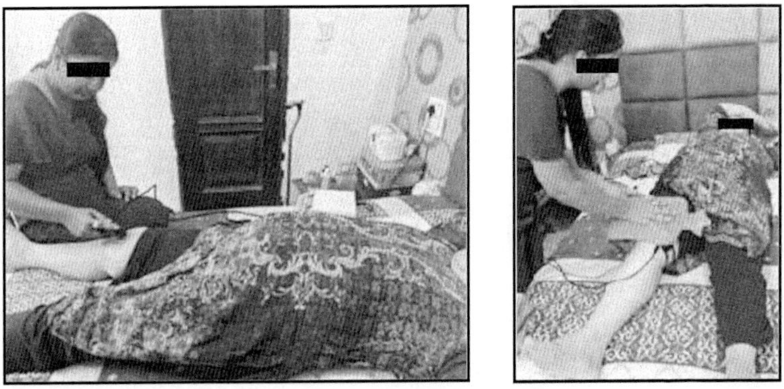

Plate 1.5: Ultra sound machine and heat pads used for relieving pain in the knees.

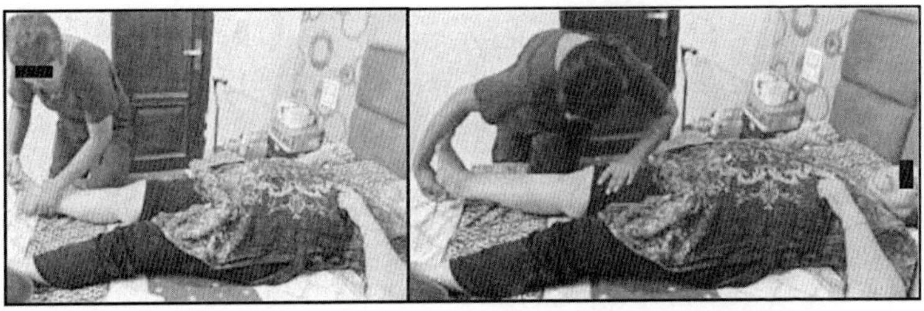

Plate 1.6: Leg strengthening and stretching exercises at home.

1.6.9 Basic Food Preparation for the Patient, Shopping and Recreational Activities

A caregiver helps the family in preparing meals for the patient. Basic food includes dalia, khichdi, tea, milk, bread, boiled eggs etc. They bring groceries and other food items, take them to the park, play board games for memory development, give an ear to their life experiences and act as their companions.

1.6.10 Naso-Gastric Tube Feeding

It is the introduction of complete liquid formula directly into the stomach or small intestine *via* a narrow, specially designed tube, in the presence of a functioning gut. Feeding through the tube is administered by both nurses and caregivers in home care.

Indicators

- Patients are unable to maintain adequate oral intake to meet metabolic demands.
- Surgical cases.
- Patients on ventilator.
- Cases of neurological dysfunction.

Feeding Position

- The patient should be elevated to an angle of at least 30-45 degrees during and after feeding for at least one hour (Plate 1.7).

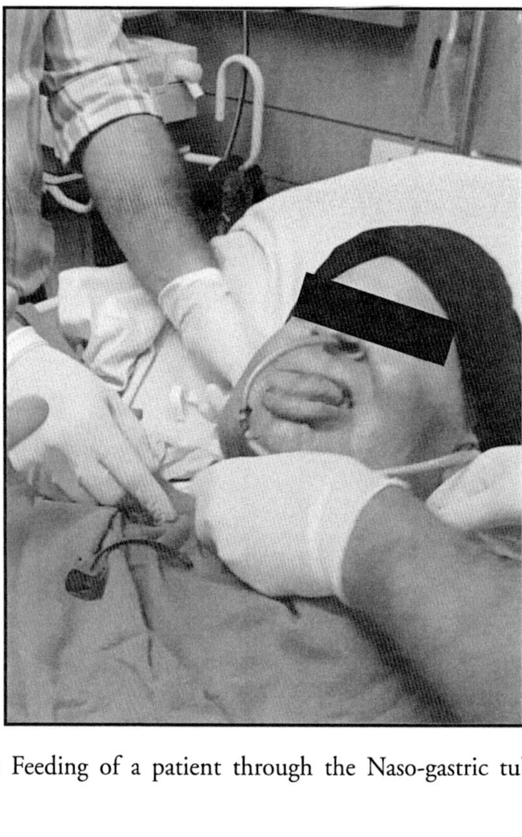

Plate 1.7: Feeding of a patient through the Naso-gastric tube.

Procedure

- Wash hands and put on clean gloves.
- Note the type, amount, and frequency of feedings.
- Assess residual feeding contents – aspirate all the stomach contents, and measure the amount prior to administering the feeding.
- Attach a feeding bag to the ryle's tube.
- Feed is to be given after every 2-4 hours as advised by physician.
- Client comfort and safety to be ensured.
- After each feeding bag along with the tube is to be cleaned with lukewarm water and changing the bag is to be ensured as per protocol.

1.7 Role and Responsibilities of Nurses

Based on the initial assessment of the elderly patient's requirements, a nurse officer prepares a patient care plan that includes a meditation plan, meals plan, exercise, massage, recreation, and daily routine. Their responsibility also includes addressing any issue that the family may have regarding the home care attendants or the conduct of the nursing staff. Various procedures are handled by home care nurses in patients' homes, depending upon the underlying condition of the patients. These nursing home care services include helping the patients with IV cannula care, blood sampling, feeding through a nasogastric tube, urinary catheter care, tracheostomy, medication administration, oxygen administration/concentrator, and checking on the vital parameters – Temperature, assessment of pulse, respiration, blood oxygen level, blood pressure, and blood sugar. Nurses monitor the patient vitals to ensure the well-being of the patient and document the same in the vital check sheet. The patient care plan outlines the patient personal details, monitoring of vital parameters, caregiver services to be provided or any special instructions to be given, and medication management. Table 1.2 presents a layout for the patient care plan prepared by the nurse manager/nursing staff.

Table 1.2: Patient Care Plan

Patient Personal Details		
Name		
Age		
Gender		
Important Contact Number		
Patient's Condition and Illness		
Allergy (if any)		
Any Infectious Disease		

a. Vital Chart

Vitals	**Date**	**Value**	**Tracking Frequency (Monthly/ weekly)**	**Acceptable Range**
Blood Pressure		mmHg		
Temperature		F		
Heart Rate/Pulse		Breaths per minute (bpm)		
Respiration Rate		Beats per minute (bpm)		
sPO_2		%		
Random Blood Sugar		Mg/dl		

b. Care Schedule

Time	**Services to be Provided**	**Notes**	
Caregiver Special Instruction			

(*Contd.*)

c. Medicine Management

S. No.	Timing	Medicine Name and Dose (Example: Tab Dolo 650 mg)	Dose (1 Tab or 1 Capsule or 1 spoon or 1 Repulse)	When Medicine is taken after breakfast/after lunch/before lunch/empty stomach/before breakfast/at bedtime

Source: Life circle Senior Services.

1.7.1 IV Cannulation and Drug Administration

Peripheral intravenous cannulation (Plate 1.8) is the most commonly used procedure for patients. They are primarily used for therapeutic purposes such as the administration of medications, fluids, and/or blood products as well as blood sampling. It is the insertion of a flexible tube containing a needle into blood vessels, usually the peripheral blood vessels.

Purpose

- To maintain fluid and electrolyte balance.
- To provide a large volume of fluid.
- To inject continuous or intermittent medications.
- To provide nutrition.

Indications

Fluid and electrolyte replacement, administration of medicines, administration of blood/blood products, and administration of total parental nutrition.

Cannula Related Factors

When considering the choice of the cannula, consideration should be given to the following:

- Minimizing discomfort to the patient.
- Ensuring good flow rates.
- The cannula to be used clinically should preferably be the safety cannula.
- Select the cannula based on the intended purpose and duration of use.
- Select the cannula based on the size of the vein to be cannulated.

Preparation of Patient

- Hands should be clean, having been washed before the procedure, and/or using alcohol-based hand rub applied to the hands before donning a pair of gloves.
- Explain to the patients about the procedure and purpose of the therapy.
- Assess for the ability to avoid movement of arms or hands for the duration of the procedure.
- Allergic history should be enquired.
- The patient should be positioned comfortably with the arm on a flat surface.
- Ensuring a no-touch technique for any part of the needle or cannula which is to puncture the patient's skin.

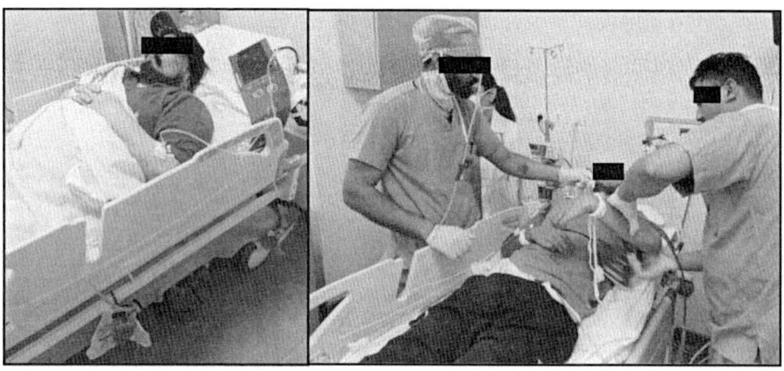

Plate 1.8: IV cannula care at home in the presence of a nurse supervisor and trained nurses.

Resting or Removal of Cannula

- Perform hand hygiene.
- Wear gloves.
- Use sterile gauze.
- Apply pressure for approx. 2-3 minutes.
- Inspect the cannula to ensure it is complete and undamaged.
- Apply appropriate dressing.
- Dispose of the cannula into the bin.
- Perform hand hygiene.

1.7.2 Blood Sampling

It is the collection of blood by pricking the skin and drawing blood from one of the veins/arteries are blood vessels that are present under the surface of the skin.

Principle

Collection of the blood sample from patients by venipuncture or by the arterial puncture.

One has to identify and prepare the patient, where the patient is an adult, and consciously follow the steps outlined are discussed as follows:

- The patient should be made comfortable in a supine position (if possible).
- A clean paper or towel should be placed under the patient's arm.
- The patient's condition should be verified. Fasting, dietary restricts, medications, timing and medical treatment are all of concern.
- The patient should be checked for any allergies to antiseptics and adhesives.
- They should not be pricked on the same side when they have an AV fistula (for dialysis)/Mastectomy (Cancer of the breast).
- Hands should be washed with soap and water and dried.
- The used needle and syringe should be discarded in a separate bag.

- At last, the blood sample should be sent to the labouratory.

1.7.3 Tracheostomy Care

Tracheostomy (Plate 1.9) is the formation of an opening into the trachea usually between the second and third rings of cartilage.

Indications

Prevention/treatment of trachea-bronchial secretions, chronic upper airway obstruction (cancer of upper airway, i.e. vocal cords, trachea), bypass acute upper airway obstruction (severe allergic reaction).

Types of Tracheostomy

1. A temporary tracheostomy can be formed when patients require long-term respiratory support or are unable to protect their airways. A tracheostomy tube will be inserted to maintain the patency of the airway. This can be removed when the patient recovers and it may become long-term if the patient's condition requires this.
2. A permanent tracheostomy is created where the trachea is bought out to the surface of the skin and sutured to the neck wall. A stoma is kept open by the rigidity of the tracheal cartilage. The patient will breathe through this stoma for the rest of his/her life.

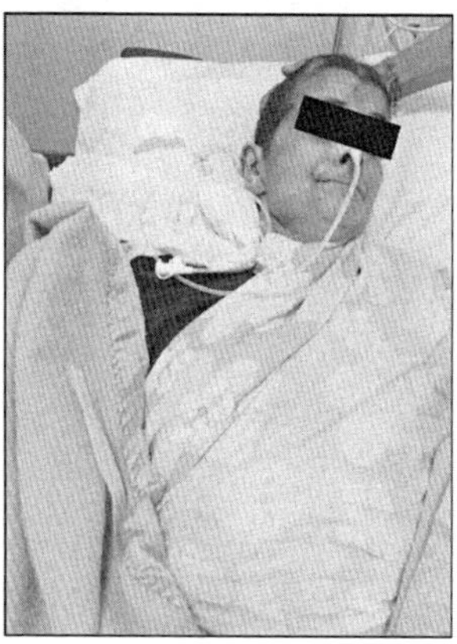

Plate 1.9: Tracheostomy care at home.

Risks

- Tube dislodgement leading to loss of airway.
- Hemorrhage.
- Infection.
- Communication problem.

Precautions

- Two lengths of tape must be used when securing the tube. Use double knots without bows or any padding.
- Tapes that are well secured should allow two fingers to pass freely around the inside of the tapes.
- Must check that airway remains patent.
- There may be blockage due to an increase in secretions or the tube slipping out of the trachea.
- The inner tube has to be removed and cleaned as required.
- Cotton should never be used, instead, use of gauze should be made for tracheostomy dressings.
- The dressing around the tracheostomy should be changed at least twice a week.

1.7.3.1 Suctioning

- Prepare the patient and administration of saline.
- Insertion of catheter and suction to be applied (Plate 1.10). The pressure setting for tracheal setting is 80-120 mmHg to avoid tracheal damage. The suction pressure should not exceed 120 mmHg.
- Guide the catheter gently into the tracheal tube until the patient begins to cough or until it stops and cannot go any further.
- The catheter should be pulled back a little before suction is applied which should make the patient more comfortable.
- Suction should not be applied for longer than about 10 seconds.

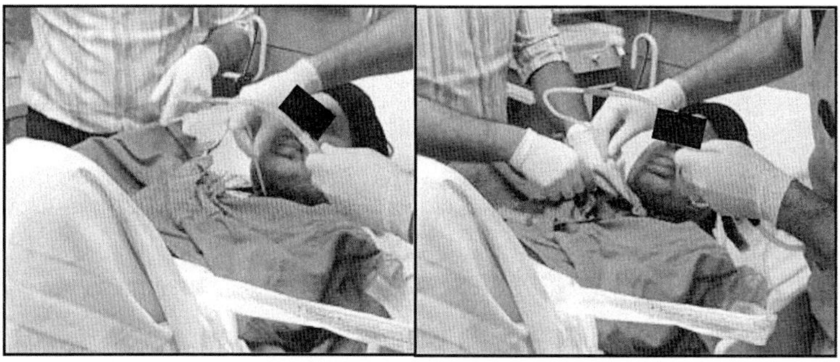

Plate 1.10: Suctioning being done by the Home care team.

1.7.4 Urinary Catheterization and Catheter Care

Urinary catheterization (Plate 1.11) is the insertion of a specially designed tube into the bladder to drain urine, removal of the clots, and instillation of medication.

Indications

Bladder drainage, acute urinary retention, and accurate fluid balance.

Procedure

- The procedure should be explained to the patient.
- Articles should be arranged.
- The bed has to be raised to an appropriate height and ensure a good light source.
- The privacy should be ensured.
- The patient should be positioned (assistant will perform) and expose the genital area to place a disposable sheet beneath the patient.
- Hand hygiene should be maintained, and sterile gloves to be used.
- After opening the catheter, pour the betadine solution in a bowl (by an assistant).

- Open the urine bag and arrange it on the side of the bed, ensuring the attachment tip is accessible and remains sterile (by an assistant).
- The sterile dressing towel should be placed between the patient's legs and over the patient's thighs.
- The perineal area should be cleaned using a new gauze swab.
- The catheter drainage bag should be then attached.
- Maintain the closed system.
- Do not allow the bag or tubing to touch the floor.
- The drainage bag should be kept below the level of the bladder.
- It has to be ensured that the catheter and drainage tubing free of kinks.

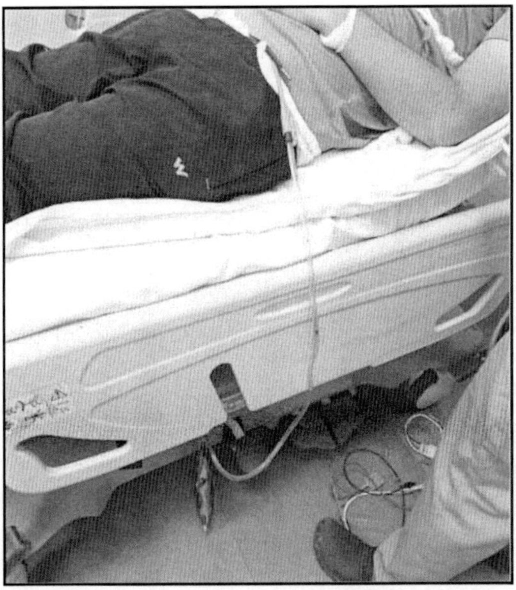

Plate 1.11: Urinary Catheter with Drainage bag.

1.7.4.1 Catheter Care

The skin around the catheter should be washed with soap and water daily and after each bowel movement. This will help reduce the risk of infection.

- Any moisture should be dried with sterile gauze.
- Make sure that urine is flowing through the catheter into the urine beg and that the urine bag does not drag and pull on the catheter.
- One should not remove the catheter unless instructed by the physician.

1.7.5 Care of Patient on Oxygen Cylinder/Concentrator/CPAP/ Portable Ventilator at Home

Oxygen concentrator (Plate 1.12) is a device that takes in air from the room and filters out nitrogen, leaving an oxygen-enriched gas to be used by patients. Oxygen can be administered by nasal cannula and face mask (Plate 1.13).

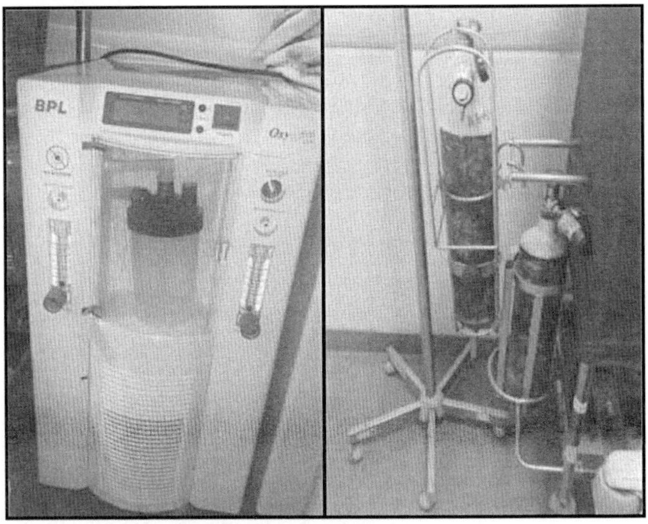

Plate 1.12: Oxygen concentrator and Oxygen cylinder.

Continuous Positive Airway Pressure machine, abbreviated as CPAP is commonly used in treatment for obstructive sleep apnea (OSA) in chronic smokers and the severely obese population.

Portable Mechanical ventilation is a supportive therapy to provide respiratory support at home for terminally ill patients who have difficulty in breathing and are neurologically weak. For example; patients on tracheostomy.

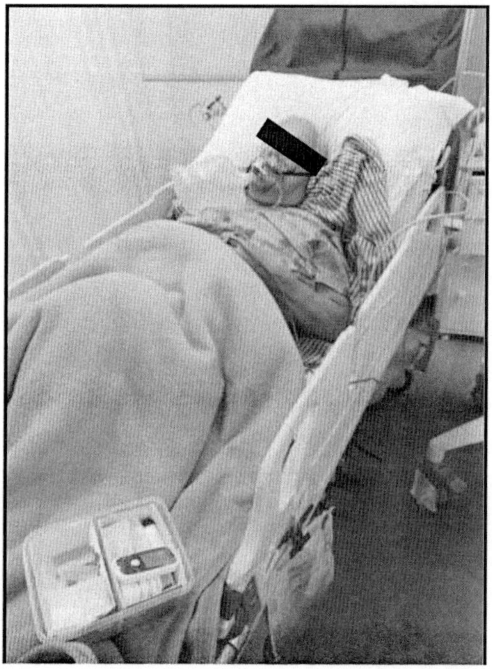

Plate 1.13: Administration of oxygen through an oxygen face mask.

Nursing Care

- The oxygen concentration should be administered as prescribed by the doctor.
- Sedatives and muscle relaxants should be administered as ordered, as may be necessary to provide adequate oxygenation and ventilation in some patients.
- Airway suctioning is to be done on an 'as needed' basis with the appropriate size of the suction catheter.
- Oxygenate before and after each suctioning.
- Cuff care should be performed every 8-12 hours to prevent necrosis (death of body tissues) and to prevent tube dislodgement.
- Patients should be monitored for any drop in BP—tachycardia (fast heart rate), bradycardia (slow heart rate),

arrhythmias (rhythm disturbance), and weak peripheral pulses.
- Continue to reposition the patient every 2 hours.
- Provide nutrition as ordered, e.g. TPN (Total parental nutrition), liquids, or eternal feeding.
- Ensure ventilator tubes should be changed as required.
- Provide oral hygiene every 4 hours and suction whenever necessary.
- Ensure maintenance of muscle strength with active/passive range of motion exercises.
- The head of the bed should be elevated 30-90 degrees, as ordered.
- The ventilator setting should be documented accurately.
- The data documentation of the events and the changes made in the ventilator settings should be documented.

1.7.6 Medication Administration

According to American Nurses Association (2006), nearly one-third of older patients are under home care are vulnerable to adverse effects as they take inappropriate drugs. The majority of the patients routinely take more than five prescribed drugs and many deviate from the prescribed regime. It was also reported that medication errors were greater in home care settings due to the unstructured environment and communication challenges in home health care. Therefore, nurses should be more vigilant for medication errors in home health care settings, and accurate documentation and review of medications for each patient in home care should be monitored (Ellenbecker *et al.*, 2006).

1.7.6.1 Administering Medications

- Before giving liquid medications bottles should be shaken.
- Using an approved measuring device, the medicine should be measured carefully. This could be a small clear plastic measuring cup, a syringe or a dropper.

- If any liquid is over poured, it should be discarded. Do not return any excess medication to the original container.
- In the case of sublingual medication, the tablet has to be kept properly under the tongue.
- Rectal medicines are medications prepared specifically for insertion into the rectum, whereas intravenous medications refer to the manual administration of a relatively small volume of a concentrated solution or medication directly into the venous system *via* peripheral or central venous access.
- The subcutaneous method of injections is pinching the skin gently between the thumb and index finger to form a fold of skin without touching the injection site. For example, insulin is given to diabetic patients.
- Inhalation administration is administering only medication at a time through the nebulizer. Several drugs used together can cause undesirable reactions. Emphasize the importance of cleaning the mouthpiece and nebulizer after each use.

1.7.6.2 Inhaler—Nasal Type

- The patient should be advised to blow the nose gently or clean nasal passages before administering drug.
- The patient should be asked to sit upright with their head tilted back.
- After inserting the tip of the nasal container into the nostril and the patient should be asked to inhale quickly and deeply while squeezing the nasal inhaler to release the spray keeping mouth closed.

Nasal Drops

The dropper should be inserted approximately one-third inch into the nares to instill the drops. Avoid touching the external nares with the dropper because this can stimulate sneezing and contaminate drops.

1.7.6.3 Eye Medications

A warm moist gauze piece should be used to remove any crusting around the eyes. Wipe from the inside part of the eye to the outer part of the eye. Use a separate gauze piece for each eye and use only warm water. For eye ointment, gently squeeze the ointment from the inner part of the pocket towards the outer part of the pocket.

1.7.7 Monitoring of Vital Parameters

Vital signs are physical signs that indicate an individual is alive, such as temperature, pulse, respiration, blood pressure, and pain. Table 1.3 indicates the different vital parameters chart.

Table 1.3: Vital Parameters Chart

SI. No.	Vital Parameters	Range	
1	Temperature	96°F	99°F
2	Pulse: adult	60/min	100/min
	Children	70/min	130/min
	Infant	80/min	160/min
	Newborn	70/min	190/min
3	**Respirations**		
	Adult	12/min	20/min
	Children	12/min	20/min
	Infant	24/min	30/min
	Newborn	30/min	60 mmHg
4	Blood Pressure	Systolic pressure (mmHg)	Diastolic pressure (mmHg)
	High Normal Blood Pressure	130	85
	Normal Blood Pressure	120	80
	Low Normal Blood Pressure	110	75

(Contd.)

SI. No.	Vital Parameters	Range	
5	SpO_2		
	Normal	95%	100%
6	Blood Sugar Level	Fasting blood sugar test	Random blood sugar test
	Normal blood sugar	99 mg/dl or below	200 mg/dl or above
	Prediabetes	100-125 mg/dl	144-199 mg/dl
	Diabetes	126mg/dl or above	<200mg/dl

1.7.7.1 Temperature

There are two ways to measure body temperature – by measuring the core temperature and surface temperature. Core temperature is the temperature of deep tissues. Measurements can be taken through the oral cavity, ear canal, rectum, and nasal cavity. While surface temperature is the temperature of surface skin tissues and the measurements can be taken through armpits. Digital thermometers are temperature–sensing easily portable instruments with a convenient digital display. It measures oral, rectal, or armpit body temperature.

Procedure

- Hands should be washed before and after taking temperature to avoid cross-infection.
- Ensure the use of a clean and disinfected thermometer with alcohol swabs after every use.
- Be alert to Fahrenheit and Celsius scales.

1.7.7.2 Assessment of Pulse

The pulse is the vibration of each wave of blood going through the arteries as the heart beats can be felt by placing fingers over one of the large arteries that lie close to the skin.

Procedure

- Before and after touching the patient, hands should be cleaned properly.
- The patient's arm and hand should be supported, press the index, middle, and ring finger of the dominant hand gently against the bone. The thumb should not be used as it has a strong pulse of its own.
- Count the pulsations for 30 seconds using a watch with a second hand. Multiply the count by 2 to determine the rate for 1 minute. If the pulse is abnormal/irregular/slow confirm the same with the nurse manager or supervisor.

Documentation

All details are to be recorded in the vital monitoring chart.

1.7.7.3 Assessing Respiration

Respiration is the exchange of oxygen and carbon dioxide in the lungs.

Procedure

- The patient's breathing pattern should be observed.
- One should count the number of times the patient inhales for 30 seconds. Multiply the count by 2 to determine the rate for 1 minute.
- When taking respirations, one should keep their fingers on the pulse so that the patient feels comforted.

Documentation

All details are to be recorded in the vital monitoring chart.

1.7.7.4 Monitoring Blood Pressure

Blood pressure is the force of blood pushing against the walls of the blood vessels.

Procedure

- Blood pressure should preferably be measured at the brachial artery.
- An injured arm should not be used.
- The patient should be in a resting position (lying, sitting, or standing as advised).
- The arm should be positioned at heart level, the cuff should be applied to the bare arm and not over clothing.
- Ensure the use of appropriate cuff size. Cuff should cover 2/3rd of the upper arm, it should completely encircle the patient's forearm about one inch.
- Position the sphygmomanometer at eye level to avoid parallax error
- Inflate the bladder/cuff and ensure the first palpating pulse disappears.
- The stethoscope should be placed over the brachial artery.
- Raise the level 20-30 mmHg above the level pulse disappeared.
- The bladder/cuff should be released slowly.
- The first sound heard is systolic, and the last sound heard is diastolic
- If the BP is surprisingly high or low, repeat the BP measuring procedure. In the case of adults who are 60 plus of age, the normal blood pressure is 134 mmHg/87 mm Hg.

Documentation

All details are to be recorded in the vital monitoring chart.

1.7.7.5 Blood Oxygen Level

The amount of oxygen in the blood is the blood oxygen level. The body needs a certain amount of oxygen to function properly, while low blood oxygen can lead to serious complications and damage to individual organ systems, especially the brain and the heart. At home, the saturation levels can be measured by pulse oximeter.

A pulse oximeter can measure blood oxygen saturation levels through a small clip that is usually placed on a finger or toe. An oximeter indicates what percentage of the blood is saturated with oxygen, known as SpO_2 level as well as heart rate.

1.7.7.6 Blood Sugar Level

At home, the staff tends to measure sugar through the fasting blood sugar test and a random blood sugar test. Fasting blood sugar level measures the blood sugar after an overnight fasting. A fasting blood sugar level of 99 mg/dl or lower is considered normal, while 100 -125 mg/dl indicates that a person is a prediabetic, and sugar levels above 126 mg/dl or higher indicates that a person has diabetes.

Random Blood sugar test measures the blood sugar at any time of the day, it can be two hours before or after your breakfast or lunch. A blood sugar level of 200 mg/dl or higher indicates a person has diabetes and requires Insulin administration as prescribed.

1.8 Wound Dressing

Wound types include surgical wounds, pressure ulcers (bedsores caused by prolonged pressure on the skin), vascular leg ulcers (long-standing diabetic patients), trauma, and burns.

Guidelines for Wound Cleansing

- Must use an aseptic technique procedure, which is a non-touch technique used to protect the affected parts. If the affected area is to be touched directly then sterile gloves must be worn.
- Cleansing should be performed in a way that minimizes the trauma to the wound.
- Irrigation is the most preferred method for cleansing open wounds. The procedure is carried out by using a syringe to produce little pressure and loosen the debris.
- Wounds are best cleaned with gauze swabs, and cotton wools with the help of sterile saline water or medical ointments at home.

1.9 Care of Vulnerable Patients

Vulnerable Patients (Plate 1.14) are all patients aged 65 years and above, infants and children (i.e. minors below the age of 18).

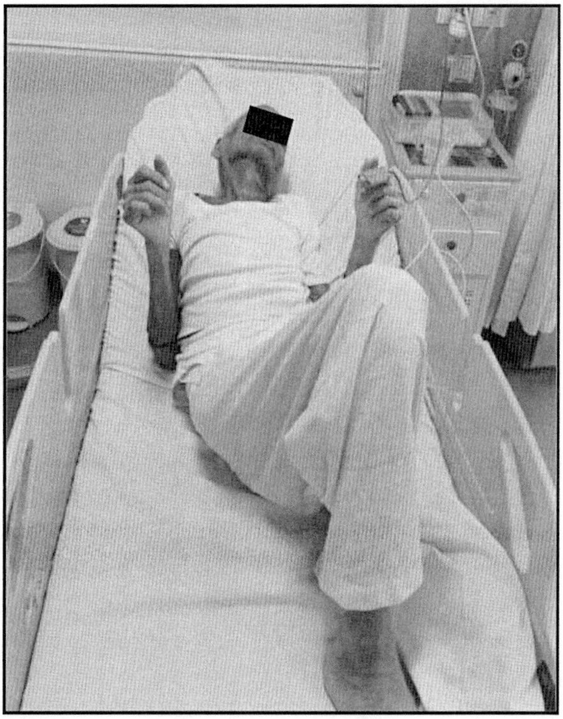

Plate 1.14: Care of elderly at home

Indications

- Patients with limited physical mobility. Especially those who cannot perform their daily necessary activities of living, i.e. going to the bathroom, eating etc.
- Patients who have impaired mental function.
- Patients who are not able to communicate (deaf or dumb) or have a language problem, e.g. a foreigner.
- Patients on wheelchairs, trolleys, walking aids etc.
- Patients under the effect of sedation or drowsy.

Policy

- To provide prompt attention and service.
- Vulnerable patients should not be left alone at any given time.
- Female patients and children of both genders will be attended for their physical interventions such as bathing and toilet by a female attendant.
- Special requests made by the patient/family will be respected.
- Regular monitoring will be ensured by the supervisory staff (nurse manager) to ensure the safety and security of vulnerable patients.

1.10 Care of Unconscious Patient

Unconsciousness is a state in which a patient is unaware of both self and external surroundings, and unable to respond meaningfully to external stimuli.

Consciousness is apparent in the patient who is not oriented, does not follow commands, or needs persistent stimuli to achieve a state of alertness. A person who is unconscious and unable to respond to spoken words can often hear what is spoken.

Consciousness is a state of being wakeful and aware of self, environment, and time.

Different Levels of Consciousness

- Alerts: - Normal Consciousness.
- Automatism.
- Aware of surroundings.
- Possibly do not remember actions later.
- A possible abnormal mood may show defects in memory and judgment.
- Loss of ability to speak and think in a logically coherent fashion.
- Responds to simple orders.
- May be disoriented by time and space.

Causes of Unconsciousness

- Head Injury.
- Asphyxia (unable to breathe).
- Cardiac Arrest.
- Blood Loss.
- Stroke.
- Epilepsy (seizure).
- Low blood sugar.
- Low sodium level.
- Blood infection in the body.

Protecting the Client

- Ensuring the use of padded side rails.
- Looking after the patient to avoid any injury.
- Talking with the client in-between.
- Speak positively to enhance the self-esteem and confidence of the patient.

Nutrition and Hydration

- Assess the hydration status, and ensure increase in the amounts of liquid.
- Start IV line.
- Liquid diet.
- NG tube feeding.
- Consider eternal feeding to provide nutritional support.
- Monitor and record fluid balance.
- Administer IV fluids as prescribed.
- The unconscious patient depends on the health care team to deliver the correct nutritional requirement.

Maintaining Skin Integrity

- Regular changing in position of the patient.
- Passive exercises for the patient.
- Back massage for the patient.

- Use splints or foam boots to prevent foot drop.
- Special beds to prevent pressure on bony prominences for the patient.
- The physiotherapist will be of benefit from the introduction of passive limb movements that will also encourage blood flow back to the heart.
- As the patient is unconscious a urinary catheter should be inserted, and her urine output should be recorded hourly.
- The patient's bowel functions should be monitored and recorded.
- Observe and report any signs of diarrhoea or constipation.

Psychosocial Needs

- All procedures must be explained to the patient/family members even when the patient is unconscious.

1.11 Caregiver Training

If one is engaging a caregiver for the first time, the nurse manager will frame a personalized care plan that includes the patient's

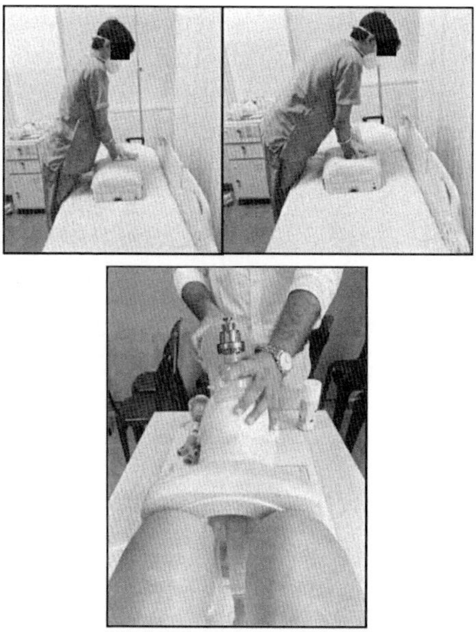

Plate 1.15: Caregiver's getting training on Basic Life Support.

condition, activities of daily living, mobility assistance – use of wheelchair/walker, toileting needs, physiotherapy, and exercise, engaging the dependents in meaningful activities, managing medication, nutrition, and diet.

Nurse Managers are expected to train the caregivers if he/she is not aware or skilled in any of the activities in the care plan. All caregivers are trained by qualified BLS instructors so that in case some patients collapse at home they can provide Cardio-Pulmonary Resuscitation (CPR) on them, which can save one's life.

1.12 Caregiver Work Shift Pattern

A caregiver can choose from work shift patterns depending on their personal preferences. Table 1.4 shows the caregiver shift pattern provided by home health care agencies.

Table 1.4: Caregiver Shift Pattern

Live In Shift	Live Out Shift
The caregiver is expected to stay round the clock with the patient for 24 hours but working hours are limited to 8 hours per day.	The caregiver is expected to stay up to 12 hours with the patient but working hours are limited to 8 hours per day.
The caregiver lives in the home of the patient and provides dedicated one-on-one care.	The caregiver operates out of their own home or hostel.
Stay with the patient.	Stay at hostel/home.
One patient care at a time.	One patient care at a time.
No commute to work.	The daily commute to work.
Food and stay provided by the patient/family.	Food to be carried.
More saving—As food and accommodation is provided by the patient/family.	Lower saving—As food and accommodation and transportation is arranged by the caregiver.
Flexible work timings that will depend on the need of the patient.	Fixed work timings—Day or Night.

1.13 Guidelines for the Health Care Staff

There are six ways by which the health care staff can make impression on the patients and their families.

- **Courtesy:** If the staff lends a smile on their face and are relaxed, the patients sense and absorb positive energy. Being generous with warm, pleasant smile is an instant winner when it arises from genuine regard for the patient. Addressing patients with respect by their name also creates a human connection and is backed by good manners and courtesy. Studies conducted by Ambady *et al.* (2002) showed that smile on the face of the physiotherapist, frowns and nods and other facial expressions were associated with short and long term improvement of the patient's physical and mental health. The study also demonstrated that patients show poor improvement in their physical, cognitive and mental functioning if their physiotherapists showed distancing behaviour.
- **Commitment to Service:** Health is the crucial part that touches the core of one's existence. The vulnerability of the patient draw their attention and compassion. Home care staff are thus expected to have high commitment towards their service and stretch themselves to adopt a can do mindset even when all formal work requirements are accomplished.
- **Presentation:** As they are representatives of their organisation or institution, the grooming and the way they present make a significant difference. It is said that "A picture is worth a thousand words". Health care nurses, personal care assistants or general duty assistants are the face of any health care agency. When they dress well, look good, creates a long lasting impression on the patients, this makes them more confident and effective in their work.
- **Attention:** Paying attention to details such as diagnosis, treatment and care are essential aspect of health care work.

As health care professionals, they should listen to patient nicely, by paying full attention to their needs by making eye contact with the patient. They should resist being preoccupied with their own personal issues, asking them precise information by giving complete attention and avoid using their own phone while on duty.

- **Competence and Training:** Maintaining professional competence is very crucial and can mean life for a patient, while incompetence knowledge can result in disability or death. The ingredients of competence include technical knowledge, trained according to the underlying condition of the patient, work management, self-organisation and time management.
- **Care Provider:** From the perspective of care providers, there are following key areas, that needs to be taken care of:

  – *Eye Contact:* The eyes are an expression of their face. The ways in which a person looks indicates a number of expressions or emotions. In many cultures, different eye contact signifies a range of emotions. Among most Asians, Arabs or Hispanics, however, it is impolite to look an elder in the eyes. Patients generally prefer that the health professional to make eye contact with them rather than just looking at the charts.

  – *Tone and Volume of Voice (Paralanguage):* Numerous number of studies suggested that a clearer tone of voice is interpreted as approval. The same word in a muffled tone conveys lack of interest or frustration. Physicians who exude warmth in their tone are less likely to have their patients switch their doctors. Moreover, health care staff should make serious efforts to learn the local language as preferred by the patients. As lack of improper communication can lead to disastrous consequences. Excessive use of Jargon (medical terminology) should be avoided. As simplifying these terms to patients will help the caregivers to understand their health needs better and this will also eliminate errors on the part of the caregiver and win their trust.

– *Colour:* Colours stimulate the nervous system, influences the human reaction and also the healing process. Fontaine *et al.* (2001) expressed that bright and vivid colours arouse automatic functions, such as blood pressure, heart rate and rate of respiration, while dim and soft colours creates calmness and repose. The Society of Critical Care Medicine recommended using calm colours in critical care units. Blue, greens and violets are appropriate for patient rooms even at home as they are thought to have healing influences.

- **Experience:** A newly health care provider should be clear on the policies and procedures followed in home care. An effective way is to ensure that staff appointed is provided trainings by the nurse manager or the experienced staff according to the underlying condition of the patient.

1.14 Expectations of the Patients

Fuscaldo (2007) expressed that friendly staff and convenience of having them are the top patient's expectations. The expectations of the patients in health care are:

- **Restoration of health:** Patients want to get better and quicker information about preventive and lifestyle modification.
- **Kindness:** Patient and his family members expect patient care plan, information about his/her health, prognosis in a cordial and kind manner.
- **Timeliness:** The staff should be punctual at their respective work places, as there is a work shift pattern and staffs are required to attend to patients on time and provide quality care.
- **Team work in the team:** Patients feel more relaxed and comfortable if they see nurse managers monitoring the patient's health and also training caregivers according to the needs and demands of the patients. For example, if

the patient is suffering from decreased cognitive function. The steps to be followed are: analyse the patient medical records, understand the severity of the disease, whether mild, moderate or severe cognitive defects. Once this has been determined, caregivers should be trained to the needs of the patient, and should understand the reasons for the patient's rude behaviour. Rather than on the contrary, should create a environment of happiness, comfort and safety (O'Toole, 2012).

- **Dignity and privacy of the patient:** Patient and his family members expect health care professionals who are working at his home should behave professionally and should treat the patient and his family decisions with respect. They should discuss about the condition of the patient with anyone except doctors or nurse managers. Privacy of the patient should be maintained.

1.15 Kano's Model for Patient Expectations

Prof. Noriaki Kano studied the factors that contributed to customer satisfaction and loyalty. Kano divided customer experience into three categories, satisfier (or performer), basic, or delighters.[6]

- **Satisfier or performer:** Every patient has a set of expectations from the hospital or health care agencies. If the expectations are met, the patient is said to be satisfied. For example: if the patient wants to know his condition, outcome or prognosis, complications with the illness, and the risks, the health care professionals should address their issues and explain them with clarity.
- **Basic:** If the expectations are met, the patient is happy but if the expectations are not met, this results in an unhappy situation. So it is expected that health care professionals should behave nicely with the patient, should be gentle and not rude. Thus, the gentle behaviour of the nurses and caregivers is not going to make the patient happy however a rude and uncooperative staff will make the patient unhappy.

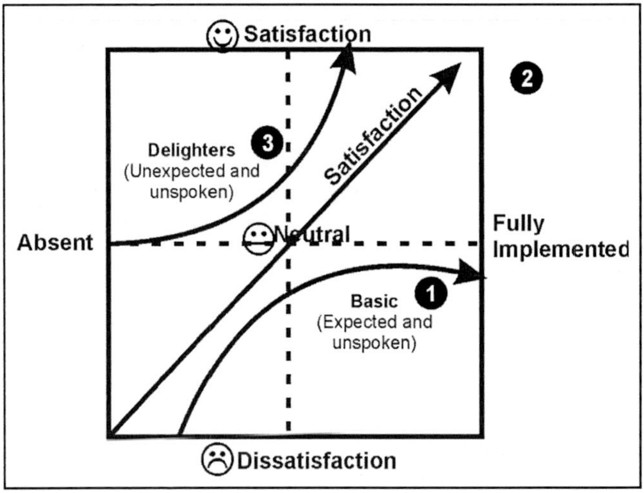

Fig. 1.1: Kano's Model of patient expectations.

- **Delighter:** Many times, the nurses and home health aides meet the unexpected requirements of the patients. Treating them as their own family members, listening to their life stories, and acting as their companions make them not only happy but also delighted.

1.16 Expectations of Caregivers

While living-in 24 hrs with the patient's family, the caregivers can expect the following in the patient's house:

- Three meals a day.
- Two times tea a day.
- Clean drinking water.
- Clean place to stay with one mattress and bedclothes, the caregivers should ensure that the sleeping area is always clean.
- Clean toilet to use, the caregivers should ensure that they always leave the toilet clean.

1.17 Caregiver's Code of Conduct

DO'S

- The caregiver must maintain good personal hygiene and grooming. They should cut nails and keep them clean; they should be clean-shaven (for male caregivers). Take a bath daily, and be dressed appropriately. Females must tie up hair adequately in a bun/For males—properly cut their hair short.
- The caregiver must keep precise and accurate medical record of patients.
- They should wear shoes or sandals and not slippers while working.
- They should greet the patient respectfully (Good Morning, Good Evening, Good Afternoon) with a smile on their face.
- They should use hand sanitizer or wash hands before feeding or touching the patient and after cleaning the patient.

DON'TS

- They should not use or disclose any confidential information about the patient or the client to anyone.
- They should not absent themselves from the workplace without the prior approval of the client.
- They should not allow their family members or friends to visit or stay over at home or hostel without the prior approval of the client.
- They should not smoke, drink alcohol, use tobacco, *paan*, etc. while serving in the patient's house.
- They should not use the mobile phone (except in an emergency), use headphones or listen to music while working with the patient.
- They should not misbehave with the patient or the family.
- They should not accept additional work requests from the client.

- They should not talk loudly during work. In any conversation, they should reply promptly to patients and not be shy.

1.18 Significance of the Study

- The study of home care is important for several reasons as it is the supportive care provided by professional nurses and general duty assistants to chronically ill and bedridden patients of which substantial numbers are immobile or suffer from chronic illnesses.
- The importance of the study lies in the fact that while there have been other studies that have analyzed the problems or single perspectives of any one of them, i.e. Caregivers/Nurses/Patients, this study is an attempt to find out the emotional experiences of the home care workers and the underlying conditions under which they perform their duties and how these workers are currently managing themselves and the kind of support they require from the clients, their family members, and agencies.
- The study also emphasizes that worker's stress was often related to role ambiguity as the families are not given clear instructions about the duties that will be carried out by caregivers. Empirical studies exist on nurses and caregivers provided the reasons why they do their jobs (feeling respectful, rewarded, and valued for their work, love with the profession, patient fate) and the challenges they face while working in home care (Lack of respect, support, trust from the patient, their family members and agency supervisors). The study also reiterates that successful retention of people working in home care is essential. Insights into the job experiences of nurses and General duty assistants were provided through qualitative findings.
- The research will contribute to a better understanding of burden experienced by family caregivers and paid caregivers as it is the most important caregiver-related variable in

care at home for the chronically ill person. The extent of subjective burden (which is borne by the caregivers) has a significant impact on the emotional and physical well-being of the family caregivers and the paid caregivers (nurses and General duty assistants).Through a thematic content analysis approach, the research would provide an insight into how the caregivers perceived their job, and the impact on their physical, mental and social health was explicitly explored.

- The research would help understand the perspective of the patients who were receiving home health care services and their satisfaction with regards to caregiver work, whether there was an improvement in their condition and the problems faced by patients and their family members concerning caregiving and nursing services.
- The study also tries to understand the journey of the patients as narrated by their family caregivers and how this formal care has helped them through the years.
- Finally, the study would provide insight into the training and support from the agencies and its need as felt by the families is discussed.

Notes

1. http://www.albrightstonebridge.com/health care_india/
2. http://www.health-policy-systems.com/content/9/1/42
3. http://health care.financialexpress.com/201101/anniversaryspecial09.shtml
4. http://silverinnings.blogspot.ae/2011/05/support-for-our-elders-1298-senior.html
5. www.lifecircle.in
6. https://www.merriam-webster.com/dictionary/nurse
7. www.kanomodel.com

2

Literature Review

Elderly Health, Illnesses and Home Health Care Services

2.1 Introduction

A literature review is a comprehensive summary of the previous research related to the topic. It provides a critical and evaluative analysis of the literature relevant to a research area or topic. The literature review surveys scholarly articles from the books, journals, newspapers, and other sources relevant and related to the area of research under study. It acknowledges the work of previous researchers and creates a landscape to understand the strength and weaknesses of the research and identifies gaps if any in the literature and the selected area of study.

This chapter discusses the literature review of the studies focusing on elderly population and their health ailments. Furthermore, the researcher has paid direct attention and elaborated on studies within the home health care sector highlighting the role of nurses and personal care assistants in home care.

2.2 Elderly Population

According to UNDESA data on projected age structure of the population (2008), The total number of the elderly in India was more than 91.6 million in 2010 with an addition of 2.5 million elderly (annually) between 2005 and 2010. The number of elderly population in India is expected to reach 158.7 million in 2025 (United Nations Department of Economic and Social Affairs, 2008). It is further projected that by 2050, this population will surpass the population of children below 14 years (Raju, 2006).

It has been projected that the population estimates for North India in 2025 will retain a "pyramidal" shape, while for southern part of India, the share of the senior population is expected to expand considerably. Linear growth is expected to be seen for the senior population in the next 100 years, having a steeper gradients of increase in the elderly population in the central and eastern part of India while in the north, south, west, and northeast, there will be levelling off absolute numbers of elderly, i.e. there will be no rise or fall in the population level, rather the growth of population will stay at the same level (Aiyar and Rajan, 2008). Table 2.1 shows the data on elderly population, as per census data.

Table 2.1: Elderly Population aged (60 years & above) in India

Source	Total			Rural	Urban
	Person	Female	Male		
Census 1961	24.7	12.4	12.4	21.0	3.7
Census 1971	32.7	15.8	16.9	27.3	5.4
Census 1981*	43.2	21.1	22.0	34.7	8.5
Census 1991**	56.7	27.3	29.4	44.3	12.4
Census 2001***	76.6	38.9	37.8	57.4	19.2
Census 2011***	103.8	52.8	51.1	73.3	30.6

Source: Census Data (2011).

* The 1981 Census could not be held in Assam owing to disturbed conditions. The population figures for 1981 of Assam were worked out by 'interpolation'.

** The 1991 Census was not held in Jammu & Kashmir. The population figures for 1991 of Jammu & Kashmir were worked out by 'interpolation'.

*** The figures include the estimated population of Mao Maram, Paomata and Purul sub-divisions of Senapati district of Manipur.

Over 7.5 per cent of the total elderly population, two-thirds of them live in villages and nearly half of them are from poor socio-economic status (SES) (Lena *et al.*, 2009). Often due to various reasons like widowhood, divorce, or separation, half of the senior population are dependents, of which a majority of the elderly are women (70%) (Rajan, 2001). It has been also observed that a smaller percentage (2.4%) of the elderly living alone, there are more number of women (3.49%) than men (1.42%) (Rajan and Kumar, 2003). Thus, the majority of elderly population who resides in rural areas, belongs to low socio-economic status, and are dependent upon their families.

In India, most of the southern states (Andhra Pradesh, Karnataka, Kerala, and Tamil Nadu) are considered to be the biggest drivers of ageing, notably other states are also experiencing an elderly population boom, (Haryana, Himachal Pradesh, Maharashtra, Odisha, and Punjab) largely in rural areas (Alam and Karan, 2010). The elderly population, however, most frequently suffers from cardiovascular illness, cancer and circulatory diseases, while the non-elderly population faces mortality due to infectious and parasitic diseases (Alam 2000; Kosuke and Soneji 2004; Shrestha 2000). There is rise in communicable diseases as well as chronic non-communicable diseases, particularly, cardiovascular, degenerative and metabolic disorders (Ingle and Nath, 2008). In the elderly, cardiovascular disease is the leading cause of death (Jha *et al.*, 2006). Multiple chronic diseases afflict the elderly population: chest pain, kidney problems, digestive disorders, vision problems, diabetes, chronic bronchitis (Angra *et al.*, 1997; Kumari, 2001; Raju, 2000; Roy, 1994; Shah and Prabhakar, 1997).

2.3 Multiple Diseases Afflicting the Elderly

The elderly population suffers from neurological diseases particularly, Alzheimer's, Stroke and Parkinson's disease leading to progressive disorder of the nervous system, cancers (where there is abnormal growth of cells), respiratory disorders, cardiovascular diseases, kidney problems, musculoskeletal diseases, skin diseases, liver infections and wounds.

2.3.1 Diseases of the Nervous System

Neurological disorders are the diseases of central and peripheral nervous system, that occurs usually in the brain, spine and multiple nerves that connects both brain and spine. The most common neurological diseases are Alzheimer's disease, Parkinson's disease and Stroke.

Alzheimer's Disease is a neurodegenerative disease that starts slowly but worsens with time. It is the cause of progressive dementia in older adults. The most common symptoms visualized are difficulty in remembering what has happened recently. With progression of this disease, symptoms include loss of memory, problems with language, mood swings, disorientation, loss of interest, aggressive behaviour and other behavioural issues. As the patient condition deteriorates, they lose interest in life and withdraw themselves from family and friends. To create awareness towards this disease, 21st September is observed as World Alzheimer's day around the world as a part of World Alzheimer's Month. This initiative by the Alzheimer's Disease International has taken place to raise the awareness about the disease. According to World Health Organisation (WHO), Alzheimer's disease is the most common cause of dementia. Dementia is a general term used for the severe decline in mental ability. It is generally the family members and friends, who tend to visualize the worsening of symptoms. In the present study, it was found that it took few years for many families to analyse that the patients are suffering from this disease, as there is mild to moderate to severe memory loss. As a result, patient needs 24 hours monitoring which is together managed by the care givers and families at home.

Parkinson's Disease: Parkinson's disease is a progressive disorder of the nervous system and also affects other parts of the body that are controlled by nerves. Early symptoms are tremors in one hand. The disorder may also cause muscle stiffness, slowed movement (difficult to get out of chair), impaired body balance, slurred speech, little or no facial expressions and changes in writing as it becomes hard to write.

Stroke: A stroke is also called brain attack. It occurs in two ways: A blocked artery happens when a blood clot blocks the flow of blood in an artery within the brain also known as ischemic stroke. A ruptured artery also known as hemorrhagic stroke occurs when a blood vessel bursts within the brain. The common symptoms of stroke includes trouble in walking and speaking, blurred or blackened vision, severe headache followed by vomiting and dizziness.

2.3.2 Cancer

It is a type of disease that occurs when there is abnormal growth of cells and thus these cells divide and spread to other tissues and organs. The rapidly growing cells are also called neoplasms and may cause tumors. There are general four types of cancer. Carcinoma is a cancer that starts in the skin, sarcoma is a cancer of connective tissues such as bones, muscles and cartilage. Leukemia is a cancer of bone marrow while lymphoma and myeloma are cancer of the immune system. Other types of cancer are appendix cancer, bladder cancer, bone cancer, breast cancer, cervical cancer, liver cancer, lung cancer, oral cancer, ovarian cancer, prostate cancer, stomach cancer and vaginal cancer. According to an article published by (Iyer, 2022) in *The Times of India* showed the number of cancer cases (Plate 2.1) in 2020 by a study conducted by Dr. Rajendra Badwe.

The study reflected that in a population of 1.3 billion, total number of active cancer cases was 13,24,413 of which 10.3 per cent were suffering from breast cancer, 13.5 per cent were suffering from lip and oral cavity, 9.4 per cent were suffering from cervix uteri and a major 56.5 per cent were suffering from other types of cancer. Parth (2022) asserted that the treatment for cancer, which often goes on for years, drain the families of the patient mentally and take a toll on their finances (Plate 2.2). Taking cognizance of these issues, the Union for International Cancer Control (UICC), the international body to collabourate global efforts has launched the Access to Oncology Medicines (ATOM). Prof. Anil D'Cruz from India said that India was one of the 170 odd members of the union and will have access to cheaper medicines in future.

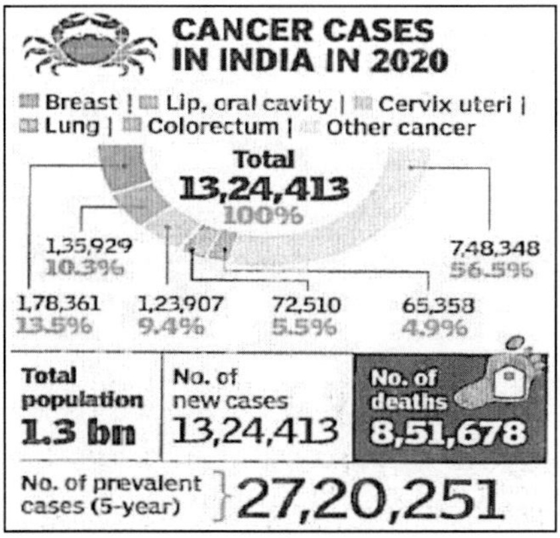

Plate 2.1: The number of cancer cases in 2020 (Iyer, 2022).

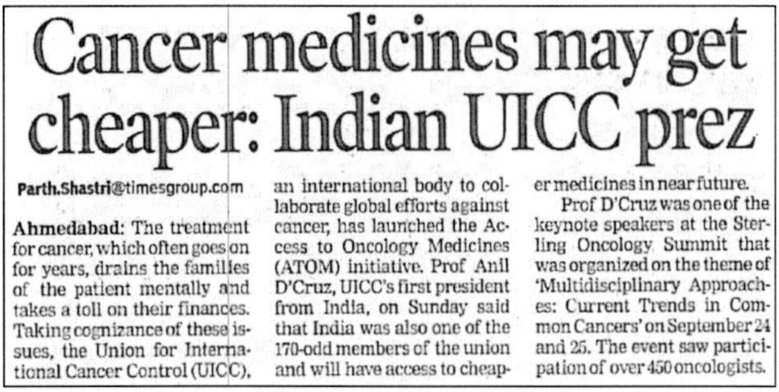

Cancer medicines may get cheaper: Indian UICC prez

Parth.Shastri@timesgroup.com

Ahmedabad: The treatment for cancer, which often goes on for years, drains the families of the patient mentally and takes a toll on their finances. Taking cognizance of these issues, the Union for International Cancer Control (UICC), an international body to collaborate global efforts against cancer, has launched the Access to Oncology Medicines (ATOM) initiative. Prof Anil D'Cruz, UICC's first president from India, on Sunday said that India was also one of the 170-odd members of the union and will have access to cheaper medicines in near future.

Prof D'Cruz was one of the keynote speakers at the Sterling Oncology Summit that was organized on the theme of 'Multidisciplinary Approaches: Current Trends in Common Cancers' on September 24 and 25. The event saw participation of over 450 oncologists.

Plate 2.2: Cancer medicines may get cheaper (Parth, 2022).

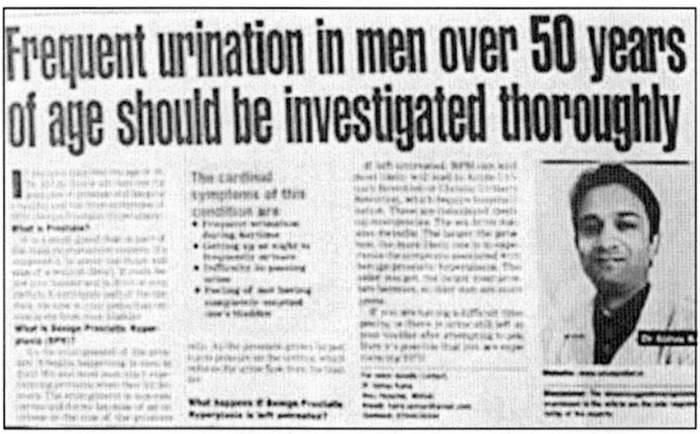

Frequent urination in men over 50 years of age should be investigated thoroughly

The cardinal symptoms of this condition are

Plate 2.3: Frequent urinary in men should be investigated thoroughly over 50 years, (Kalra, 2022).

Kalra (2022) advises the men over 50 years of age to take good care of prostrate and keep it healthy and free from symptoms of BPH (Benign Prostatic Hyperplasia) (Plate 2.3). Prostate is a small gland that is a part of male reproductive system and is supposed to be the size of walnut. BPH refers to the enlargement of prostate gland. If left untreated, it can lead to symptoms like frequent urination, difficulty in passing urine and feeling of not completely emptied one's bladder.

McCorkle *et al.* (2000) examined the impact of home care by advanced practice nurses and found that the older patients who were surgically treated for cancer and were receiving home care services lived about 7 months longer than the usual care group. Also, the survival rates among the patients in the late stages have 2-year survival rates than those in the usual care group. Post-surgery, the patients are discharged with highly complex problem which are often accompanied by catheters, wound dressings and equipments such as pain infusion pumps. Additionally, the patients also need assistance with fall prevention, bathing, grooming and preparation of meals and for some patients who are discharged early, and in some geographical areas, they are not available and not affordable also (Oberst and James, 1985; Federal Register, 1997; Harris, 1998).

2.3.3 Diseases of the Respiratory System

Respiratory diseases refer to the disorders of the airways and the lungs that affect human respiration. Respiratory diseases include the asthma, chronic obstructive pulmonary disease, cystic fibrosis, acute bronchitis and chronic bronchitis.

Asthma: The airways (windpipe) are consistently inflamed causing wheezing (whistling sound while breathing) and shortness of breath. Infections, allergies or pollution can excavate these symptoms.

Chronic obstructive pulmonary disease: In this condition, the patient shows trouble in breathing and can't exhale properly.

Cystic fibrosis: In this type of condition, one has trouble clearing the mucus out of the bronchi. This leads to repeated lung infections.

Acute Bronchitis: There is a sudden infection of the airway and caused by a virus.

Chronic Bronchitis: In this form of COPD, the person suffers from long term wet cough (Hoffman, 2020).

Neff *et al.* (2003) examined the effect of home care on patients with respiratory issues and suggested that the patients with chronic obstructive pulmonary diseases (COPD) who received advanced practice nursing transitional care also experienced fewer hospital admissions. Patients also experienced an increase in the performance of their functional abilities and showed fewer depressive symptoms than the patient receiving the usual care.

2.3.4 Disease of the Endocrine System

The endocrine system is a network of glands that produce and release hormones that help to control various body functions including body's ability to change calories into energy that powers cells and organs. It plays a vital role in whether or not a person develops diabetes, thyroid diseases, growth disorders, sexual disorders and other hormonal related disorders. The most common endocrine diseases are diabetes and thyroid disorders in India. The prevalence of diabetes is estimated to be about 11.8 per cent in the Indian population accounting for 72.9 million cases in adult population.[1]

2.3.5 Diseases of the Circulatory System

Circulatory system diseases also called cardiovascular diseases are conditions that affect our heart and blood vessels and make it harder for the blood to flow throughout the body. These diseases can cause a number of issues that includes problem with the heart's pumping actions, change the structure of heart, blocked or narrow blood vessels and also weakening of blood vessels. Malik (2022) asserted that the India is known as the diabetes capital of the world and about 30 million people in the country suffer from heart diseases (Plate 2.4). Over one million people in India are expected to be suffering from this silent disease. According to the World Health Organization, cardiovascular diseases which includes heart attack, stroke and hypertension are the biggest cause of death globally, which estimates that 20 million people die from cardiovascular disease every year compared with about 17.5 million people a decade ago.

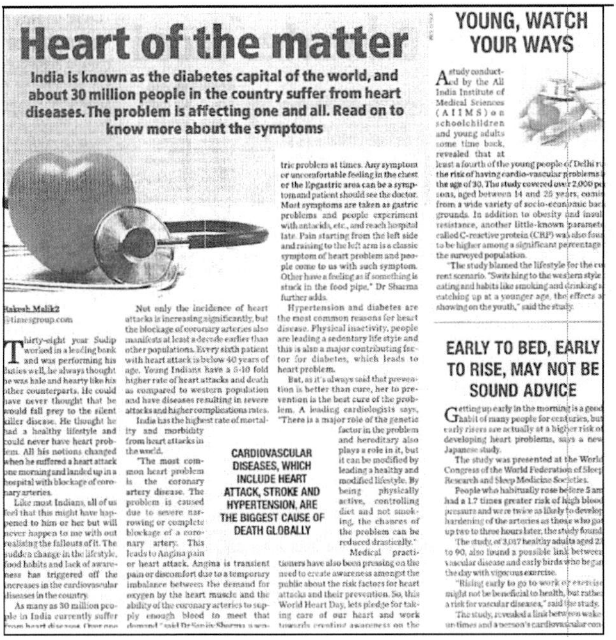

Heart of the matter

India is known as the diabetes capital of the world, and about 30 million people in the country suffer from heart diseases. The problem is affecting one and all. Read on to know more about the symptoms

Rakesh Malik2
@timesgroup.com

Thirty-eight year Sudip worked in a leading bank and was performing his duties well, he always thought he was hale and hearty like his other counterparts. He could have never thought that he would fall prey to the silent killer disease. He thought he had a healthy lifestyle and could never have heart problem. All his notions changed when he suffered a heart attack one morning and landed up in a hospital with blockage of coronary arteries.

Like most Indians, all of us feel that this might have happened to him or her but will never happen to me with out realising the fallouts of it. The sudden change in the lifestyle, food habits and lack of awareness has triggered off the increases in the cardiovascular diseases in the country.

As many as 30 million people in India currently suffer from heart diseases. Over one

Not only the incidence of heart attacks is increasing significantly, but the blockage of coronary arteries also manifests at least a decade earlier than other populations. Every sixth patient with heart attack is below 40 years of age. Young Indians have a 5-10 fold higher rate of heart attacks and death as compared to western population and have diseases resulting in severe attacks and higher complications rates.

India has the highest rate of mortality and morbidity from heart attacks in the world.

"The most common heart problem is the coronary artery disease. The problem is caused due to severe narrowing or complete blockage of a coronary artery. This leads to Angina pain or heart attack. Angina is transient pain or discomfort due to a temporary imbalance between the demand for oxygen by the heart muscle and the ability of the coronary arteries to supply enough blood to meet that demand," said Dr Sanjiv Sharma, a sen-

tric problem at times. Any symptom or uncomfortable feeling in the chest or the Epgastric area can be a symptom and patient should see the doctor. Most symptoms are taken as gastric problems and people experiment with antacids, etc., and reach hospital late. Pain starting from the left side and raising to the left arm is a classic symptom of heart problem and people come to us with such symptom. Other have a feeling as if something is stuck in the food pipe," Dr Sharma further adds.

Hypertension and diabetes are the most common reasons for heart disease. Physical inactivity, people are leading a sedentary life style and this is also a major contributing factor for diabetes, which leads to heart problem.

But, as it's always said that prevention is better than cure, her to prevention is the best cure of the problem. A leading cardiologists says, "There is a major role of the genetic factor in the problem and hereditary also plays a role in it, but it can be modified by leading a healthy and modified lifestyle. By being physically active, controlling diet and not smoking, the chances of the problem can be reduced drastically."

Medical practitioners have also been pressing on the need to create awareness amongst the public about the risk factors for heart attacks and their prevention. So, this World Heart Day, lets pledge for taking care of our heart and work towards creating awareness on the

CARDIOVASCULAR DISEASES, WHICH INCLUDE HEART ATTACK, STROKE AND HYPERTENSION, ARE THE BIGGEST CAUSE OF DEATH GLOBALLY

YOUNG, WATCH YOUR WAYS

A study conducted by the All India Institute of Medical Sciences (AIIMS) on schoolchildren and young adults some time back, revealed that at least a fourth of the young people of Delhi r[un] the risk of having cardio-vascular problems [by] the age of 30. The study covered over 2,000 pe[r]sons, aged between 14 and 25 years, comin[g] from a wide variety of socio-economic back[]grounds. In addition to obesity and insul[in] resistance, another little-known paramet[er] called C-reactive protein (CRP) was also fou[nd] to be higher among a significant percentage [of] the surveyed population.

"The study blamed the lifestyle for the cu[r]rent scenario. "Switching to the western style [of] eating and habits like smoking and drinking a[re] catching up at a younger age, the effects a[re] showing on the youth," said the study.

EARLY TO BED, EARLY TO RISE, MAY NOT BE SOUND ADVICE

Getting up early in the morning is a good habit of many people for centuries, but early risers are actually at a higher risk of developing heart problems, says a new Japanese study.

The study was presented at the World Congress of the World Federation of Sleep Research and Sleep Medicine Societies.

People who habitually rose before 5 am had a 1.7 times greater risk of high blood pressure and were twice as likely to develop hardening of the arteries as those who got up two to three hours later, the study found.

The study, of 3,017 healthy adults aged 2[] to 90, also found a possible link between vascular disease and early birds who began the day with vigorous exercise.

"Rising early to go to work or exercise might not be beneficial to health, but rather a risk for vascular diseases," said the study.

The study, revealed a link between wake up times and a person's cardiovascular con

Plate 2.4: Newspaper article highlighting the severity of heart diseases in India (Malik, 2022).

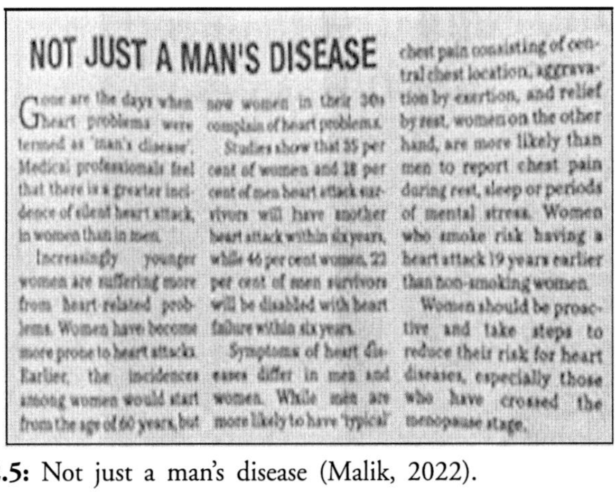

NOT JUST A MAN'S DISEASE

Gone are the days when heart problems were termed as 'man's disease'. Medical professionals feel that there is a greater incidence of silent heart attack in women than in men.

Increasingly younger women are suffering more from heart-related problems. Women have become more prone to heart attacks. Earlier, the incidences among women would start from the age of 60 years, but now women in their 30s complain of heart problems.

Studies show that 35 per cent of women and 18 per cent of men heart attack survivors will have another heart attack within six years, while 46 per cent women, 22 per cent of men survivors will be disabled with heart failure within six years.

Symptoms of heart diseases differ in men and women. While men are more likely to have 'typical' chest pain consisting of central chest location, aggravation by exertion, and relief by rest, women on the other hand, are more likely than men to report chest pain during rest, sleep or periods of mental stress. Women who smoke risk having a heart attack 19 years earlier than non-smoking women.

Women should be proactive and take steps to reduce their risk for heart diseases, especially those who have crossed the menopause stage.

Plate 2.5: Not just a man's disease (Malik, 2022).

Not only this, the incidence of heart attacks is increasing significantly. The most common heart problem is the coronary heart disease. The problem is caused due to severe narrowing or blockage of the coronary artery. This leads to Angina pain or heart attack. The classic symptoms of the problem are chest pain in the epigastria (stomach) area, which is taken as gastric problems at times (pain starting from the left side and raising to the left arm is a classic symptom of heart problem. Malik (2022) has further explained that hypertension and diabetes are the most common reasons for heart diseases and elaborated that it is no longer a man's disease, more number of women are also now-a-days prone to heart attacks.

To create awareness amongst the public about risk factors for heart attacks and their prevention, World Heart Day is celebrated on 29th September. Another study showed that roughly 25 per cent of the patients suffering from heart failure require hospital re-admission within 30 days. Such incidences can be avoided and prevented by assisted care provided by the professional nurses and caregivers that provides a variety of services that helps the patients to regain their lost strength and develop a healthier lifestyle with greater independence.

Patient with the congestive heart failure (CHF) have been shown to have long survival times with regard to their first admission (Fortinsky *et al.*, 2006; Naylor *et al.*, 2004; Hughes *et al.*, 2002; Jerant *et al.*, 2003). It was reported that the patients who received advanced practice nurse transitional care, team-based home based primary care or a multidisciplinary specialty team intervention also had fewer unplanned hospital admissions. Team managed home based primary care has been the most effective for the severely disabled patients (Hughes *et al.*, 2002).

2.3.6 Disease of the Kidneys

Kidney diseases are the ones that affect the kidneys, where they are damaged and cannot filter the blood. The disease is called chronic as the damage to the kidneys happen over a period of time. The job of the kidneys is to filter extra water and waste out of our blood to make urine. The kidney also balances the salts and minerals in the body such as calcium, phosphorous, sodium and potassium in the blood. The symptoms of chronic kidney disease are pain in chest, itching, feeling tired, headaches, loss of appetite, nausea, vomiting and increased or decreased urination. McDowell *et al.* (1999) tested behavioural management interventions for treating urinary incontinence in older patients and reported positive results who were self monitored and had bladder training.

According to Centre for Disease Control and Prevention (2019) chronic kidney problems are common among adults in the United States, it was estimated that more than 37 million American adults are suffering from CKD. Additionally, kidney diseases also increase with age the longer the person is suffering from diabetes, high blood pressure and heart disease as they tend to damage the blood vessels in the kidneys.

2.3.7 Diseases of the Skin

Skin diseases are the conditions that affect the skin and causes rashes, itchiness and discolouration of the skin. Common skin diseases seen in elderly population are eczema (means dry, itchy skin leads to swelling or cracking), psoriasis (scaly skin), Vitiligo (white patches develop on the skin due to lack of melanin), Dermatitis (inflammation and skin irritation of the skin). To provide effective care, it is important that caregivers are trained with needed specialized knowledge and diagnostic skills to make clinical decisions. It is unlikely that specialised dermatological care will be delivered in the growing long term care sector.

Hahnel *et al.* (2017) reported that the burden of skin diseases also increases with age, thus, implying a direct relationship of the variables, age and disease.

2.3.8 Diseases of the Liver

Liver diseases are the condition that damages the liver and prevents its proper functioning. Common liver diseases are Jaundice caused by viral infections, problems with the immune system, when our immune system is attacked by liver, inherited diseases, alcoholic fatty liver disease (cased of consuming excess of alcohol) and non-alcoholic fatty liver disease (caused by consuming too much fat). Chronic liver disease is a disease marked by gradual destruction of liver tissues over time such as cirrhosis and fibrosis.

2.3.9 Disease of the Musculoskeletal System

Musculoskeletal diseases are characterized by impairments in the muscles, bones, joints and adjacent connective tissues leading to temporary or lifelong limitations in functioning. Musculoskeletal conditions are typically characterized by pain that is persistent, limitation in mobility reducing people's ability to work. Musculoskeletal conditions includes conditions that affect the joints (arthritis), bones (osteoporosis), muscles and multiple body areas such as back and neck pain.

A Global burden of Disease (GBD) 2019 data showed that approximately 1.71 billion people live with musculoskeletal conditions including lower back pain, neck pain, fractures, other injuries, amputation and rheumatoid arthritis. Musculoskeletal conditions are also the biggest contributors to years lived with disability (YLDS) worldwide with approximately 149 million YLDs accounting for 17 per cent of all YLDs worldwide (Cieza *et al.,* 2021).

Care for any injury caused due to fall or accident is very prominent among home care patients (Centres for Medicare & Medicaid Services, 2006). Thirty per cent of the people aged 65 or above fall each year and one in every five patients needs medical attention (Gillespie *et al.*, 2003). Falls are leading cause of injury related deaths (National Centre for Injury Control and Prevention, 2006). For the older population, evidence suggests that the individualized home care programmes for muscle strengthen; balance restraining, health/environmental risk factor screening, medication reviews, and home hazard assessments can reduce the occurrence of falls (Gillespie *et al.*, 2003).

2.3.10 Wounds

According to National Pressure Ulcer Advisory Panel, a pressure injury is a localized damage to skin and underlying soft tissues. It can be present as intact in the skin or an open ulcer and may be painful. It occurs due to the intense or prolonged pressure on the skin. Wound types included the surgical wounds, pressure ulcers (bedsores caused by prolonged pressure on the skin) and vascular leg ulcers (in case of long standing diabetic patients). Corbett (2003) analyzed that the individualized education in foot care for the diabetic patients improved the overall effective self-care. Over 60 per cent of the wounds in home care are surgical, however just one quarter of the wounds seen are vascular leg ulcers and are pressure ulcers (Weaver *et al.*, 2003).

Rodriques and Megie (2006) found that 37 per cent of wounds in home health care were pressure ulcers which can prolong for duration of 27 months. Further they investigated and reported that 1 in 10 patients who were admitted had pressure ulcers and about one-third were at additional risk of developing new ulcers. Reasons associated with the development of pressure ulcers are limitations in performing ADLs, mobility impairment, fractures, anaemia, use of oxygen and recent discharge from any hospital (Ferrell *et al.*, 2000; Bergquist, 2001)

2.4 Studies on Home Health Care

According to Centre for Medicare and Medicaid Services (2006) Medicare beneficiaries who are in poor health, have low income, and those who are 85 years of age or older have relatively high rates of home health care use. Among the home health care patients, 31 per cent of patients suffer from circulatory disease, 16 per cent of them suffer from heart diseases, 15.9 per cent (injury and poisoning), 14.1 per cent are affected with musculoskeletal and connective tissue disease, while 11.6 per cent are diagnosed with respiratory disease problem (Kaiser Family Foundation, 2005).

Research showed that older Americans overwhelmingly articulate a desire to age in place and receive care at home rather than in institutional settings. A survey conducted by the American Association of Retired Persons found that nearly three quarters of a survey population of those age 45+ strongly agreed with the statement, "what I'd really like to do is stay in my current residence for as long as possible" (Keenan, 2010). This is echoed in the last stages of life, where the Dartmouth Atlas researchers found that more than 80 per cent of patients say that they "wish to avoid hospitalization and intensive care during the terminal phase of life" (The Dartmouth Atlas of Health Care, 2012).

In 2013, in the context of Medicaid long-term services and supports, there were more home-and-community-based service providers than institutional providers, which was an 18 per cent increase since 1995 (Terence *et al.*, 2012). Approximately 3.4 million people receive Medicare skilled home health care, which supports homebound patients by providing coverage for intermittent skilled nursing and therapy services that are provided by Medicare-certified home health agencies subject to a physician's plan of care. In 2014, Medicare spent $17.7 billion on home health care (Medicare Payment Advisory Commission, 2016).

According to Centre for Medicare and Medicaid Services (CMS), there are 8,090 home health care agencies in the United States providing care to more than 2.4 million senior population and disabled people annually.[2] There has been significant rise in the expenditures for Medicaid for home and community-based services, doubling from $25.1 billion in 2002 to $55 billion in 2012, reflecting the growth in use of home-based care services as compared to institutional care (AARP, 2015).

The Medicare Payment Advisory Commission (MedPAC) estimates that the enrolment in Medicare is expected to increase by more than 50 per cent over the next 15 years, reflecting a rise from 54 million beneficiaries today to more than 80 million in 2030 (Medicare Payment Advisory Commission, 2016).

These figures reflect an overall aging of the United States population and it is estimated that by the Census projects that the proportion of U.S. residents who are older than 65 years will almost be doubled from the year 2010 by the year 2030 (20% *vs.* 13%) (Ortman *et al.*, 2014). Among the oldest population of Americans, the Census also predicts that the population who are 85 years and above will double by 2036 and will triple by 2049 (Medicare Payment Advisory Commission, 2016).

The professional workers in the home health care are important for good medical care of the patients (Stone and Dawson, 2008). When patients leave the hospital and return home with the home nursing care, they get highly supportive medical environment with many nurses, aides and other medical professionals in home environment with formal and informal caregivers with support received from home care nurses (Romagnoli *et al.*, 2013). These workers who are directly involved in the care are described as the centre part of our long-term care (Stone and Wiener,2001). These support workers are the vital members of the health work who are actively involved in the care of older adults.

Demand for the home care services has become more complex with the growing of aged population, more people are discharged from hospitals with multiple health issues and there is a need for advance nursing care (Kerkstra and Hutten, 1996; Thome *et al.*, 2003; Modin and Furhoff, 2004). The treatment of patients in their homes has become a common model for the health care in the Western world (Duke and Street, 2003; Magnusson and Lutzen, 2002). Technological advances have allowed for more medical treatments to be carried and monitored in private homes (Ward-Griffin and McKeever, 2000) such care is sometimes called "hospital at home" is often put into practice and handled by team of nurses delivering complex care (Temmink *et al.*, 2000).

Review studies have indicated that home care workers have a purpose hidden in their jobs of helping people, feel good about the mission of serving the people and appreciate the variety and flexibility in their Job (Eustis *et al.*, 1993; Feldman,1997). Studies undertaken by (Benjamin and Matthias, 2004) examined various reasons on recruiting and retaining personal care assistants in home care has been difficult. Wages are low, while the benefits are poor or non-existent and the hours are often long and inconsistent (Kemper *et al.*, 2008; Morris, 2009). Workers also highlighted the challenges they face in home care (Low wages, Job insecurity, lack of respect, inconsistent hours, benefits and recognition) (Ashley *et al.*, 2010). Past research has highlighted the poor working conditions; work overload, inadequate training and lack of opportunity for advancement were also related to retention of staff (Brannon *et al.*, 2007; Jorgensen *et al.*, 2009). All health care workers involve some kind of emotional labour or relational work required to bring trust with the patients and ensure them comfort. Majority of the home care services are delivered by home care aides and personal care assistants who shoulder the bulk of responsibility required for patients (Butler *et al.*, 2012; Rodat, 2014). Home care workers report a high level of stress caring for the ill, dying and aggressive patient and prioritizing patient's emotional needs and happiness above their own. It was examined that the home care hourly wage rate is less as compared to other jobs in the health sector. (Arts *et al.*, 1999; Hakanen *et al.*, 2008; National Institute for Occupational Safety and Health, 2010).

Banijamali *et al.* (2014) highlighted problems while working in home care as well as the reasons for discontentment in such jobs which included insufficient pay, not receiving enough paid hours, inconvenient and inconsistent hours of work and longer hours of work. There is scarcity of benefits and often the work-life balance is hard to maintain.

Home care models are such that the staff has to prioritize tasks like helping the patient in bathing, eating, dressing and grooming, the emotional labour is invisible in this work for which the workers receive no training, compensation or support (Stacey, 2011). However, many home health care aides report their relations are very rewarding part of their job and allow them to find value and meaning in their job (Banijamali *et al.*, 2012; Blustein *et al.*, 2004; Blustein, 2008; Butler *et al.*, 2010; Russell *et al.*, 2013). Research in nursing home care is also suggestive that a culture of 'companionate love' can improve patient's outcome and job satisfaction (Barsade and O'Neill, 2014). Understanding a worker's emotional stress is important and critical as it helps to maintain a skilled, qualified workforce, and will improve patient care (Franzosa *et al.*, 2019).

2.4.1 Conceptual Model

Across different industries, workers were facing problems of depression, stress, burnout and exhaustion and this has led workers to feel disinterested in their jobs (Karimi *et al.*, 2015) and it is a reported fact that workers who receive support at work place tend to function and flourish more productively both on and off the job (Huppert and So, 2013).

Schulte *et al.* (2015) proposed a unified concept of worker well-being, the study addressed all factors that affect the health of workers and the quality of their working lives with the goal to find out who are enjoying a fulfilling work life and are benefiting from the safe, supporting work place. The study focused not only on the objective factors such as wages and benefits but also on the subjective factors such as performing valued work.

Franzosa *et al.* (2019) model identified three primary domains (the economic, physical and emotional work environment) that contribute to overall well-being of the workers. Traditionally, workforce well-being focused on economic domain like wages, benefits as well as control over the physical work force. These factors are often driven at the organizational level generally funded by agency (public or private). The study also tends to incorporate the unaddressed emotional domain. The centre of this domain is the aide-patient relationship.

The present study tries to build a model (Fig. 2.1) that focus on the experiences of home care workers, the emotional stress they face at their work place, the conditions under which they perform their duty, and what support they requires from the client's, their family members and agencies. These relationships are driven by four factors: emotional, economic, physical and social work environments that contributes to their well-being or stress. The

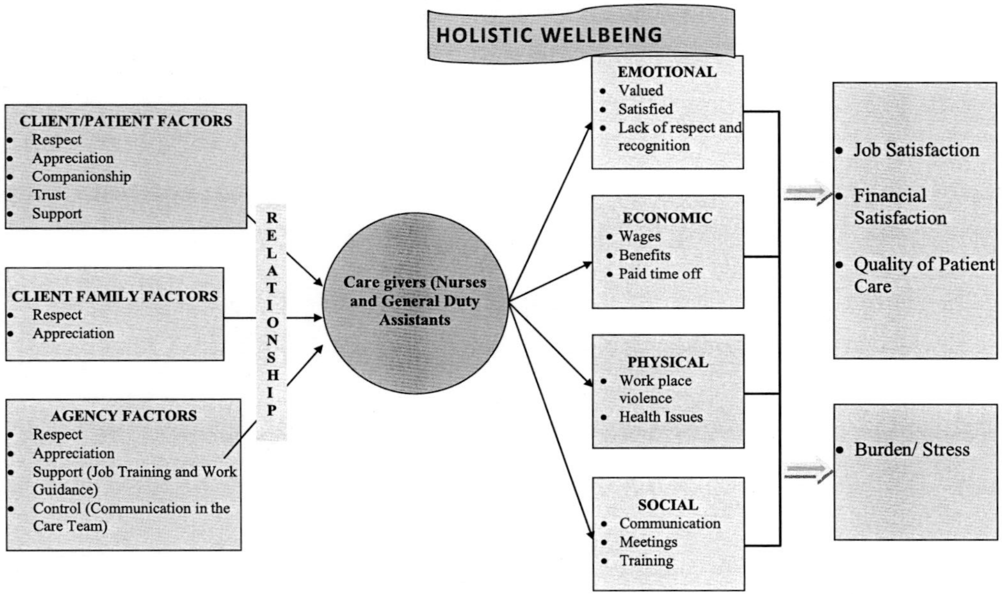

Fig. 2.1: Factors affecting Home Care Workers in Tricity (Chandigarh, Mohali, Panchkula) adapted from (Franzosa *et al.*, 2019)

emotional domain which incorporates the sense of being valued, rewarded and satisfaction at their work place or the lack of respect or recognition adding to depression or turnover, economic domain which is influenced by wages, benefits or paid leaves, physical domain is related to the workplace violence or the health hazard. The social domain has been added in the study which incorporates the need of communication, meetings and trainings in the care team which are generally driven at an organizational level and are funded by agencies (public or private) and the independent work where the employees are directly employed by the families. These factors would together contribute to their holistic well-being through job satisfaction, financial satisfaction and quality of patient care or burden/stress which is caused by additional amount of workload or responsibilities on staff leading to disturbed mental state.

2.5 Studies on Personal Duty Assistants

Grunfeld *et al.* (1997) undertook a study in Canada, about caring for elderly people at home and their consequences for the caregivers. It was noted that caring for a patient with dementia is one of the most difficult challenges being faced by caregivers. The cognitive problems thus impair the social skills of the patient and lead to changes in personality and disruptive behaviour of the caregiving staff. People with advanced dementia require 24-hour surveillance and many patients suffer physical disability as well. Further studies have shown that the stress felt by the caregiver increases with the patient's health deterioration and the stress of caring for a patient with dementia is typically worse than cancer (Clipp and George, 1993).

It has been interpreted in many studies that caring for an elderly family member at home suffering with dementia may create a situation of chronic stress, which may also adversely affect the caregiver's emotions along with his physical health (Morris *et al.*,1988, Schulz *et al.*, 1990, Chappell and Penning, 1996). However, it was noted that in case of terminally ill patients, family caregivers experience significant psychosocial, (Chappell and

Penning, 1996; Hinton, 1994; Hinds, 1985) physical and economic burdens, which effect their life negatively (McMillan, 1996).

Ashley *et al.* (2010) examined the job experiences of home care workers in Maine. The qualitative data was collected from 131 participants. The respondents gave reasons like love for their job, feeling rewarded, valued for their work, work adding meaning to their life, however, many challenges existed for home care workers/personal support specialists (PSS) which are low wages, unpredictable work schedules, job security, can not make ends meet, no health insurance, lack of benefits was also reported such as no paid time for vacations, no holidays, lack of respect and recognition. There were participants, who asserted that the existence and support from friends, agency and staff add to their job satisfaction. The staff expects paid sick leaves and paid vacations from the agencies and giving this would reduce their stress and burn out.

Varela *et al.* (2011) have explored home care prospects for patients with Alzheimer's disease, emphasizing on the caregiving strain. They highlight that living with Alzheimer's disease affects the person's cognitive, emotional, and physical well-being and also that of the caregiver. It is the most common type of dementia that results in brain cell damage and those diagnosed eventually need assistance in their daily living. Because of this prolonged nature of the disease, care is provided at home is delivered by caregivers that are mostly family members who may range from spouses, extended family, friends and sometimes health care personnel such as doctors and nurses. This home care supposedly puts up a lot on the shoulder of the ones looking after. At times because of the severity of the disease, a person may have to be institutionalized and home care may not be the ideal solution, but in other cases where ever home care is required one has to be acquainted with the skills and ability to look after the patient because care for such patients is consistent.

The time and efforts take up a lot from both the patient and the caregiver, affecting both identically. While some may find acceptance eventually others may be more emotionally affected displaying variety of emotions ranging from shock to a state of anger, leading to grief. Sansoni *et al.* (2004) have confirmed the presence of both physical psychological illnesses among the caregivers due to the stress that comes with the job. The 'round the clock' nature of caregiving for such patients leaves behind little time for self-care and social activities for oneself and one may feel emotionally, physically and mentally drained, similar findings presented by Ferrara *et al.* (2008) confirm this assertion. Findings of stress and pressure among caregivers are consistent across cultures (Ferrara *et al.*, 2008, Grant *et al.*, 2002 and Lutgendorf *et al.*, 2009), because of the severity of the disease, a caregiver is required to do much more than just looking after the patient. To name a few, getting the patient in and out of bed, feeding them, dressing them, getting them to and from the toilet, bathing them etc. are few of the many duties that a caregiver performs, along with providing necessary medical attention. This leads to consequences for the caregiver in forms of physical and psychological distress. The stress incurred is so powerful that caregivers of Alzheimer's patients have an association with poor immunity, cardiovascular issues such as higher blood pressures and decreased wound healing mechanisms, sleep patterns overall reflecting poorly on their quality of life, well-being and health.

Ugur *et al.* (2014) have emphasized on the need of studying the challenges of the home care providers owing to the lack of training and planning in home care services sector and have tried to ascertain the reasons for the same. They emphasize that although with the advancement in medical technology and health care, there are a variety of options available for caregiving, home care still remains a significant practice. Some reasons being, lack of staff, accommodation facilities and economic difficulties (Bektas and Akdemir, 2006, Romito *et al.*, 2013). Their study was based on 137 voluntary caregivers of cancer patients who seemed to be involved in all kinds of activities along with medical care such as changing clothes, cooking for the patient, shopping for them, maintaining their personal hygiene, taking them to the hospital and bringing them back etc. Thus, home care not only puts up a responsibility of looking after on the shoulders of a caregiver, in some ways, it holds the caregiver accountable for all tasks related to the patient under care. This includes management, health care organization, and other related duties such as physical care and basic in-house activities, which sometimes they are not prepared for because of lack of formal training of such kind.

Chamber *et al.* (2001) in their study have stressed that home caregivers do not receive any formal training about patient handling and related activities, and it is through their own methods and mistakes they learn the process of caregiving.

Some challenges encountered by home caregivers as highlighted by Ugur *et al.* (2014) are patient's lack of mobility, difficulty in handling the patient, patient's risk of falling or the fear of dropping them while looking after their hygiene-based needs, lack of knowledge about medicine management and pain management for the patient. The lack of practice and skill about handling a patient whose body has been weakened by the chronicity of a disease such as cancer is a challenge for home caregivers. Therefore, they need to be informed about the severity, management, issues and strategies required to handle such patients to be able to help them reduce stress and increase efficacy in looking after the patient keeping the cultural and structural factors in mind (Given *et al.*, 2001, Henderix *et al.*, 2006).

The role of health professionals in this arena is crucial. They should define the physiological, social and emotional needs of caregivers and train caregivers prior patient discharge to improve their integration in their new role as home caregivers (Meeker *et al.*, 2011; Serfelova, 2012).

Banijamali *et al.* (2014) studied the characteristics of home care workers and surveyed 402 former home care workers in the Washington state, who tend to leave their jobs in lieu of poor pay and low status. The researchers proposed a conceptual model and hypothesized that job satisfaction was influenced by extrinsic awards such as wages, benefits, fringes and training and career development by opportunities for advancement, basic training and continuing education. The respondents gave different reasons for entering home care was the rewarding work, feeling of obligation to care for their particular clients. Insufficient pay, not receiving enough paid hours of work, inconvenient hours of work, and pursuit for better career opportunities (wages and benefits) was the most predominant reason for leaving home care jobs was for better wages and benefits. Moreover, the workers who claimed to be very satisfied with their home care jobs tends to be less educated, to be older by 5.5 years (from average age), have fewer dependents and were earning more than $10 per hour and were working full time.

Franzosa *et al.* (2019) examined the effect of emotional labour on home health aides. The study was conducted on 4 worker focus groups (n = 27). Building a close relationship with client was the main central focus of emotional well-being of health workers. This well-being was also influenced by their relationship with clients/ patients and their family members and agency supervisors, the level to which their work was being valued. The aides were alone in managing their job stress as sometimes they felt that family members perceive them as housekeepers or maids and desired more communication care and support from clients, agency supervisors and peers as these relationships add value and meaning to their work. The emotional well-being is important and this well-being would improve aides' sense of confidence, will provides happiness and work-life balance.

2.6 Studies on Nurses

Romagnoli *et al.* (2013) conducted a study on home care and asserted the importance of home care nurses who provide a valuable service to their patients by helping them stay healthier, reducing costs, and avoid hospital stays and providing the patients with long term care facilities in Pittsburgh, US. Home care nurses either sometimes receives lot of information like all the clinical documentation, detailed discharge summaries or too little information (demographic details, primary discharge diagnosis and reason for caring at home). Nurses who are not provided with some actionable information have to rely on caregivers and patients for beneficial, reliable and hopefully accurate information. However, caregivers and patients were not able to provide accurate information because of poor memory, miscommunication and misinterpretation. Moreover, discharge summaries are rarely available to home care nurses as this paperwork is often times either discarded or lost. When nurses make decisions with incomplete information, often this contributes to adverse events because of in appropriate information. Home care providers, physicians, and hospitals need to better engage nurses so that they better understand the information of their patients. Developing interventions for nurses improves caregiver communication and training in the proper care of patient which minimize the risk care givers introduce.

Fatemi *et al.* (2019) conducted a study on challenges faced by nurses in home care settings using a content analysis qualitative method in Iran. Semi-structured interviews were conducted on 33 nurses. Purposive sampling and snowball sampling method were used for data collection. The results of the study showed that nurses were experiencing several economic, psychosocial and bureaucratic problems. They were experiencing physical and mental stress at work. Regarding the economic problems, the nurses believed that home care services are not affordable in Iran as these are not covered under health insurance. Moreover, families receive help from unauthorized persons who are unskilled and uneducated and provide services at low cost. This aspect could endanger the well-being of patients. Issues such as power status change, lack of social security, reduction of social status, extreme bureaucracy were the social difficulties and challenges which were faced by home care nurses in Iran.

Andersson *et al.* (2017) conducted a study on nurses' competencies in home health care. Ten nurses were interviewed and data was analyzed through qualitative technique using content analysis. It was highlighted that nurses in home care wanted to take care of the patients by developing their competencies. Sometimes, they feel as their competencies are being wasted because they are made to be involved in lot of administrative work which they actually consider as time consuming and stealing time from actual nursing care. Moreover, they felt that managers should provide sufficient recognition and support to nurses in their competence development otherwise working in an unstructured and chaotic environment can increase the risk for staff turnover.

Oresland *et al.* (2008) examined the role of nurses as guests or professionals in home health care. Ten nurses were interviewed using discourse analysis. The findings interpreted that nurses working in home care constructed position as guests and as professionals. The participants were nurses working in home health centre in Sweden who provided care to patients at home. Almost all the nurses used the term guest to explain their relationship with the patient. They asserted that nurses are more committed at in home care than in hospitals. They also believed that in patient homes, patient act as daily routine and not the nurses. They have to live by the guest behaviour, ask for permissions, and imitate the patients' way of talking. Although nurses preferred their position as guest, but occasionally they took position as professionals as a part of their responsibility, the nurses also gave advice to the patients regarding medication, nutrition and technological equipment. They made decisions for the patients, taught and supported their relatives and even patient helpers. They were clear to express that in their relationship with patients, they have to maintain a distance. They further said that especially in home care, nurses have to make a choice between two positions. However, the two positions creates different ethical appeals and encourages nurses to act and perform in diverse ways.

Chhugani and Merlin (2017) analyzed the challenges faced by nurses in the health care system in India. It is evident that nurses play an integral role in the care of patients. There are certain challenges faced by nurses that include workplace violence which is caused by the additional amount of workload and responsibilities on the staff leading to stress and disturbed mental state. Workplace mental violence can be in the form of verbal abuse, harassment and threats caused by patients, visitors, and even the co- workers. Shortage of staff also leads to unmanageable patient care and thus inefficient care. Furthermore, the nurses are also confronted with high risk of developing occupational health hazards at their workplace. The authors also elaborated on the long working hours and double shifts carried by nurses. Thus, it is quite difficult to provide nursing care with exhausted mind and body. Lack of teamwork and recognition at workplace is also an emerging challenge in health care. It is noted that in almost all health care settings, nurses are the ones spending more time on the non-nursing work for example: record keeping, laundry, physiotherapy, diet thereby reducing time for patient care. If at any point of their work, there is any fault, they have to bear the burden in the form of salary deductions and cancellation of leaves. It is of utmost importance to not only recognize and understand their problems but find solutions to resolve them.

2.7 Studies on Patients

Welch *et al.* (1996) conducted a study on the use of Medicare home health care services. The programme consisted of home visits by nurses and health care aides as a means to facilitate patients after hospital discharge. As home health care is considered as one of the fastest growing Medicare expenditures. The study examined the relation between home care visits and the hospital discharge. The researchers also investigated about the number of months clients received home health care services on enrollees living in 310 U.S metropolitan areas and determined whether with areas of higher home health care have short length of stay in hospitals or lower admission rates. It was found that about 3 million people received over hundred and sixty million home care visits. Seventy eight per cent of the visits happened after more than after hospital discharge. Sixty one per cent of the visits were to enrollees who received home care services for a period of six months or a year. Four per cent of them who received home care for about a month. The majority of the respondent diagnosis reported were chronic condition such as diabetes and cardiovascular diseases but there was no evidence that home health care can be substituted for hospital care. With regard to the geographical variation, five states (Tennessee, Mississippi, Louisiana, Albama and Georgia) has visualised more than 9500 visits per 1000 enrollees. Three states (Minnesota, Hawaii, South Dakota) have less than 2000 visits per 1000 enrollees. Overall, it was analyzed that home care visits are used primarily to provide long term care to patients suffering from chronic conditions. Home health aides play a larger role in providing companionship, assisting with the personal hygiene or performing activities of daily living or helping the families in household chores. Such visits are the substitutes of care earlier provided by the family members or friends.

Dey *et al.* (2012) have pointed towards the demographic transition and the rising population of the elderly in the country. The rise in population is bound to bring more challenges and unprecedented burdens of morbidity and mortality which will impose a great burden on the country's public health care system. Although there are local studies that point towards high prevalence of various risk factors, the rise in ailments and utilization of health care services among the elderly but in general, there is a scarcity of large scale studies affirming this for the growing subset of population. Multiple studies under the scope of this review emphasize that the elderly are more prone and likely to suffer from chronic illnesses than from acute illnesses and even though there is a sharp rise in non-communicable, communicable and infectious diseases, the leading cause of death among the elderly is cardiovascular disease.

There is a gap in the accessibility and affordability of health care because of social and physical barriers in the presence of social inequality. Accessibility is limited by various factors both social and physical. Social factors such as gender, marital status, religion, caste, education, economic independence and sanitation also do have a bearing on the health of the elderly. Patterns of living, property ownership and kin-based caregiving were also factored to be affirmative factors affecting the health of the elderly in India. It is to be noted that social ties and strong social support additionally do have a health protective impact, no matter what their source is. The impact of traumatic events such as marital or familial exploitation, financial deprivation, verbal, psychological or emotional humiliation tends to impact the elderly negatively, compromising their health in the longer run. Stigma around ageing and associated events such as widowhood, dementia, depression etc. is also a social barrier faced by the elderly depriving them of quality life. The ignorance towards mental health in our society in general has not left the elderly unaffected and they are not acknowledged under the purview of health care in India.

Physical barriers include access to home-based care which is needed due to illness related confinement; this is consistent in both rural and urban areas in India. This confinement is directly related to increasing age that hinders the mobility of the elderly and thereby directly hindering health seeking, however, with increasing age, health needs tend to increase and not *vice versa*.

The review does not fall short on highlighting how affordability is a constraint even today because of limited income, lack of financial protection and unavailability of mechanisms of social security. The urge and need to work in order to support themselves has a direct impact on the health of the individual. In the Indian scenario, there is disparity in the availability of insurance and pension schemes. Not every stratum in the workforce has equal access to these which pushes a considerable proportion of the elderly to work. Sometimes, limited remuneration is also a limiting factor, this imposes a burden on their pockets, often leaving a little for their health needs. In such a scenario, security in old age is assured through movable or immovable property assets which in a patriarchal society as ours, is more accessible to the men of the household.

Inability to pay for health care is also a major barrier towards the health care of the elderly, the inefficiency of the health care system has led to a boom of private health care system which puts people into a vulnerable position both financially and health-wise. With a rise in the burden of chronic diseases, the elderly require long term care which increases the likelihood of large sum of expenditures being utilised on health care in these private sectors, posing direct bearing on their pocket and long term effects on their health. The need for financial protection in such a scenario becomes crucial. In India, this is provided either by a person's own savings or by insurance, both of which are not equally accessible to all. Such benefits are often limited to and enjoyed by the privileged sections of the society. Therefore, the different patterns and priorities of the elderly can be examined by careful examination of this section of the population. The study strongly points out the various challenges to access and affordability, the likely determinants of such challenges and the incompleteness of data on these burdens of health care for the elderly.

McCorkle *et al.* (2000) conducted a study on how specialized home care intervention improves survival among older post-surgical patients. The study was undertaken on 375 patients aged between 60 to 92 years diagnosed with solid cancer, and were surgically treated between February 1993 and December 1995. One hundred ninety patients were randomized to the intervention group and 185 to the usual care group. The study undermines that changes in the health care system have resulted in shortened hospital stays, moving the focus of care from hospital to caring at home. Patients who are discharged post-operation have their ongoing needs. However, their recovery and survival rates are influenced by nursing care post hospitalization. Post-surgical patients are discharged with highly complex problems, accompanied by catheters, dressings, and high technology equipment, including pain infusion pumps. Most of patients after their surgery need monitoring for their healing of wounds, pulmonary complications, fever and pain. In addition to this, most of them need assistance in performing activities of daily living like ambulation (assisting in walking), basic hygiene (bathing, dental care, dressing, grooming) and preparation of meals. Unfortunately, for some older patients who are discharged early, they are not able to afford home follow ups and in case of some geographic areas, this service is not even available (Oberst and James, 1985; Federal Register, 1997; Harris, 1998).

It was found that the patients who received home care lived 7 months longer than the usual care patients and the invention group have twice survival rates than the usual care group. It was further investigated that specialized home care nurses works on a standard nursing protocol by providing direct physical care, education, an ongoing psychosocial support, and further help the patient in the management of surgical complications, if any. Moreover, caregivers involved in the home care are taught to provide direct care to the home patients. Overall, the specialized home care intervention group was found to have increased survival among patients.

Yaffe *et al.* (2002) underwent a study on patient and caregiver characteristics and nursing home placements for patients with dementia. The primary indications are severe impairment of the cognitive system for nursing home patients. About 90 per cent of the patients requires institutionalized care before their death. The decision whether to place the patient in long term care depends upon the characteristics of the patient and the primary caregivers along with their socio-cultural context. Thus, the home care nursing placement intervention aims at long care placements would ultimately reduce health care cost and would possibly improve the quality of life of patients by maintaining their independence also (Michel *et al.*, 2001). A prospective study model was framed for 5788 dementia patients with ethnically diverse characteristics living in community and were enrolled in Medicare Alzheimer Disease and Demonstration and Evaluation (MADDE) in United States to predict which patients and their caregivers needed home nursing placement during the 3-year period. The patients who were recruitment were based on physician recruitment and self-referral. The baseline characteristics of difficult behaviour visualized were psychotic symptoms, anger, aggressiveness, dangerous to self and others and wakes caregiver up at night. The patient's cognitive Status was assessed with a 30-point Mini-Mental State Examination (MMSE). Patient's functional status was measured with the help of Katz activities of daily living such as bathing, dressing, eating, transferring and helping with the commode (Katz *et al.*, 1963). They also recorded medical co morbidities such as hearing impairment, arthritis, diabetes, hypertension, artery disease, pulmonary disease and vision impairment. The baseline characteristics of caregivers caring for dementia patients were analyzed. Along with that caregiver burden was assessed with the use of Zarit Scale with specific items assessing caregiver sense of control, stress, anger, and time constraints. Additionally, the findings of the study suggested that caregiver burden is associated with nursing home placements for patients with dementia. However, caregiver stress and depression can be prevented. A comprehensive counselling intervention for the caregivers helps to teach the caregiver behavioural management techniques to reduce difficult patient behaviour. So this training can bring about a delay in nursing home care placements needs for patients which could produce large health system cost savings. Unfortunately, physicians fail to notice the caregiver stress and depression and the caregiving services are not always accessible. The lower rate of nursing home use by some caregivers is also associated with economic hardships. The demands and cost associated with caregiving will always become a matter of concern.

Dias *et al.* (2008) conducted a study on the effectiveness of home care programme for supporting caregivers who are taking care of dementia patients. The purpose of the study was to evaluate the effectiveness of home care intervention in reducing behavioural problems in elderly persons with dementia and reducing caregiver burden and promoting their mental health. The study was conducted in Goa on 89 patients and their caregivers. It was concluded that home based support for caregivers of persons who are caring for dementia patients emphasize the use of locally available and low cost human resources. This has led to the significant improvements in caregiver mental health and also helps in reducing their burden of caring.

Caregiver mental health was measured through General Health Questionnaire, caregiver burden (Zarit Burden Score) and activities of daily activities of elderly with dementia was measured with Everyday Abilities Scale for India (EASI). While distress and severity of the behavioural problems was measured with (NPI-D, NPI-S). One of the major findings was that the intervention led to significant improvement in caregivers' mental health and perceived burden as the model aimed to improve the knowledge and awareness of family caregivers regarding dementia, in addition to provide emotional support to caregivers thus improving their caregiving skills. Further non-significant reductions were observed for behaviour disturbances and functional ability and a 64 per cent reduction in the risk of death in the intervention arm.

Suk Jung *et al.* (2013) evaluated the quality of life in home health care patients between the start of care and discharge. The sample consisted of 100 home health care patients who are receiving health care services from home care agency in the United States. The data was collected through using the World Health Organization, Quality of life scale-brief used for measuring quality of life, activities of daily living and instrumental ADL. The study showed that home care services which were provided care by registered nurses using the OASIS items showed improved clinical outcomes and improved quality of life after 60 days of home care. Major improvements were seen in specific caregiving areas such as dressing lower body and bathing. In case of IADL, improvement was seen in preparing light meals, shopping and house-keeping. Overall, the findings showed that quality of life, general health and 3 domains, i.e. physical, psychological and environmental but not same in the social domain that showed signs of improved at the discharge or 60 days of care. It was concluded that home care nurses should focus on improving the functional abilities of patients and this would play an important role in improving the lives of these patients which receive care at home.

Wang *et al.* (2014) analyzed the review studies on world aging problems. It has been intercepted that the world is facing tremendous problem with tremendous growth of older population. Older people are discharged from hospitals with complex medical problems as they are not able to manage their health needs during the transitional period. Many older people have no family members who could take care of their needs. Nurses are expected to take full responsibility for the patient's health care needs. Therefore, effective discharge planning was very important to ensure continuity of care for the older population. The transitional period is defined as period after hospital discharge for a major health disorder for recovery of patients in a home setting. The review studies highlighted the need for continuing care. Discharge planning was thoroughly discussed and the follow up intervention implementation in China. It was further analyzed that inadequate discharge planning and follow up were the factors that were associated with readmission of older patients. Further, it was important that nurses led discharge plan should be implemented in China.

Nelson *et al.* (2018) examined the home-based kidney care in rural communities in Zuni Indians living in United States. To develop the intervention, the authors worked with the Zuni tribal leadership to improve health literacy about diabetes and kidney disease in the community. A 12-month clinical trial was performed in 98 adults suffering from CKD to examine the efficiency of home-based kidney care. After initial lifestyle lessons, the intervention group received additional information by the community health representatives about their diet, exercise, alcohol abuse, smoking, management of diabetes and hypertension. The participants were also trained to used blood pressure and glucose monitor machines. Highest scores for the patients in the intervention group predicted improved quality of life. Thus, the patient in the intervention group showed confidence in managing their health.

Prinja *et al.* (2018) investigated the cost of intensive care treatment for liver disorders. The study was undertaken to assess the health care cost, out of pocket expenses and the financial risk related with the treatment of liver disorder. The present study was carried out in intensive care units (ICU) of a tertiary hospital in North India. Data on out-of-pocket expenditure and indirect cost related to liver disorders was collected from 150 patients. Result indicated that in the year 2013-14, health care cost per patient treated in ICU and HDU (high dependency unit) were Rs. 1,63,644 and Rs. 1,17,985 respectively. The mean OOP expenditures for treatment in the ICU and HDU were Rs. 1,42,297 and Rs. 1,05,093 respectively. Indirect cost accounted to about Rs. 9,952 and Rs. 10,903 respectively. Overall, it was investigated that the treatment of chronic liver disorders poses an economic burden for the patients and the health care system. There is an utmost need to focus on the prevention of liver disorders and finding additional ways to treat patients without exposing their households to the effect of out-of-pocket expenses.

Kumari *et al.* (2020) explored and identified the practices of self-management by heart failure patients and the home management of heart failure symptoms by their family caregivers and health care providers. The qualitative study was conducted in North India on total 41 participants (15 patients, 12 caregivers, 10 nurses and 4 doctors). It was found that the patients and their family members were not able to manage heart failure symptoms. Nurses and doctors faced various barriers to provide specialized care to the patients. It seemed very important to develop self-care management protocol for the heart failure patients. Health care professionals must find a solution to overcome the barriers to train patients and their family caregivers for self-care at home.

Mathur (2022) outlined the role of home health care in the treatment of kidney patients. In India, diabetes and hypertension accounts for about 40-60 per cent cases of CKD, Chronic Kidney Disease. As per the data sources of Indian Council of Medical Research, the prevalence of diabetes has risen to 7.1 per cent. With the rising prevalence of these diseases in India, the prevalence of CKD is also going to rise. Patients with kidney diseases faces multiple issues such as sudden deterioration of kidney function (Acute Kidney Failure), severe UTI (Urinary Tract Infection), dehydration due to poor intake or loss from the body. Home health care services providers support to patients to help to manage their disease at home. The independent treatment for peritoneal dialysis, PD (type of dialysis which is used to remove excess fluid and remove toxins in patients with kidney failure) is some suitable alternative to hospital treatments. One of the advantages of home care is the avoidance of hospital borne infections which can lead to morbidity and mortality. Additionally, the cost of caring patients at home is lower than in a hospital. A part of regular monitoring is keeping tab of sugar and blood pressure by the health care professionals keep the disease under control by modifying medication as per the requirement of the patients. Advanced home care services are available in India for the sick and ailing patients. An ICU set up can be created in the home with complete medical equipment such a facility at home could cost less than half of the cost of being in an ICU of hospital. All the treatment is monitored by trained nursing staff, doctors and nurse supervisors at home. All aspects of kidney care, dialysis kidney transplant care can be provided in the comfortable surroundings of the home. The patient care plan also includes monitoring of vital parameters, A.V. fistula care and catheter care along with the infection controlled diet and medication management. This entire care continuum can go a long way in preventing further deterioration and adds to improved patient care.

Desai (2019) elaborated that the home based health care is not just convenient and time saving for the patient, but could also be the solution to the shortage of hospital beds. The health care landscape in India is expanding and is projected to reach $6.2 billion by 2020 and could replace up to 65 per cent hospital visits and reduce hospital cost by 20 per cent, according to CMR's India Home Healthcare Report 2016.

Though in a nascent stage in India, and largely serviced by unorganized players, start-ups and recent hospital initiatives, the market stood at around $3.20 billion in 2016, and is expected to grow to around $4.46 billion by 2018 and $6.21 billion in 2020, according to Cyber Media Research (CMR) Ltd. analysis and industry estimate[3].

Patel *et al.* (2011) asserted that India has one of the most fragmented and commercialized health care systems in the world, where world-class care is greatly outweighed by unregulated poor quality health services. India can no longer accept a health care system that is frequently exploitative, almost completely unregulated, and so poorly performing. The health conditions for

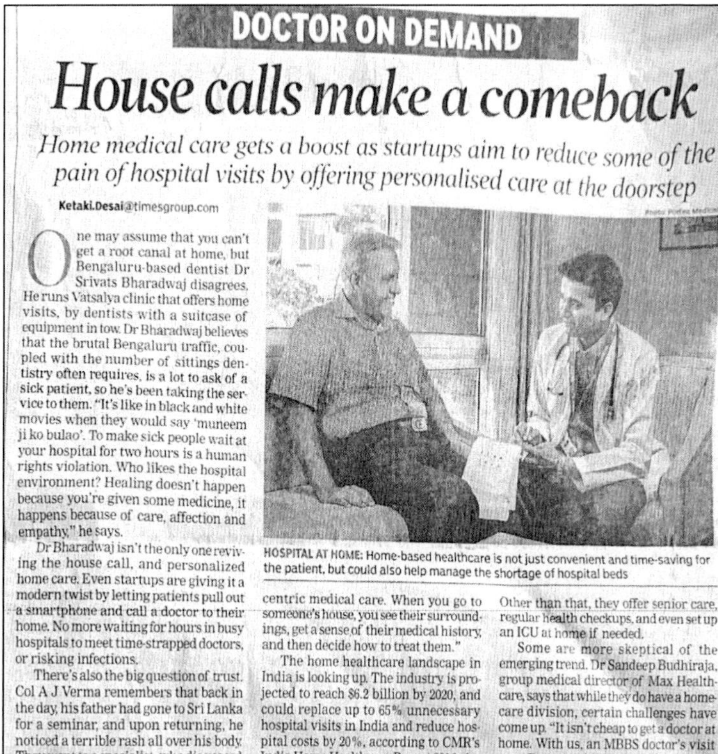

DOCTOR ON DEMAND

House calls make a comeback

Home medical care gets a boost as startups aim to reduce some of the pain of hospital visits by offering personalised care at the doorstep

Ketaki.Desai@timesgroup.com

One may assume that you can't get a root canal at home, but Bengaluru-based dentist Dr Srivats Bharadwaj disagrees. He runs Vatsalya clinic that offers home visits, by dentists with a suitcase of equipment in tow. Dr Bharadwaj believes that the brutal Bengaluru traffic, coupled with the number of sittings dentistry often requires, is a lot to ask of a sick patient, so he's been taking the service to them. "It's like in black and white movies when they would say 'muneem ji ko bulao'. To make sick people wait at your hospital for two hours is a human rights violation. Who likes the hospital environment? Healing doesn't happen because you're given some medicine, it happens because of care, affection and empathy," he says.

Dr Bharadwaj isn't the only one reviving the house call, and personalized home care. Even startups are giving it a modern twist by letting patients pull out a smartphone and call a doctor to their home. No more waiting for hours in busy hospitals to meet time-strapped doctors, or risking infections.

There's also the big question of trust. Col A J Verma remembers that back in the day, his father had gone to Sri Lanka for a seminar, and upon returning, he noticed a terrible rash all over his body. They went to a specialist, who diagnosed it as herpes. When days of medication led to no improvement, they finally turned to a family physician who, after some extensive questioning, realized it was just an allergic reaction to seafood and cured him in no time. So, when Delhi-based Col Verma, 65, found himself with an excruciatingly painful skin condition, he decided to turn to FamPhy, an app that brings a doctor to your doorstep through a call or a click.

Col Verma says, "When Dr Kalita of FamPhy came to my house, he spent 2-3 hours trying to understand my history, because I am also a cancer patient. He took a very holistic view, and has become someone whose opinion I really trust."

Initiatives like FamPhy are looking to revive home-based healthcare in India, not just for the elderly or bedridden, but anyone — the busy, the lazy, and the hospital-detesting. Dr Soumik Kalita, founder of FamPhy, says, "My parents were family doctors, and looked after people in the remotest areas of the country. Today, there is a problem of over-specialization, and a lack of person-centric medical care. When you go to someone's house, you see their surroundings, get a sense of their medical history, and then decide how to treat them."

HOSPITAL AT HOME: Home-based healthcare is not just convenient and time-saving for the patient, but could also help manage the shortage of hospital beds

The home healthcare landscape in India is looking up. The industry is projected to reach $6.2 billion by 2020, and could replace up to 65% unnecessary hospital visits in India and reduce hospital costs by 20%, according to CMR's India Home Healthcare Report 2016. An increasing number of players offer everything from post-operative care to physiotherapy, and lab tests to post-natal assistance. Some are startups looking to disrupt the medical ecosystem, while others are hospitals like Apollo that have expanded to home-care to tackle overcrowding of hospitals.

> **When you go to someone's house, you see their surroundings, get a sense of their medical history, and then decide treatment**
>
> **DR SOUMIK KALITA** | Founder, FamPhy

Portea Medical has treated over 3.5 lakh patients in their homes in 16 Indian cities. Their CEO Meena Ganesh says, "As a country, we have been focussing on investing in hospital care, but nothing else. People in their 30s and 40s are getting chronic diseases like diabetes and hypertension more often now, and we're looking to cater to this population." Other than that, they offer senior care, regular health checkups, and even set up an ICU at home if needed.

Some are more skeptical of the emerging trend. Dr Sandeep Budhiraja, group medical director of Max Healthcare, says that while they do have a home-care division, certain challenges have come up. "It isn't cheap to get a doctor at home. With us, an MBBS doctor's visit costs Rs 3000, while a specialist charges Rs 5000. When people are paying that much money, they want the logistics to be according to their own liking, which is difficult. Specialists are busy and want to optimise their time."

CEO of Healthcare at Home Vivek Srivastava likens the rise of home healthcare to e-commerce. "People want everything to be delivered to their homes. Why should healthcare be any different?"

Also, in terms of cost, Srivastava argues that it is cheaper — according to their calculations, a home-based ICU stay is 30% cheaper than what it would be in a hospital.

Dr Bharadwaj believes in outcome-based pricing rather than a pre-determined fee to rebuild the doctor-patient trust that rising rates and over-prescription have gotten in the way of. One of his patients is Ajay Parikh whose family of three have all received dental care at home. "You're busy during the week, and dread the traffic on the weekend, so you keep postponing the appointment. By the time you finally go to the doctor, the problem has gotten worse. This way, you're able to intervene a lot faster."

Plate 2.6: Home medical care offering personalized care at the door steps (Desai, 2019).

most have to improve if all Indians want to enjoy the freedoms that lend value to their lives.

With a rapidly aging population, the demand for home care aides is projected to increase by over 50 per cent in the next decade (National Advisory Committee on Rural Health and Human Services, 2009). These aides, frequently called home care aides (HCAs) or personal care attendants (PCAs) and whose work is coordinated and overseen by nurses, provide assistance with personal care, activities of daily living, transportation, and light housework. Recruiting and retaining reliable HCAs/PCAs has been an ongoing challenge for home health care agencies throughout the country, a challenge which will only increase as the demand for the services performed by these workers continues to climb. The short supply of direct care workers has been labelled by some as a public-health crisis, because the ultimate victims of this care gap are the elder consumers of services (Wilner and Wyatt, 1999).

2.8 Relevance and Anticipated Outcomes

The market for home health care services in India is a cheaper and more comfortable option for patients which is set to double in a year's time, as per the health economists. However, large-scale studies of the health behaviours of this growing elderly Indian population are still scarce.

Information gathered from numerous surveys and regional and local studies point to the high prevalence of several risky behaviours, such as tobacco and alcohol use (Goswami *et al.*, 2005; Gupta *et al.*, 2005; Mutharayappa and Bhat, 2008), and physical inactivity (Rastogi *et al.*, 2004; Vaz and Bharathi, 2004). With these stressors, predictably, aggregate data comparing the 52nd (1995-1996) and 60th Rounds (2004) of the National Sample Survey (NSS) suggest a general increase in the reports of ailments and utilization of health care services among the elderly (Alam and Karan, 2010; Rao, 2006). Access to services, however, remain uneven across the country.

With advancements in information technology and integration

with medical electronics, it is now possible to provide high-quality care at home at an affordable price. Additionally, home health care services mean more beds available for needy patients. Home health care services are an extension of hospital services into the patient's house and providing personalized care by competent professionals. "Home health care companies work with hospitals to widen their reach, by freeing the beds for new patients while covering almost 70 per cent of all health care requirements of a consumer and extending to management of lifestyle and chronic diseases like diabetes, hypertension etc. over a consumer's lifetime," said Vivek Srivastava, CEO and co-founder of Noida-based "Health Care at Home", a home health care provider.

The advantages of home health care include cost effectiveness with excellent clinical outcomes as customers end up saving 20-50 per cent costs as compared to regular hospital treatment depending upon the services taken. For instance, ICU services are 50 per cent cheaper than those provided in hospitals. There is tremendous pressure on hospitals in delivering services at their facility, especially in critical care. As per government and private hospital statistics, about 40 per cent of patients admitted in hospitals suffer from chronic diseases such as heart diseases, diabetes, stroke and chronic obstructive pulmonary disease (COPD).

The typical cost of stay in an ICU in a hospital could range between Rs. 5,000 to Rs. 50,000 a day. By contrast, setting up an ICU facility at home with equipment and medical expertise would range between Rs. 7,500 to Rs. 10,000 a day. Even hospitals are entering the home health care market. Max Health care, a health care provider, recently introduced 'Max@Home', its home-based health care service offering programme. Max@Home has been launched as a specialized continued care programme, backed by Max Healthcare's 12-hospital network.

The programme facilitates real-time patient monitoring by connecting doctors, dedicated case managers, trained nursing staff and emergency services through an efficient technology infrastructure created by Western India Products (WIPRO), a multinational IT consulting and system integration Service Company.

The state of geriatric care is still at a very nascent stage in India where the population outnumbers the health care service providers. Although there has been an entry of home health care in both private and public sectors in India, it is still in its early years of conception and is a growing industry. Most home health care services are clustered in southern part of the country. Some of the major stakeholders of the market are India Home Health Care, Portea Medical, Nightingales, Apna Care, Health Heal etc. With an upward rising trend and preference of home health care in India, there have been investments by many big investors such as Angel Investment, Marquee Angel Investors, Accel Partners, Venture East, Qualcomm Ventures etc. Therefore, the growth of such service providers is evidence of the fact that integrated home care is an urgent requirement for caregiving of the elderly in India, which can be a lucrative and successful market in the country (Singh, 2017).

Various studies have called for attention to the scenario of home health care in India. They talk about the rise in costs and inflated health care which is a matter of concern for aging populations, especially those coming from developing countries. In such scenarios, there is humungous scope for growth of the home health care sector which is a seemingly less costly option than availing regular institutional care.

There has been an elaborate effort in understanding the extensions to home health care, first are the organizations that are involved in the manufacturing, supplying, and monitoring, of therapeutic and interventional devices for health care, and second are the organizations that provide home care services concerning health to the patients and needy. These both are essential components of comprehensive health care in developing countries like India. Home care in India consists of both small and large organizations which remain organized, semi-organized, and unorganized. The organized sector is formed of hospitals, nursing homes, and old age homes whereas the semi-organized sector represents the various home health providers in different cities. The largest sector is the unorganized sector where semi-trained male and female house helpers are kept for caregiving directly by the patient and perhaps provided on-the-job training by the family or the visiting staff.

It is not to be missed that home care is mostly needed by the elderly and by patients suffering from chronic diseases who require constant and consistent medical care and monitoring. The acute shortage of hospital beds and rising costs of these kinds of services are driving factors behind this demand rise. Thus, home care seems to be the best alternative for patients requiring persistent care.

It has also been highlighted that home care and care by family members are preferred by Indians contrary to Western countries where post-retirement homes, long-term insurance, and advanced at-home care form the backbone of health care. This difference could be attributed to the difference in the cultural backdrop and also to cut costs on large hospital bills. Whatever may be the reason, this has led to an increase in home care trends across the country in one form or another. With this trend, it is now possible for people to remain in the comfort of their homes rather than use institutional or hospital-based care. Home care also comes with its own set of benefits such as more personalized care, living within the comfort of own home, freedom to move around in the home etc. which are important to the happiness of the patient and aid recovery. It allows the patient to assume a feeling of independence.

Keeping this in consideration, a comprehensive list of home health care provider services in India and detailed information on them can be helpful for needy patients. However, even the most beneficial of services do not come without challenges, therefore, due attention has also been paid to call out the challenges in the home care sector.

The problem of home health aides and nurses in comparison to the demand, lack of proper training, lack of quality products, difficult working conditions, stressful work environment, difficulty in reaching isolated places, investment in travel costs, apprehensions of family members, and doubts about service providers are some of the many challenges put across these home health care providers. Thus, along with the many benefits, there are immense challenges in this booming industry that need to be dealt with to provide quality health care and for the growth of this sector.[4]

The state of the elderly in the country is such that they are without any social or health safety nets in the sunset years of their lives. Among this section, the most deprived are the ones who are bedbound or in need of home care round the clock. Realizing the need and urgency of this concern and its impact on our health care system HelpAge India carried out an innovative pilot in 3 locations of India that are Shimla, Leh, and Cuddalore to comprehend the concept of Community and Family Caregivers for Long Term and Palliative Care need of the elderly and published a report titled "Home care for the elderly in India—A call to action". This was an experimental study to ascertain if an approach like other Asian countries such as Thailand can be applied in India.

These places were chosen based on the problems of the elderly and remoteness which makes provision for caregiving a tough task in such areas. The sample reflected that a significant percentage, i.e. 59 per cent out of the total sample of 2500 were suffering from a long-term disease that required regular medication and long-home care. The report indicated that 62.1 per cent of the elderly require home care of the total sample included in the study. It is well highlighted that it is high time to wake up to the silent sufferings of its elderly who constitute the most marginalized and neglected section of society. As a country moving towards providing the highest quality of life for its citizen; the state of the elderly tell an altogether different story.

The lives of the elderly in the country are destitute, they suffer from ill health, neglect, and abuse at the hands of their children, families, and others. Changes with declining age such as reduced eyesight, hearing, and mobility are additional factors inducing the destitution of the elderly. There is a deepening crisis for this age group particularly due to the non-existent facilities in both public and private sectors, however, the report also highlights the provision of some governmental support services available across various states such as pension schemes, shelter for the elderly etc.

The lack of health care for the elderly is a matter of grave concern, therefore, it is suggested that a model for care provision which is effective both cost and programme-wise to the community should be taken up within the existing public health system. The results reflect that as compared with the other two places under study, Leh reported a very high need for Home care services, i.e. 55.8 per cent, in which females required more attention than their male counterparts. The study successfully demonstrated that the elderly preferred family members and someone known to them deliver the care. Wherever the caregiver was employed they visited the elderly routinely and provided various care to them at their homes.

Their ill health and low quality of life are a matter of concern and the project ensured linking the elderly to the various programmes of HelpAge which was benefiting for the elderly, as they were then able to visit doctors and seek help *via* referrals. The project ensured the utilization of the 24×7 Elderly Helpline of HelpAge India as well. The elderly were also linked to the local government health centres. The baseline data from these three places indicate the need to intervene and ensure the provision of care to the elderly at home and how it can be insured.

The project was successful in demonstrating that with the proper community mobilization and participation, it is possible to commit that the community and family members work together to ensure care and health for their elders in the true spirit of respect and caregiving.[5]

Given the large number of elderly persons who receive care from Medicare-certified home health care agencies, it is reasonable to anticipate that some patients will be in a trajectory of decline. Due to both normal aging and pathological processes that occur more frequently with advancing age, some elderly persons will experience decreasing ability to carry out activities of daily living (ADLs), even when high-quality home health care is provided. Thus, an implicit goal of home health care should be to facilitate a supported decline. This is consistent with the American Nurses Association's assertion that promoting the patient's optimal level of well-being is a legitimate goal of home health care[6]. The demand for at-home health care delivery is growing because quality post-operative care in familiar surroundings has been observed to enable faster patient's recovery.

With these perspectives in sight, present study is an attempt to highlight the state of the home health care sector highlighting the role, responsibilities, experiences and burden of patients, family caregivers, nurses and personal care assistants in home care.

Notes

1. https://www.yashodahospitals.com/blog/endocrine-disorders-symptoms-causes-diagnosis-treatments/
2. https://www.cms.gov/Medicare/Quality-Initiatives-Patient-Assessment Instruments/HomeHealthQualityInits/index.html (accessed on 15/07/2019).
3. Market for home healthcare services in India to double in a year: report (livemint.com)
4. https://www.academia.edu/5861649/Home_healthcare_In_India
5. Homecare-Report.pdf (helpageindia.org)
6. https://www.livemint.com/Politics/NfL5WsKohfFzCTcbCLdrQN/Market-for-home-healthcare-services-in-India-to-double-in-a.html(accessed on 10/06/19)

3

Research Methodology

Approaches and Techniques

Research is a scientific endeavour. It involves scientific method which serves as a means for gaining knowledge of the universe. It does not only belong to any particular body of knowledge, it is universal. It does not refer to a field of scientific subject of matter, but rather to a procedure or mode of investigation (Kothari, 2009).

Research methodology is a way to systematically solve the research problem. In the present study, the researcher has examined data through both quantitative and qualitative means. The chapter also presents the research methodology involved in investigating the role of home care agencies. The central part of the dissertation revolves in analyzing the problems faced by patients, their family members and care providers (Nurses and GDAs). It is through this work, that the researcher would elaborate the need of home care services for the ageing population who nevertheless are also suffering from multiple problems. In order to ensure a representative sample out of the total population, In-depth interviewing with a proportionate representation of age and sex variation will be ensured.

The data generation for this research work is done with the help of following techniques:

- In-depth interviews
- Focused group discussions
- Observation
- Case studies
- Schedules.

Data were collected through field research method. Information was gathered through unstructured interviews, open ended interviews and informal way of asking questions, interpreting, analyzing the context and giving representations.

The study is exploratory in nature, it is also known as formulative research. The purpose of the study is to generate new ideas about research, and to increase the research familiarity of the existing problem and to make a precise formulation of the problem or to gather information for clarifying concepts. An exploratory study as identified by Katz and Festinger (1953) tends to conceptualize two levels. At the first level, the researcher discovers the significant variables and during the second level, there is discovery of relationship between the variables.

In the present study, the researcher conducted in-depth interviews with nurses and general duty assistants and different relationships were discovered between the variables. The study is also descriptive in nature. It is a fact-finding investigation and the results are more specific. It aims at identifying various characteristics of the organisation, community, or problem under study.

Case study which is a significant method of exploring and analysing the life of a social unit, a person, be it a family, institution or community has also been employed in the present study. The case studies are gathered with a view to record the history of a social unit in its natural context and its relationships with the social factors. In the present study, the investigator recorded medical history of the patients, the scrutiny was done with a view to figure the complex set of variables in generating observed results and the intensive study unravelled the complexities of the behaviour (Xavier *et al.,* 2007).

Narratives also contribute meaningfully and form a large part of the study as they bring about a more comprehensive view of events that have occurred over a period of time. Data were collected through in-depth interviews and narratives were framed from responses recorded from the interviewee.

For evaluation of the Socio-economic status which is considered as one of the most important factors in understanding the health conditions of an individual or family. Almost all the studies done in the health-related fields require the assessment of the socio-economic status during the process of data-analysis. In the present study, the researcher has made use of the Modified Kuppuswamy socio-economic scale for the year 2021 (Sheikh and Shah, 2021).

3.1 Research Design

The research design is the 'formidable problem', the conceptual structure within which the research is conducted, as it involves the collection, measurement and analysis of data with an aim to combine the relevance to the research problem (Selltiz, 1962). More explicitly, the design includes an outline of the what is the research study about, what is the actual purpose of study, where the

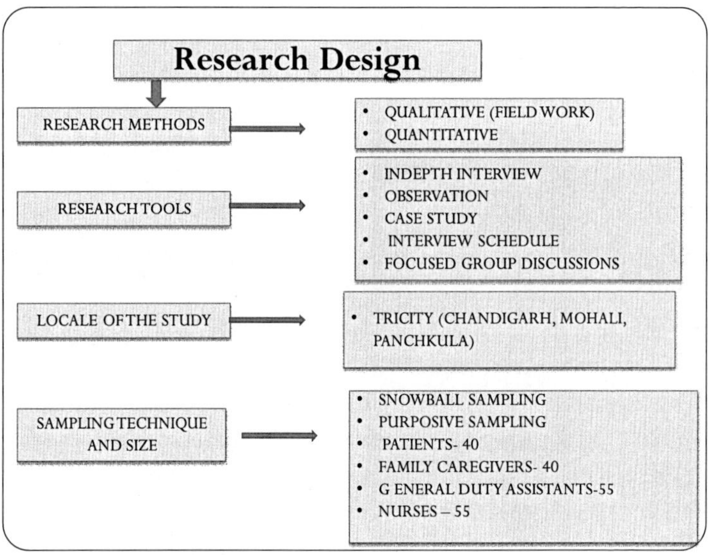

Fig. 3.1: Research Design.

research will be carried, what type of data is required, from where can the data be found, how much is time period of the study, what will be the design of sample, what techniques of data collection are employed, how will the data be analysed by qualitative and quantitative means and how the report will be prepared (Kothari, 2009).

The research design followed in the present study is presented in Fig. 3.1.

3.1.1 About the Study Area, Sample and Duration

Literature was reviewed for a thorough understanding of the research problem and for framing aim and objectives. After formulating the aim and objectives of the study, a pilot study was conducted in the months of June 2020 and July 2020. The main focus of pilot study was to demarcate the area of study and establish a rapport. The researcher visited Max Hospital, Mohali and Hauz Home Health Care Services, Panchkula and 10 per cent (19) of the respondents were taken for this purpose of pretesting and finalizing the Interview schedule.The interview schedules were pre-tested during course of the pilot study by interviewing 15 nursing staff and 15 general duty assistants who are employed and working in home care. After this, necessary modifications were made in the schedule, repetitive and irrelevant questions were deleted.

Snowball sampling method was used to gather further information about more respondents who could be a part of the study. A total sample of 40 nurses, 40 general duty assistants, 40 patients and 40 family caregivers comprised the total sample of the study who were interviewed to analyse altogether tries to understand the problems and perspectives of general duty assistants, nurses and the patients in home health care.

Additionally, 30 focused group interviews were conducted with 15 nursing staff and 15 general duty assistants working in various agencies in Mohali, Chandigarh and Panchkula to get an insight of the overall problems faced by caregivers in home health care. Data were gathered through in-depth interviews, focused group discussions and case studies.

28 case studies were generated through in-depth interviews with the family caregivers. These case studies helped to analyse the medical history of patients.

The present study analysed the overall problems faced by nurses and general duty assistants with respect to the agencies and patients. Additionally, the problems faced by respondents, their family members with regard to the caregiver services provided by (nurses and caregivers) were examined too.

3.1.2 Preparation of Interview Schedules

Three interview schedules were prepared as shown in Annexure-I, Annexure-II and Annexure-III) were developed with the help of information collected through pilot study and secondary sources:

1. Nurses who were working round the clock in various agencies and providing skilled home care services to patients suffering from neurological disorders, cancer, illness and post-surgical care. The minimum educational qualifications of a nurse providing home nursing services are ANM, GNM or B.Sc. Nursing.
2. A schedule was also prepared for the general duty assistants who perform professional caregiving services and are called home health aides, geriatric home health aides (relating to old people), bed side assistants or individuals who have adequate work experience.
3. Patients who were suffering from multiple and chronic illnesses and are receiving care services at home, patients who are bedridden and post-surgery patient in need of transitional care from hospital to home care, patients with disabilities and chronic illness.
4. The fourth and fifth comprised questions related to their relationships.

Interview Schedules

1. In the *first schedule* information was sought *via* questions were framed to know about their current residence, whether they stay in the hostel provided by the agencies

or in a rented accommodation or with the patient. Further questions were asked about their source of income, job structure, number of patients cared for, types of patients handled and years of experience in home care.

To understand about the relationship with the patients, their family members and the agency supervisors, nurses were also interviewed. The variables were further researched to understand the challenges faced by nurses with regard to their emotional well-being at work place. Problems related to the food they were being served, safety issues faced by the respondents were also analysed. Moreover, their satisfaction with the remuneration was also factored in. Henceforth, 28 questions were framed for analysing nurses' burden at their workplace. Burden Scale for Family Caregivers (Grasel, 1995) was used to analyze the burden felt by nursing staff working for the patients in home care and the socio-economic status of the respondents was examined through Modified Kuppuswamy's Scale (Sheikh and Shah, 2021).

2. In the *second schedule*, questions related to the demographic profile of General duty assistants (name, address or place of birth, age, gender, marital status, and religion). Additionally, questions were framed with regard to obtaining information about their current residence, whether they stay in the hostel provided by the agencies or in a rented accommodation or with the client. Information on education, occupation and family income of the respondents were gathered. Further questions were asked about their source of payment, job structure, number of patients cared for, types of patients handled and years of experience in home care. The researcher also interviewed the bed side assistants regarding their relationship with the patients, their family members and the agency supervisors. The variables were helpful for the researcher to understand the challenges faced by home health aides with regard to their emotional well-being at work place. Problems related to the food being served, safety issues faced by the respondents were also analyzed. Moreover, their satisfaction with respect to remuneration was also studied. They were also interviewed to obtain information regarding professional caregiving services performed in home health care and the benefits and adverse effects of working in home care. Henceforth, 28 questions were framed for analyzing caregiver's burden at their workplace. Burden Scale for Family Caregivers (Grasel, 1995) was used to analyse the burden felt by caregivers working for the patients in home care.

3. The *third schedule* was used for collecting information from patients. Questions were framed and the patients and their family members were interviewed. Questions were framed to gather detailed information about the medical history of respondents that included information on name, address, age, gender, marital status and religion. Additionally, they were asked questions regarding their current residence, whether they are staying in their own place, or in a rented accommodation or with any of their relatives. Further questions were framed to know about the primary caregiver, home settings of the patient, whether the patient is suffering from any infectious disease, protective equipments provided to them, length of engagement of caregivers, services preferred, number of health care personnel preferred, gender preferred, language and religion preferred. At the same time, patients and their family caregivers were also interviewed to know about their preference for caregiver shift patterns, performance of daily activities and instrumental activities of daily living required by the patients as per the underlying diseases they suffer from. However, they were also interviewed to know whether they were satisfied with the caregiver duties and the problems and challenges faced by them with regard to caregiver and nursing services. Zarit Burden Interview

(ZBI) Scale was used in order to identify family caregivers at risk for depression (Zarit *et al.*, 1980).

4. The *fourth* and *fifth schedules* mainly focused on collecting information about the health care staff relationship with the patients and their family members. Additionally, information was also collected about their benefits and drawbacks of working in home care.

On the basis of information collected through pilot study and literature reviewed, some changes were incorporated in the schedules and thereafter the schedules were finalised after making necessary modifications.

3.1.3 Universe and Unit of the Study

The universe for the research comprised the home care agencies and hospitals situated in Chandigarh, SAS Nagar and Panchkula and because universe of the study is too large, the nurses, General duty assistants and patients were recruited through snowball sampling technique to gather maximum information. Purposive sampling method was also used both of which are explained later in this chapter.

The researcher visited various agencies and hospitals that provided home care services. The unit of the study were nursing supervisors, nursing staff, general duty assistants, patients and their family caregivers. The family caregivers were interviewed in order to gather required information from the patient.

3.2 Sample Size

This refers to number of items to be selected from the universe of the study. The size of the sample should be optimum, should be neither too large nor too small. The sample size for the present study consisted of 55 nursing staff, 55 general duty assistants, 40 patients, 40 family caregivers. A total of 190 respondents were thus interviewed for the study. The sampling was carried out in stages.

Stage I: Initially nurses who are working as home care staff were approached for being interviewed. To ensure diversity in the sample, nurses from different states and religions were included in the study. In-depth interviews were conducted to gain deeper insight into their behaviour and to understand the problems and challenges and the benefits of working as home care staff. To further analyse the scope of home care, the nurse managers who were responsible for supervising the staff were interviewed as well.

Stage II: General duty assistants also known as bed side assistants, home health aides, or geriatric home health aides. Such caregivers who worked in Tricity and ranged from different states and religions were interviewed. Those caregivers were selected who have received professional training and have prior experience in providing caregiving services to chronically ill and bedridden patients.

Table 3.1: Total Sample size

<table>
<tr><th>Unit of the study</th><th>Sample size</th><th>Locale of the study</th></tr>
<tr><td>Nurses</td><td>40</td><td rowspan="4">Home care agencies, hospitals, Patient's homes, Chandigarh, Mohali (SAS NAGAR) and Panchkula</td></tr>
<tr><td>General Duty Assistants</td><td>40</td></tr>
<tr><td>Patients</td><td>40</td></tr>
<tr><td>Family Caregivers</td><td>40</td></tr>
<tr><td>Nurses</td><td>15</td><td rowspan="2">Home care agencies</td></tr>
<tr><td>General Duty Assistants</td><td>15</td></tr>
</table>

Stage III: Additionally, visit to other agencies were made to collect data from the patients and family caregivers who were seeking home care services.

3.3 Duration of the Study

The field work was carried out for 12 months in four phases. The researcher visited various agencies and conducted in-depth interviews with the nurses, general duty assistants, clients and their family caregivers in the months of September 2020-November 2020, February 2021-April 2021, May 2021-June 2021, September 2021-October 2021.

Focused group discussions were conducted in the months of February 2022- March 2022.

3.4 Sample Design

Sample design is a plan for obtaining a sample from a given population. It refers to the technique adopted by the researcher in selecting items for the sample (Kothari, 2009). For the present research work, purposive sampling, snowball sampling and focused group interview methods were used for the research study.

(a) **Purposive Sampling:** It means interviewing people or the selection of sample units that confirm to specific purpose or are selected on the basis of predetermined criteria. This type of sampling is also known as judgement sampling as the selection depends upon the subjective judgement of the researcher. The researcher purposely chooses the nurses, general duty assistants, patients and their family members who in her judgement are related to the research study and also holds some characteristics relevant of the sample.

(b) **Snowball Sampling:** This is the name of technique for building up a list or sample of a special population by using an initial set of members as its informants (Xavier *et al.*,2007). In the present study, the nurses, general duty assistants were selected by this method. Suppose, as the researcher tends to interview one nursing staff, the investigator used to get phone number for the other two nurses. Even more as the GDAS and the nurses were working together, the researcher was able to contact all of them. This sampling was very helpful in diffusion of information among professionals of various kinds. Further, the name of patients and their addresses were also generated through this method. Nurses and General duty assistants were working with the clients and thus, the researcher was able to find patients.

3.5 Research Questions

Research questions are formulated keeping in mind the objectives of the study, they are backbone of any research. Following questions were formalized for the present study:

1. What is the role of socio-economic status in the home health care?
2. Whether the patient is in a position to bare the expense of home care services?
3. What is the medical history of the patient?
4. Are there any benefits and drawbacks of home health care?
5. What are the problems faced by the patients and their family members?
6. Whether the client is able to provide a safe and secure environment to the care providers?
7. Are they treating them as paramedical professional and are not utilising him/her for jobs outside the scope of work?
8. What are the factors which compel them to take the services of care providers?

The study was undertaken with the following aim and objectives.

3.6 Aim and Objective of the Study

3.6.1 Aim

To understand the home health care services provided by the home health aides and the socio-medical perspective of patients receiving care at home.

3.6.2 Objectives of the Study

1. **To study the demographic profile of the nurses, nurse managers, and general duty assistants**
   To fulfil the first objective, the socio-economic status of the respondents was analysed using the Kuppuswamy's socio-economic scale and the data were collected with regard to their education, occupation and family income. The respondents were asked about their age, gender, place of birth, marital status, and religion.

2. **To study the adjustment between the respondents, their family members, caregivers and agencies**
   For the purpose of this objective, Questions were prepared regarding the current residence of the nurses and general duty assistants, payment source (whether they are being paid by the agencies or by the clients) and their relationship with the patient, their members and the agencies. All these aspects were under analysis.
3. **To examine the emotional well-being and challenges faced by health care staff in home health care**
   Respondents were asked questions about the job structure, number of patients handled, types of patients cared, years of experience in home care. Further, questions were also put up on problems faced with respect to food, job, safety issues and their remuneration at workplace. More questions were included in understand the services performed by home care staff. At the same time, to understand their emotional well-being, questions were framed and were analysed using the caregiver burden scale.
4. **To understand the job experiences of nurses and general duty assistants working in home health care**
5. **To gather in depth data about the demographic profile of the patients**
   Questions were framed regarding the name, address and current residence of the clients. Further, questions were asked such as who is the primary caregiver, disease they are suffering, home setting of the patient, i.e. whether he is staying alone or with spouse or family. The researchers further investigated whether the patient is suffering from any infectious disease and if the families are providing personal protective equipment to the caregiver.
6. **To study the problems faced by respondents (patients), their family members and care providers (nurses and caregivers)**
   Questions were framed to comprehend about the services required for caregivers and length of engagement, preference of services required (professional caregiving or

home nursing), number of health care personnel required, gender, language, and religion preferred. Additionally, the respondents were also interviewed on the work shift pattern preferred, performance of activities of daily living depending upon the condition and severity of the disease and instrumental activities of daily living. However, whether the patients and their families were satisfied with the caregiver work, if there is an improvement in the condition of patient and the problems faced by patients and their family members with regards to caregiving and nursing services at home were studied.

8. **To understand the life styles borne/adopted by the patients and their care providers to cope up with the disease**

   Case studies were generated with the help of in-depth interviews from the client and their families.

3.7 Tools and Techniques

A number of tools and techniques are employed for collection and analysis of data. It is the prerogative of the researcher as to what sort of methods would be employed for collection of data. The method of collecting primary and secondary data differs. In the present study, the primary source of data collection was done from the patients, their family members, nurse managers, nursing staff and General duty assistants. While the secondary data was gathered with respect to the research topic through books, journals, manuals and supplementary material such as home care booklets, home care pamphlets, NCERT course books available in Libraries such as A.C. Joshi Library, PU Chandigarh, Hauz Home Care Agency, Panchkula, MAX Hospital, SAS Mohali, Life Circle Senior Services, Delhi. Additionally, various databases were searched for in-depth understanding of the topic and to establish a framework for conducting the research.

3.7.1 Qualitative Approach

The first and foremost task was to decide the method of data collection. For preparing a structured interview schedule, exploratory research tool was used to generate new ideas and to increase the researcher familiarity with the problem. Since, the research is descriptive in nature, it tends to identify the various characteristics of community or institution as in the present study the health care employees were interviewed to analyse their problem in home care sector. There are various methods of data collection. A method is different from a tool, while the method refers to the way or mode of gathering data, a tool is an instrument used for the method. Here in the study, the schedules are used for interviewing (Xavier *et al.*, 2007). The important methods employed in the present study are: Observation method, In-depth interviews, Field research method and narratives were employed for collection of data.

(a) **Observation Method:** Observation means viewing or seeing. It may be defined as systematic viewing of a particular or specific phenomenon in its proper setting for the specific purpose of gathering data for a particular study. In qualitative research, the observer is a part of the phenomenon or group and he/she acts both as an observer and a participant. In the present research, the researcher worked with Hauz Home Health Care Services, Plot No. 303, Industrial Area, Phase-2, Panchkula which is franchise of Life Circle Senior Services, Delhi. The researcher worked with the home care staff for a period of about 1 year. This helped the researcher to understand the emotional reactions of the observed group, i.e. patients, their family members, nurses, nurse managers and general duty assistants.

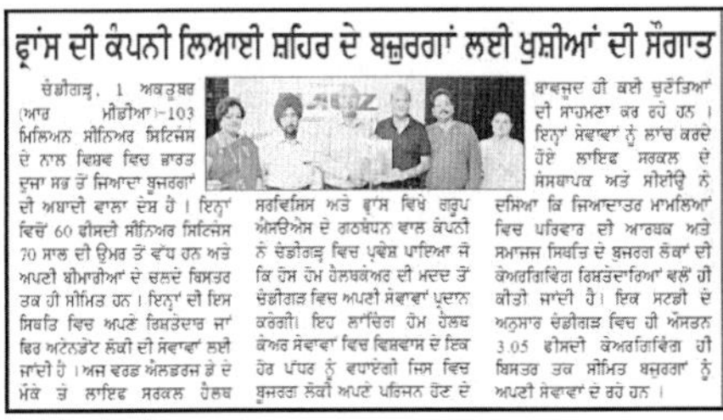
ਫ੍ਰਾਂਸ ਦੀ ਕੰਪਨੀ ਲਿਆਈ ਸ਼ਹਿਰ ਦੇ ਬਜ਼ੁਰਗਾਂ ਲਈ ਖੁਸ਼ੀਆਂ ਦੀ ਸੌਗਾਤ

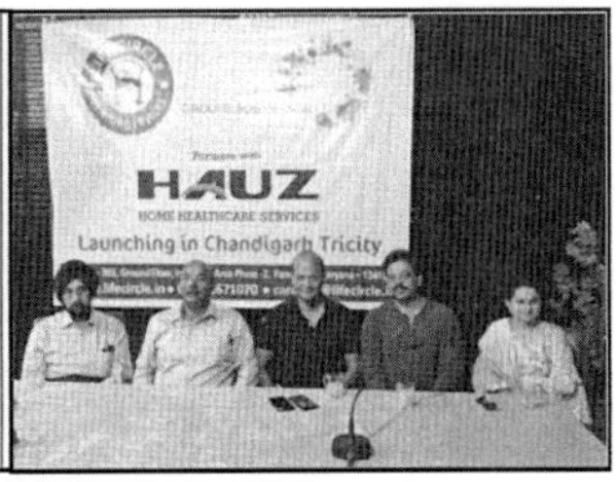

Plate 3.1: Researcher with the HAUZ Healthcare Team.

(b) **In-depth Interviews:** Interviewing is one of most important and significant method of data collection. It is one of the prominent methods for collecting wide range of data from factual demographic data to highly personal and intimate information related to person's attitude, opinion, values, past experience and future prospects. Data was gathered through standardized detailed schedule. The same questions were put to all the respondents and in the same order. However, the interviewer encouraged the respondents (Nurses and GDAs) to speak about home care agencies, their working scenario and their relationship with patients and their family. Additionally, detailed interview schedule was framed for gathering patient information.

(c) **Case Study:** In the present research, the patients and their family members were interviewed to gather information on sensitive topics such as difficult behaviour in case of Alzheimer patients, problems with Parkinson's disease and the problems, adjustments and relationship with the caregivers. The problems were explored were explored in an unrestricted manner. Non-directive and unstructured interviews were conducted. For this purpose, a broad interview guide was used. This type of interviewing is more useful in generating case studies.

(d) **Focused Group Discussions:** Here the researcher attempts to focus on the discussing the actual effects of the given experience to which the respondents have been exposed. The focused discussions were conducted with a team of 30 members (15 nurses and 15 GDAs). Each group comprised 5 members who were subjected to same experiences. The discussions permitted the interviewer to obtain details of their emotional experiences, personal reactions, and specific emotions regarding the situation under study.

(e) **Narratives:** Narratives are written or spoken accounts of connected events or stories. In the present study, the respondents were given a chance to speak freely about their experiences and the same were framed in the form of narratives.

3.7.2 Quantitative Approach

Questions were clear, multi-choice, relevant, short, logically arranged and were in tune with the objectives of the study so that the responses could be statistically tested. This method involves drawing statistical inferences about the population under study through mathematical values. A wide variety of techniques were used such as Frequency, percentage, Chi-square using Software Package for Social Sciences (SPSS 16) are used and the results are presented in the form of tables and graphs.

(a) **Chi-square Association:** The Chi-square was used to test the relationship between variables. In the present study, the influence of different demographic variables such as education, family income, occupation of the head, religion, marital status, gender and religion of the respondents (nurses and general duty assistants) were analysed to study the burden and socio-economic status of respondents. This test was used to determine whether or not there is any or significant association between these variables.

Assumption of Chi-square test

p-value	Significance Level
0.000 to 0.001	Highly-significant (***)
0.001 to 0.01	Moderately-significant (**)
0.01 to 0.05	Significant (*)

In case where the results were non-significant that means statistically, there was no association between the variables under study.

For references, the researcher has used Current Anthropology, Vol. 60, Suppl. 20, August 2019.

3.8 Data Analysis

The preparation of data involves the identification of data, coding of data and the grouping of data for preliminary research interpretations. It is also called processing of data. The data gathered in the form of interview schedules, focused group discussions, field notes, and transcripts is mostly the data in large forms. In the data preparation step, the data are prepared in the Excel Sheet or in a format which allows the researcher to statistically analyse data.

(a) **Editing of Data:** The next step in the processing of data is editing of data instruments. Editing is generally done to detect errors and omissions which occurs during data preparation. It ensures that the data is complete in all respects. The first step of editing is to see whether the answers to all questions that were sought, are complete in all senses or are there any omissions. Apart from omissions, accuracy of recorded answers should be checked. In addition, another lookout is looking for uniformity in data. The final step in editing of data set is to maintain a log of all correction and documentation helps to retain the original data set.

(b) **Coding of Data:** The edited data is then subjected to classification and codification. The coding process consists of assigning numerals or symbols to the responses of sets of data. In the present study, the variables when they are categorised also need codification. The coding sheet need to be prepared carefully. In the present study the scoring is done on the basis of revised scales.

(c) **Content Analysis:** It is a method of social science research that aims at analysis of content both qualitative or quantitative data from documents, newspapers, magazines, transcripts and any written material. In the present research focused group interviews were conducted with 15 nurses and 15 GDAS. Responses were written in the form of transcripts. The questions were asked in the same way and order as mentioned in the interview schedule. Respondents spoke freely about their job, problems faced and about their relationship with the patients, their family members and agency supervisors. Themes were generated and the data was classified on the basis of recordings.

(d) **Classification:** In many cases, the researcher is not able to code data because of the exhaustive nature of the data. They need to classify it and then code them. Classification is necessary where the responses are open-ended (Xavier *et al.*, 2007).

(e) **ATLAS ti:** Software ATLAS ti was chosen to analyse the qualitative data. After the finalisation of the Discussion Guide, Codebook development is the next step before data collection. As it is a lengthy process and is also time-consuming, it is a good method for quick check of the correct numbering of the questions or sections. Data analysis is primarily the coding of transcripts in Atlas ti.

(f) **Tabulation of Data:** The data is further summarised and arranged in compact form for analysis. This process is called Tabulation. In this study, the data is presented in the form of tables, bar graphs, line graphs and pie chart to have a precise view of the findings and trends.

3.9 Scales used in the Study

(a) **Modified Kuppuswamy Scale for the Year 2021:** The scale was devised by Kuppuswamy and is the most widely used scale for determining the socio-economic status of an individual or a family in urban areas (Bairwa *et al.,* 2012) Initially, the scale was developed for determining SES of an individual, but later on, it was modified to determine SES of a family rather than an individual. The scale was initially formulated by Kuppuswamy in the year 1976 including index parameters like education, occupation, and total income which was further modified in later years to include head of families' educational status, occupational status and overall aggregate income of the whole family, pooled from all other sources (Kuppuswamy, 1981). The Kuppuswamy SES has 3 parameters, and each parameter is further classified into subgroups and scores have been allotted to each subgroup. The category of occupation is grouped into ten categories (unemployed; elementary occupation; plant and machine operators; craft and related trade workers; skilled agriculture and fishery workers; skilled workers and shop and market sales workers; clerks; technicians and associate professionals; professional and legislators, senior officials and managers and the scores have been allotted from 1 to 10. The updated monthly family income in rupees ranges from INR < 6174 to INR > 1,23,322 and the scores have been allotted from 1 to 12. The scoring is calculated on the basis of the education of the head of the family, irrespective of whether he/she is the subject or not. The category of education is grouped into seven categories (Illiterates to Profession or Honours). The scoring ranges from 1 to 7. The total score of Kuppuswamy SES ranges from 3 to 29 and it classifies families into 5 groups, "upper class, upper middle class, lower middle class, upper lower and lower socio-economic class."

(b) **Burden Scale for Family Caregivers:** The Burden Scale for Family Caregivers (BSFC) (Grasel, 1995) is a 28-item questionnaire that was initially developed to measure the level of perceived burden of family caregivers. The extent to which the family caregivers feel burdened has a significant influence on the caring style, as well as upon the continuation of home care. A total of 28 statements determine the burden felt by caregivers working for the patients.

(c) **The Zarit Burden Interview Scale:** The Zarit Burden Interview Scale is a popular assessment tool for evaluating caregiver burden that is widely used around the world. It was originated as a 29-item questionnaire (Zarit *et al.*,

1980). The revised version contains 22 items (ZBI-22) which was later developed in 1985 (Zarit *et al.* 1985). Each item on the interview is a statement which the caregiver is asked to endorse using a 5-point scale. Response options range from 0 (Never) to 4 (Nearly Always). The scores ranging 0-21 predicts little or no burden, 21-40 (mild to moderate burden), 41-60 (moderate to severe burden), and 61-88 severe burden identifying caregivers at risk for depression.

3.10 The Field Area, Hospitals and Home Care Agencies

The city Chandigarh was declared Union Territory in 1966 with joint capitals of both the states Panjab and Haryana. Since 1971, Chandigarh has progressed in terms of urbanisation, from 2 towns to 6 towns and a decline from 24 villages in 2001 to 5 villages in 2011. The total population of Chandigarh according to Census in 2011 was 1,054,686, (rural: 29,004 and urban: 1,025,682). The Union Territory recorded a population of 10,54,686 in 2011 with much lower decadal rate of increase in population with only 154051 people being added to the Chandigarh UT during the last decade. The growth rate of merely 17.10 per cent between 2001-2011 is the slowest since its inception. This is perhaps due to the rapid pace of urbanization taking place in the neighbouring towns of Mohali, Panchkula, Zirakpur, Kalka, Kharar etc. falling within the 16 km periphery control area (Census, 2011).

3.10.1 Density of the Population

The population density during the last 5 decades (1961-2011) has increased multi-fold, from 1051 to 9252 persons per sq. km. With the latest census data becoming available, the density recorded for the Chandigarh UT is now placed at 9252 persons per sq. km in 2011 (Census of India, 2011). The sex ratio among elderly people was as high as 1028 in 1951, subsequently dropped and again reached up to 1033 in 2011. The life expectancy at birth during 2009-2013 was 69.3 for females as against 65.8 years for males. At the age of 60 years average remaining length of life was found to be about 18 years (16.9 for males and 19.0 for females) and that at age 70 was less than 12 years (10.9 for males and 12.3 for females).

The old-age dependency ratio climbed from 10.9 per cent in 1961 to 14.2 per cent in 2011 for India as a whole. For females and males, the value of the ratio was 14.9 per cent and 13.6 per cent in the last census that was conducted in 2011 (Elderly in India, 2016).

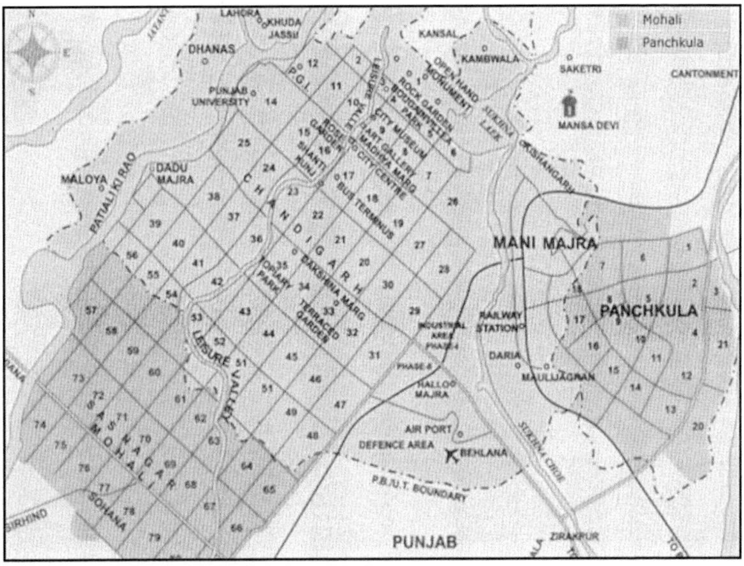

Map 3.1: Map of Chandigarh, Panchkula and Mohali[1].

Table 3.2: Size of Elderly Population (aged 60+) and their Share in Total Population in Chandigarh, Punjab and Haryana

States/UT	Percentage of elderly people in total population	Number (in thousand) of persons aged 60 & above for different sub-population in the state				
		Total			Rural	Urban
		Persons	Male	Female		
Chandigarh	6.4	67	32	35	1	66
Punjab	10.3	2866	1422	1444	1958	908
Haryana	8.7	2194	1105	1089	1513	681
India	8.6	103849	52777	51072	73294	30555

Source: Population Census, 2011.

State-wise data on elderly population indicates that Kerala has maximum proportion of elderly people in its population (12.6%) followed by Goa (11.2%) and Tamil Nadu (10.4%) as per Population Census, 2011. This may be due to the lifestyle and better medical facilities in respective states. Chandigarh falls somewhere in the middle, the least proportion is in Dadra & Nagar Haveli (4.0%) followed by Arunachal Pradesh (4.6%) and Daman & Diu and Meghalaya (both 4.7%). The phenomenon of population ageing is becoming a major concern for the policy makers all over the world, both for developed and developing countries. Industrialisation, urbanization and migration of population have brought the concept of nuclear family, as a result of which a section of the family, primarily the elders, are confronting the problems of financial and physical support. There is an emerging need to pay greater attention to ageing related issues and to promote holistic policies and programmes for dealing with ageing society (Elderly in India, 2016).

3.10.2 Hospitals and Home Care Agencies

Various field visits were made to several hospitals that are listed as follows:

- Alchemist Hospital, Sector 21, Budanpur, Panchkula (Haryana).
- Ojas Hospital, Sector 26, Panchkula (Haryana).
- Government Multi-Speciality Hospital, Sector 16, Chandigarh.
- PGIMER, Sector-12, Chandigarh.
- Max Hospital, Phase 6, Sector 56, Sahibzada Ajit Singh Nagar (Punjab).
- Fortis Hospital, Sector 62, Sahibzada Ajit Singh Nagar (Punjab).

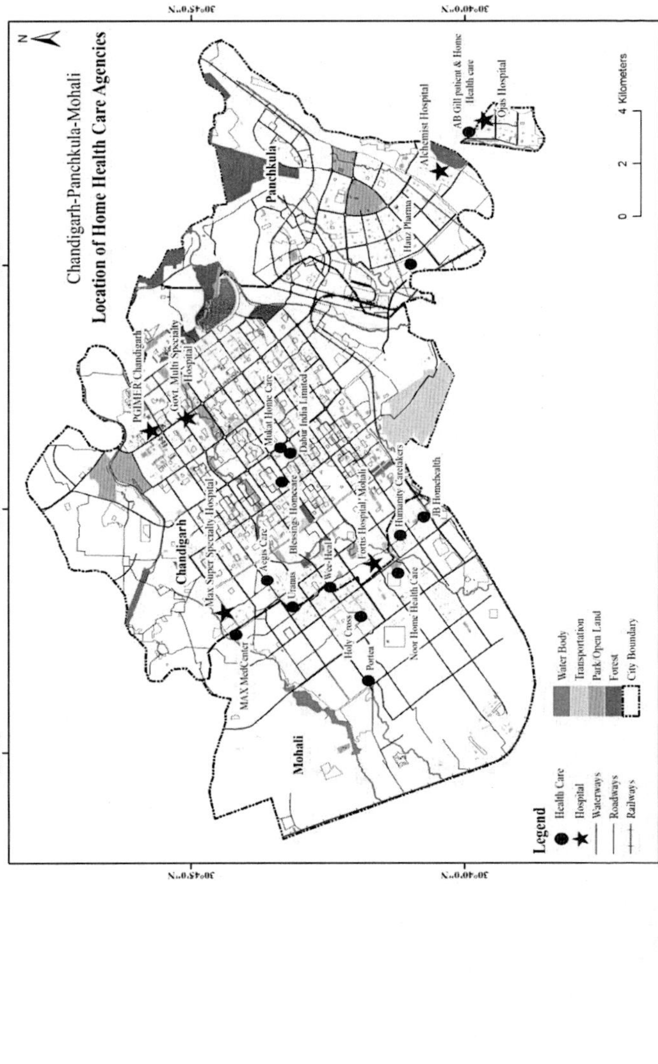

Map 3.2: Hospitals and Home Care Agencies in the Field Area.

Visit to various agencies was also made which included agencies such as:

- AB Gill patient and Home-Health Care Services, Sector 24, Panchkula (Haryana).
- Aegis Care at Home Pvt. Ltd., Cabin No. 1, Franco Road, Phase 1, Sahibzada Ajit Singh Nagar, Mohali (Punjab).
- Blessings Home care, Sec-46C, Chandigarh.
- Dabur Healthcare at Home, Chandigarh.
- Hauz Home Health Care Services, Plot No. 303, Industrial Area, Phase-2, Panchkula (Haryana).
- Max@Home Healthcare, Phase 6, Sector 56, Sahibzada Ajit Singh Nagar, Mohali (Punjab).
- Mukat Home Care, 49, Dakshin Marg, Sector 34-A, Chandigarh.

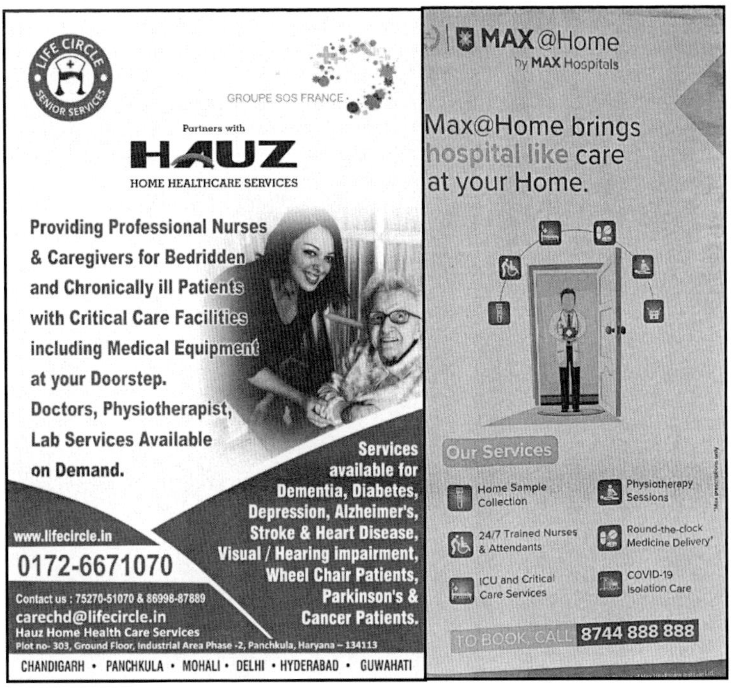

Plate 3.2: Home Health Care Services provided by different Agencies.

- Portea Home Health Care, E-309, Sector 75, Industrial Area, Mohali (Punjab).
- Zorgers-Home Health Care, SCO 12-13 Phase-11, Sahibzada Ajit Singh Nagar, Mohali (Punjab).
- Additionally, visit to other agencies were made to collect data from the patients who are seeking home care services.
- Holy Cross Home Health Care, SCO-1013, 2nd Floor, Sector -70, Sahibzada Ajit Singh Nagar (Punjab).
- Humanity Caretakers Home Health Care Services, SCF 60, 2nd floor, Sahibzada Ajit Singh Nagar (Punjab).
- JB Home Health Care Services, 100, Phase 11, Sector-65, Sahibzada Ajit Singh Nagar (Punjab).
- Noor Home Health Care, Shop 1, 2nd Floor, Sector-68, Sahibzada Ajit Singh Nagar (Punjab).
- Uranus Home Health Care, 155, Mohali Stadium Road, Phase 4, Sector-59, Sahibzada Ajit Singh Nagar (Punjab).
- Weeheal Home Health Care, H.No. 2876, Phase 7, Near Chawla Hospital, Sahibzada Ajit Singh Nagar (Punjab).

Note

1. https://chandigarhmetro.com/chandigarh-panchkula-mohali-tricity-better/(accessed on 14/07/2019)

4

Home Care Staff, their Adjustments and Challenges at Workplace

God gave burdens, but he also gave helping hands

Advancements in technologies and changes in the health care system have resulted in shortened hospital stays, moving the focus of care from hospitals to homes. These services include nursing care, professional caregiving to chronically ill and patients of which substantial numbers are bedridden, immobile or suffer from chronic illnesses like dementia, cancer, heart, lungs, liver, kidney etc. However, home care services range from basic support on activities of daily activities to complex nursing services like feeding through a naso-gastric tube, catheter change, injection, and tracheostomy. The goals of home health care services include helping individuals to improve function and live with greater independence; to promote the client's optimal level of well-being; and to assist the patient to remain at home, avoiding hospitalization or admission to long-term care institutions. The present study will focus on the importance and need of caring for patients at home by care providers. This study would further analyze the problems faced by the care providers (nurses and caregivers) providing home care.

According to (U.S. Bureau of Labour Statistics, 2009), Home care worker's average hourly wage rate is considered lower than other jobs in the health care sector. A national survey reported that 75 per cent of the states named recruitment and retention of home care workers as a major policy issue (National Clearinghouse on the Direct Care Workforce, 2005).

4.1 Demographic Profile

The socio-economic status of the respondents was analyzed using the Modified Kuppuswamy socio-economic scale for the year 2021 (Sheikh and Shah, 2021) and the data were collected with regard to their education, occupation, and family income. The first objective focused on studying the demographic profile of the nurses, nurse managers, and general duty assistants. The respondents were asked about their age, gender, place of birth, marital status, and religion.

4.1.1 Education of the Head

The scoring is calculated on the basis of the education of the head of the family, irrespective of whether he/she is the subject or not.

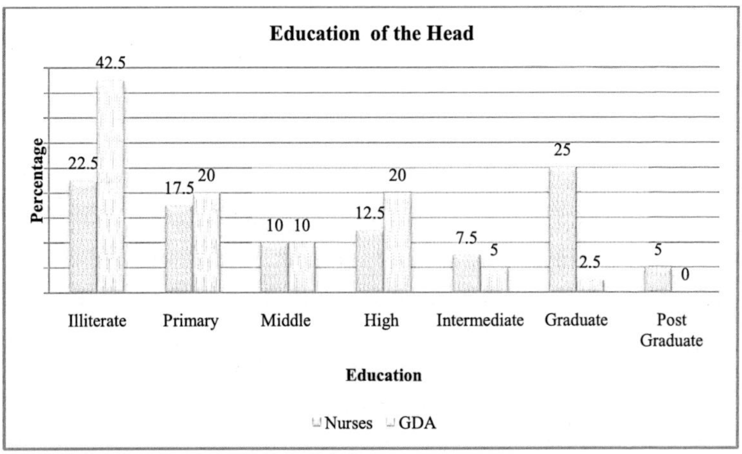

Fig. 4.1: Education of the Head of the Family [Nurses and General Duty Assistants (GDA)].

Note: Chi-square test value = 12.7*, among above categories with p-value = 0.04.
Source: Primary Data Collection.

Data on education were analyzed as it is an important factor in understanding the socio-economic status of respondents. The maximum level of education attained by the respondents was considered. Fig. 4.1 indicates the education of the head of the family.

With respect to the education of the head of the family, overall it was analyzed that 32.5 per cent of the heads of the family fall under the category of illiterates (42.5% GDAs and 22.5% nurses), while 20 per cent GDAs and 17.5 per cent nurses family heads have achieved primary education, followed by 10 per cent who have achieved middle school education. It was noted that 12.5 per cent of nurses and 20 per cent GDAs family heads are 10th pass (High School Certificate). Only 7.5 per cent of nurses and 5 per cent GDAs are intermediates. Interestingly, it was found that about 25 per cent of heads of the nursing family are graduates while only 2.5 per cent of heads are graduates from GDAs families. Henceforth, only 5 per cent of heads are postgraduates from nursing staff, while none of the heads are post-graduates from the GDAs family.

The results analyzed were significant ($p<0.05$) as is evident from the Chi-square value (12.7*) which is a clear indicator that the level of education of the head of the family does have an effect on the socio-economic status of the family which recognized as one of the important factor affecting the health condition of the individual or family.

4.2 Education of the Respondents

To know about the maximum level of education attained by the nursing staff and general duty assistants, they were interviewed and the data is represented in Table 4.1.

It was analyzed that with regard to nurses, 70 per cent of the respondents were intermediates, i.e. they have passed 10+2 education followed by 30 per cent who were graduates. However, in the case of general duty assistants, 55 per cent were intermediates followed by 30 per cent who have passed high school certification, followed by 5 per cent who have attained primary and middle school education and are graduates respectively. However, none of the respondents in either category were postgraduates.

Table 4.1: Education of the Respondents (Nurses and General Duty Assistants)

Education of the respondents		**Group**		**Total**
		Nurses	**GDAs**	
Primary School Certificate	Count	0	2	2
	% within Group	0.0%	5.0%	2.5%
Middle School Certificate	Count	0	2	2
	% within Group	0.0%	5.0%	2.5%
High School Certificate	Count	0	12	12
	% within Group	0.0%	30.0%	15.0%
Intermediate	Count	28	22	50
	% within Group	70.0%	55.0%	62.5%
Graduate	Count	12	2	14
	% within Group	30.0%	5.0%	17.5%
Post Graduate	Count	0	0	0
	% within Group	0%	0%	0%
Total	**Count**	**40**	**40**	**80**
	% within Group	**100.0%**	**100.0%**	**100.0%**

Note: Chi-square test value = 23.8***, among above categories with p-value < 0.0001.

Source: Primary Data Collection.

Similar results were observed in a study conducted on New York home health workers (Chichin, 1992). It was found that half of them were without high school diplomas. Henceforth, the results of the present finding are highly significant ($p < 0.0001$) as it is evident from chi-square value (23.8***) showing a strong association of level of education with the socio-economic status of the respondent, i.e. the maximum level of education one achieves is reflective of their status.

4.3 Specialized Education of the Nurses

Nurses were interviewed to know their degree/level of education.

Nurses pursued courses in General nursing midwife (GNM), Auxiliary nurse midwife (ANM), and bachelor of science in nursing (B.Sc. Nursing). The general nursing midwife is a three-year and six-month diploma course designed for candidates who are interested in pursuing a career in clinical nursing. An auxiliary nurse midwife is a 2-year undergraduate diploma course in nursing with a specialization in maternity care and they are educated in providing assistance to new mothers during pregnancy and post-delivery. They are also educated on the various aspects of medicare that aim at improving the health of patients, families, and society at large. B.Sc. in nursing is an undergraduate course that all medical aspirants can pursue in different nursing colleges in India. It is offered as a 4-year undergraduatc programme for all students who have passed post high school from the stream of science. The course can be availed from any recognized institution.

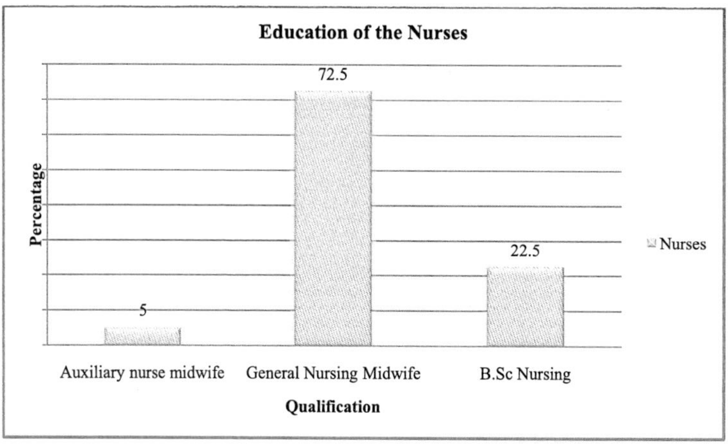

Fig. 4.2: Education of the Nurses.

Source: Primary Data Collection.

It is evident from Fig. 4.2 that 72.5 per cent of respondents were GNMs, while 22.5 per cent of them were graduates in nursing having availed B.Sc nursing degree and just 5 per cent of them were ANMs. No Statistics were computed because this group is constant.

One of the respondents narrated her journey of becoming a nurse, she goes on saying:

> 'I am a nurse by profession. I completed B.Sc. nursing post attaining my high school education. I used to attend classes in the morning and completed my studies at night. Now I am working as a nurse manager' (R62/26/NM/H/U/Exp. 7 years).

4.4 Occupation of the Head of the Family

The occupation here refers to the occupation of the head of the family. In case the head of the family is retired, their last job held is taken into consideration. The scoring of the occupation is from unemployed to legislators, senior officials, and managers. This broad category of occupation is grouped into ten further categories (unemployed; elementary occupation; plant and machine operators; craft and related trade workers; skilled agriculture and fishery workers; skilled workers and shop and market sales workers; clerks; technicians and associate professionals; professional and legislators, senior officials and managers). Data is represented in Table 4.2.

Table 4.2: Occupation of the Head of the Family (Nurses and General Duty Assistants, GDAs)

Occupation of the Head		Group		Total
		Nurses	GDAs	
Unemployed	Count	0	3	3
	% within Group	0.0%	7.5%	3.8%
Elementary occupations	Count	4	4	8
	% within Group	10.0%	10.0%	10.0%
Plant and machine operators and assemblers	Count	2	1	3
	% within Group	5.0%	2.5%	3.8%
Craft and related trade workers	Count	3	11	14
	% within Group	7.5%	27.5%	17.5%
Skilled agriculture and fishery workers	Count	14	14	28
	% within Group	35.0%	35.0%	35.0%

(*Contd.*)

Occupation of the Head		Group		Total
		Nurses	GDAs	
Skilled workers and Market sales workers	Count	6	5	11
	% within Group	15.0%	12.5%	13.8%
Clerks	Count	3	1	4
	% within Group	7.5%	2.5%	5.0%
Technical and associate professionals	Count	6	1	7
	% within Group	15.0%	2.5%	8.8%
Professionals	Count	2	0	2
	% within Group	5.0%	0.0%	2.5%
Legislators, senior officials & Managers	Count	0	0	0
	% within Group	0.0%	0.0%	0.0%
Total	**Count**	**40**	**40**	**80**
	% within Group	**100.0%**	**100.0%**	**100.0%**

Note: Chi-square test value = 14.5, among above categories with p-value = 0.06.
Source: Primary Data Collection.

Interestingly, in the case of general duty assistants, a very small percentage, i.e. 7.5 per cent of the head of the family were unemployed. 10 per cent each of the heads of the families of GDAs were elementary workers who were working as a watchman and domestic workers or any other such job that requires no education or training. While in the semi-skilled category (a job that requires some training and is related to plant and machine operators and assemblers), 5 per cent of family heads of families of nurses and 2.5 per cent of heads of families of GDAs were working as factory labourers. While 27.5 per cent of family heads from the GDAs family and 5 per cent of heads from the nurse's family are involved in craft-related trade workers, who are working as carpenters, brick layers, electricians, floor layers, and tile settlers. In the skilled worker category (a job that requires long training in complicated work), however, the majority of the heads, i.e. 35 per cent each from nurses and from the GDAs families were working as farmers. Moreover, 7.5 per cent of heads from families of nurses and 2.5 per cent of heads from families of GDAs are involved in arithmetic skill jobs (that require some training in arithmetic and also involves reading and writing) and are working as clerical staff.

The technical and associate professionals were 15 per cent and 2.5 per cent respectively. Interestingly, this percentage is higher in the case of heads of the families of nurses as they are employed as high school teachers, junior administrators, and junior medical practitioners. While 5 per cent of the heads from the nurse's families were professionals in their field, none of the heads from the GDAs families were not working as professionals.

4.5 Family Income per Month

Family income is to be assessed as total family income (per month) and not the per capita income.

From Table 4.3, it can be seen that with concern to nurses, the maximum number of respondents i.e. 27.5 per cent respondents fall in the income bracket of (Rs. 18,497-30,830) followed by 22.5 per cent in the income bracket of Rs. 30,831-46,128). While in the case of GDAs, the majority of respondent's i.e. 42.5 per cent of their family earnings was between the category of Rs. 18,497-30,830 which is almost the same when compared to the family income of nurses.

Table 4.3: Family Income of the Respondents (Nurses and General Duty Assistants)

Family Income per Month		Group		Total
		Nurses	GDAs	
≤ 6174	Count	1	0	1
	% within Group	2.5%	0.0%	1.3%
6,175-18,496	Count	7	12	19
	% within Group	17.5%	30.0%	23.8%
18,497-30,830	Count	11	17	28
	% within Group	27.5%	42.5%	35.0%
30,831-46,128	Count	9	7	16
	% within Group	22.5%	17.5%	20.0%
46,129-61,662	Count	7	4	11
	% within Group	17.5%	10.0%	13.8%

(Contd.)

Family Income per Month		Group		Total
		Nurses	GDAs	
61,663-1,23,321	Count	3	0	3
	% within Group	7.5%	0.0%	3.8%
≥ 1,23,322	Count	2	0	2
	% within Group	5.0%	0.0%	2.5%
Total	**Count**	**40**	**40**	**80**
	% within Group	**100.0%**	**100.0%**	**100.0%**

Note: Chi-square test value = 9.67, among above categories with p-value = 0.139.
*R—Respondent, *N—Nurse,*GDA—General Duty Assistant, U—Unmarried, *M—Married, *S—Sikh *H—Hindu, *C—Christianity, *MU—Muslim, *Exp.—Experience.
Source: Primary Data Collection.

One of the respondents who is working as a GDA elaborated on her family's financial condition.

> "My father is a farmer, but as my brother is not keeping well and there are financial issues in the family so unwilling I have to work as a home care staff" (R76/24/N/H/U/Exp.6 years).

However, for the family income of nursing staff, just 5 per cent of them have a family income greater than Rs. 1,23,322, whereas, none of the GDAs has a family monthly income even above Rs. 61,663.

Banijamali *et al.* (2014) investigated that more than 30 per cent of home care workers and families earn below the poverty threshold. Many struggle to even meet their basic needs and also make difficult choices between caring for themselves and others.

4.6 Socio-Economic Status

Socio-Economic Status (SES) is one of the most important factors for evaluating the health and nutritional status of a family. The socio-economic status may be defined as "a position attained by any individual within a system of hierarchical social structure" (Miner *et al.*, 2015).

Table 4.4: Socio-Economic Status of the Respondents

Socio-Economic Status		Group		Total
		Nurses	GDAs	
26-29 Upper (I)	Count	3	0	3
	% within Group	7.5%	0.0%	3.8%
16-25 Upper Middle (II)	Count	11	2	13
	% within Group	27.5%	5.0%	16.3%
11-15 Lower Middle (III)	Count	14	14	28
	% within Group	35.0%	35.0%	35.0%
5-10 Upper Lower (IV)	Count	11	23	34
	% within Group	27.5%	57.5%	42.5%
<5 Lower (V)	Count	1	1	2
	% within Group	2.5%	2.5%	2.5%
Total	**Count**	**40**	**40**	**80**
	% within Group	**100.0%**	**100.0%**	**100.0%**

Note: Chi-square test value = 13.4***, among above categories with p-value = 0.009.
Source: Primary Data Collection.

Table 4.4 shows the socio-economic status of the respondents (nurses and general duty assistants). The total score of the modified Kuppuswamy socio-economic scale for the year 2021 (Sheikh and Shah, 2021) ranges from 3-29 and it classifies the families into 5 groups, "upper class, upper middle class, lower middle class, upper lower and lower socio-economic class." With respect to nurses, the majority of respondents, i.e. 35 per cent belong to the lower middle class followed by 27.5 per cent belonging to the upper middle and upper lower class, and only a few, i.e. 7.5 per cent belong to the upper class. Whereas in the case of the general duty assistants, it was visible from the findings that the maximum respondents, i.e. 57.5 per cent of the respondents belong to the upper lower class followed by 35 per cent who were from the lower middle class. For this particular category, none of the respondents belongs to the upper-class section.

The results analyzed were highly significant ($p<0.05$) as is evident from the chi-square value (13.4***). Thus, assimilating the SES scale as the indicator of one's social status in society.

4.7 State-wise Distribution

Respondents under study were from different states of India. To see whether this variable has an effect on their socio-economic status, information on their state of belongingness was obtained which is tabulated in Table 4.5.

Table 4.5: State-wise Distribution of the Respondents (Nurses and General Duty Assistants)

State-wise Distribution			Group		Total
			Nurses	**GDAs**	
	Chandigarh	Count	1	3	4
		% within Group	2.5%	7.5%	5.0%
	Himachal Pradesh	Count	2	7	9
		% within Group	5.0%	17.5%	11.3%
	Punjab	Count	33	25	58
		% within Group	82.5%	62.5%	72.5%
	Uttar Pradesh	Count	1	2	3
		% within Group	2.5%	5.0%	3.8%
	Haryana	Count	2	3	5
		% within Group	5.0%	7.5%	6.3%
	Meghalaya	Count	1	0	1
		% within Group	2.5%	0.0%	1.3%
Total		**Count**	**40**	**40**	**80**
		% within Group	**100.0%**	**100.0%**	**100.0%**

Note: Chi-square test value = 6.41, among above categories with p-value = 0.26.
Source: Primary Data Collection.

Table 4.5 shows the state-wise distribution of the respondents. Maximum respondents (72.5%) belong to Punjab; followed by Himachal Pradesh (11.3%); Haryana (6.3%); and Chandigarh (UT) 5 per cent. Only a small number of respondents 3.8 per cent, and 1.3 per cent were from the state of Uttar Pradesh and Meghalaya respectively. Overall, only 5 per cent aides interviewed were from Chandigarh rest 95 per cent of the population were immigrants.

Similar results were intercepted by Chichin (1992) who conducted a study on home care workers in New York where the profession attracted middle age women and migrant women.

4.8 Age Group

Data on age group was collected to figure out and analyze which of age groups are more involved in providing home health care services to the sick and bed ridden patients (Fig. 4.3).

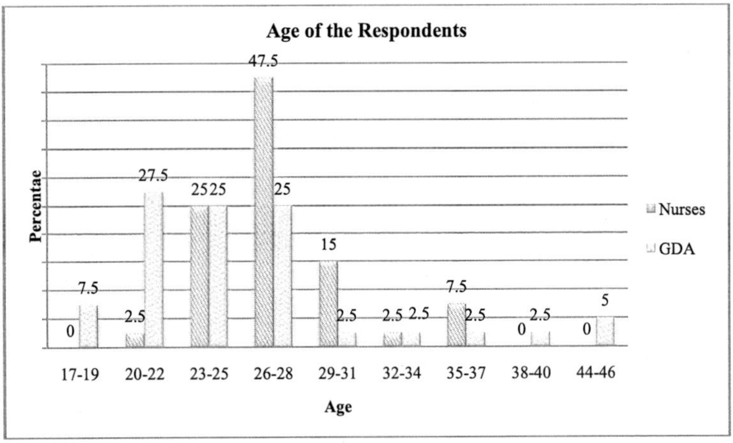

Fig. 4.3: Age Group of the Respondents (Nurses and General Duty Assistants).

Note: Chi-square test value = 21.6**, among above categories with p-value = 0.006.
Source: Primary Data Collection.

It was analyzed from the data that for nurses working as home care staff, the majority of respondents, i.e. 47.5 per cent were in the age group of 26-28 years, followed by 25 per cent in the age group of 23-25 years, 15 per cent belonged to the age group of 29-31 years while a significantly smaller percentage of respondents, i.e. 7.5 per cent were in the age group of 35-37 years, who felt comfortable to work as nursing staff in home care.

In the case of general duty assistants, the maximum number of respondents, i.e. 27.5 per cent were in the age group of 20-22 years followed by 25 per cent each in the age group of 23-25 and 26-28 years. While 7.5 per cent were from the younger segment of 17-19 years, who have completed their high school education and post-high school education and have started their career after pursuing a six-month training from different institutes. In comparison to the nurses, none of the respondents were from this age group 17-19 years as the minimum requirement for pursuing nursing is post-high school education. It was an interesting observation that people in the age group above 40 years were working as general duty assistants. Henceforth, the results analyzed were found to be moderately significant ($p < 0.05$) as is evident from the chi-square value (13.7**) showing a strong association of age group with their preference towards working in home health care. This means with increasing age people feel comfortable working as general duty assistants, but their number reduces with their increase in age, as a maximum number of them feel more comfortable when they are in their 30s or younger, as their body has more strength in their early years. However, the home care average age is 31 years in the present study, one can visualize the respondents from the younger segment, i.e. 17 years and as older as 46 years who are working for home care staff. As compared to a similar study (Montgomery *et al.*, 2005), the home care average age is 46 years, which is approximately 15 years older as compared to the present study, however, the authors ruled that the home care workers earn more than the hospital aides or nursing home aides. One of the respondents, whose father is a farmer, narrated that there is no income from farming as they do not have a bigger portion of land.

> "For 12 hours duty, I am paid about Rs.18,000 and for 24 hours duty I am paid between Rs. 30,000-32,000. Family income is very less. Salaries in hospitals are very less and salaries in home care are very good. *Majboori me karte hai kam* (Unwillingly, we have to work in home care)". (R79/26/N/S/U/Exp.3.5 years)

While in the present study, home care workers (nurses/general duty assistants) earn more than hospital staff who are working as nurses or GDAs.

4.9 Gender of the Respondents (Nurses and General Duty Assistants)

Gender was analyzed to know the ratio of males and females in the present study. The researcher interviewed 40 nurses and 40 general duty assistants working in the home care sector. In the case of nursing staff, data were collected from 80 per cent female staff and 20 per cent male staff. Analysis of home care workforce demographics found 84 per cent of the workers employed being females (Banijamali *et al.*, 2014). Concerning general duty assistants, in-depth interviews were conducted with 55 per cent of male respondents and with 45 per cent of female staff working in home care (Fig. 4.4).

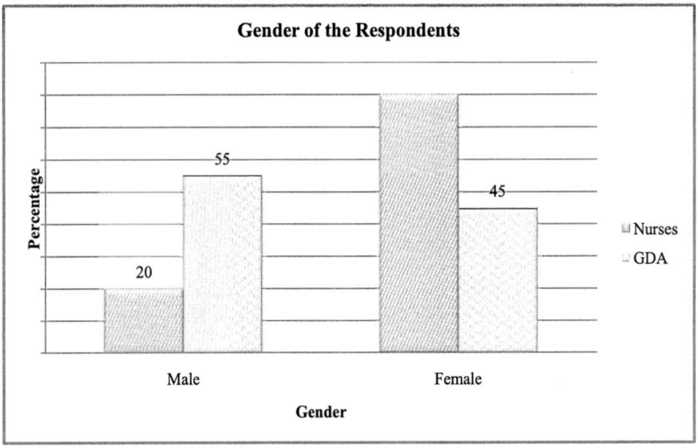

Fig. 4.4: Gender of the Respondents

Note: Chi-square test value = 10.4***, among above categories with p-value = 0.001.

Source: Primary Data Collection.

Henceforth, the results analyzed were found to be highly significant ($p < 0.05$) as is evident from the Chi-square value (10.4***). Overall, from the results, it is evident that more females are working as nursing staff, while more males are working as general duty assistants.

4.10 Marital Status of the Respondents (Nurses and General Duty Assistants)

The marital status of a person relates to marriage. Respondents working in home health care were interviewed to know their marital status.

It is clearly indicated from Fig. 4.5 that in the case of nursing staff, 27.5 per cent were married while 72.5 per cent were unmarried. While 32.5 per cent (General Duty Assistants) were married and 67.5 per cent were unmarried. From in-depth interviews, it was observed and further analyzed that most of the respondents who were interviewed felt that they can only pursue this profession till the time they are unmarried as there is a caregiver work shift pattern depending on their personal preferences (Live in shift for 24 hours and Live out shift for 12 hours) and if one is staying at patients home for 24 hours, it tends to be very difficult for them to give time to their families.

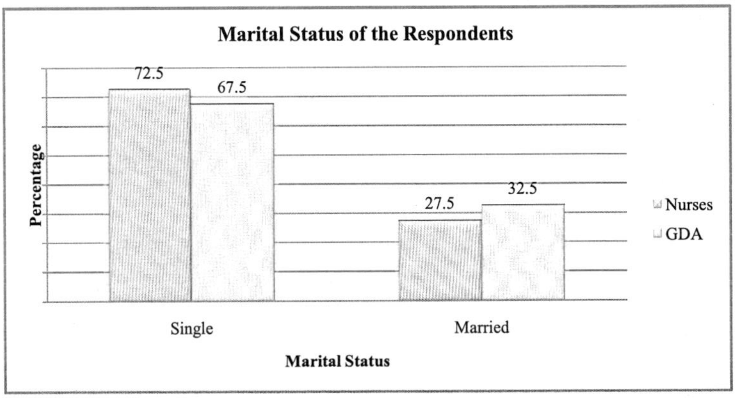

Fig. 4.5: Marital Status of the Respondents.

Note: Chi-square test value = .238, among above categories with p-value = 0.62.
Source: Primary Data Collection.

4.11 Religion-wise Distribution (Nurses and General Duty Assistants)

Data about the religion of the respondents were collected too. This data were further analyzed to study if religion had any influence on their working preferences in home care.

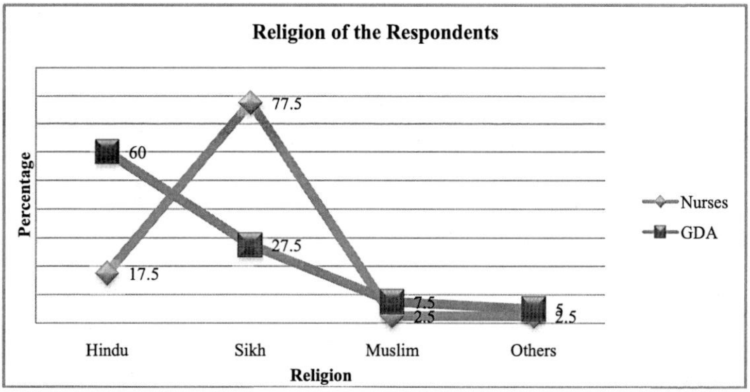

Fig. 4.6: Religion of the Respondents.

Note: Chi-square test value = 20.1***, among above categories with p-value < 0.0001.

Source: Primary Data Collection.

In the case of nursing staff, the majority of respondents were Sikhs (77.5%) followed by Hindus (17.5%), Muslims, and Christians (2.5%) respectively working at patient's homes. While in the case of general duty assistants, the maximum number of respondents belonged to the Hindu religion (60%) followed by Sikhs (27.5%), Muslims (7.5%) and others (5%) respectively (Fig. 4.6). From in-depth interviews, it was analyzed most of the families preferred caregivers belonging to Sikh and Hindu religions for their patient care, this could be attributed to the fact that the locale of the study was Tri-city (Chandigarh, Mohali, and Panchkula), there were a few families who avoided respondents belonging to the Muslim religion. Henceforth, the results found were highly significant ($p < 0.0001$) as it is evident from the chi-square value (20.1***) showing a strong association of preference for specific religion by people of the same sect.

The second objective of the study focused on studying the adjustment between the respondents, their family members, caregivers, and agencies. Questions were prepared regarding the current residence of the nurses and general duty assistants, payment source (whether they are being paid by the agencies or directly by the clients), and their relationship with the patient, their family members, and the agencies.

4.12 Residence of the Respondents (Nurses and General Duty Assistants)

Respondents were asked about their place of residence. Analysis of the data was later done to see whether there was any influence of peer group on the behaviour of the respondents who resided out of home such as in hostels. The influence of family on respondents who were staying within the family has also been analyzed.

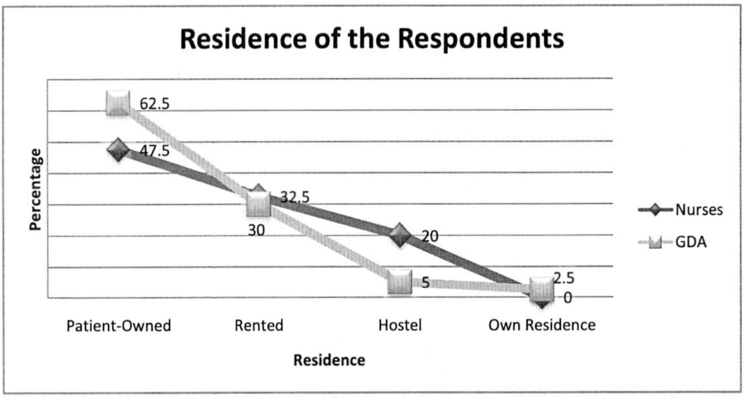

Fig. 4.7: Residence of the Respondents.

Note: Chi-square test value = 5.45, among above categories with p-value = 0.141.
Source: Primary Data Collection.

It was observed and analyzed from the data in Fig. 4.7 that concerning the nursing staff, 47.5 per cent of the respondents lived in a patient-owned residence, followed by 32.5 per cent who lived in rented accommodation, and 20 per cent of them are staying in hostels while none of them is staying at their residence. In the case of the general duty assistants, it was noticed that while a majority of them, i.e. 62.5 per cent stayed in patient-owned residences, only 30 per cent of them stayed in rented accommodation followed by 5 per cent who stayed in hostels while a meagre percentage (2.5%) stayed in their residence. It was analyzed from in-depth interviews that the respondents especially GDAs who were staying in hostels were influenced by their peer group and used to discuss the issues occurring at patient's homes with their peers, thus this factor could sometimes make them reluctant to work for 24 hours shift.

4.13 Source of Payment to the Respondents (Nurses and General Duty Assistants)

Data were collected to analyze the primary source of payment from where the payment was received by the nurses and general duty assistants. The data were further collected to find out the number of health care workers who were interested in working through agencies and the ones who were looking for direct employment (Fig. 4.8).

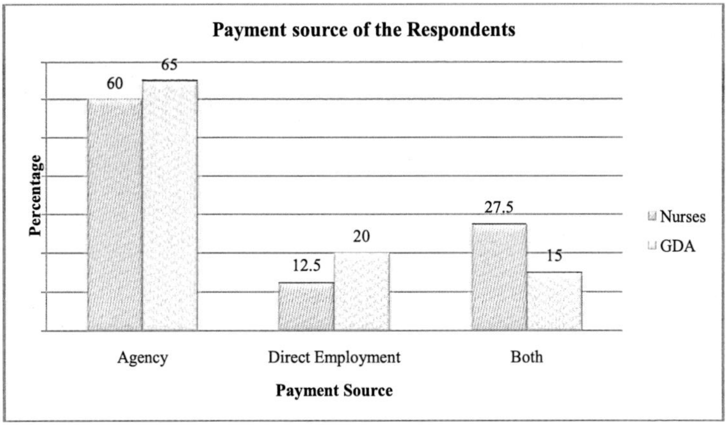

Fig. 4.8: Source of Payment of the Respondents.

Note: Chi-square test value = 2.24, among above categories with p-value = .326.
Source: Primary Data Collection.

From in-depth interviews, it was found that whether they are nursing staff or general duty assistants, about 60 per cent of them are working through agencies. They believed that if they are working through agencies, then their responsibility falls on the agencies in every regard whether it is the payment issue or their safety. However, 20 per cent of GDAs and 12 per cent of nursing staff are employed *via* a direct source. They reasoned that they are not interested in working through agencies, as the major percentage of their salaries are kept by the agencies as their commission and they earn a meagre amount. While 27.5 per cent nurses and 15 per cent of the GDAs are working through both agencies and direct sources and the results are shown in Fig. 4.8.

One of the respondents shared—

> "Some agencies solicit responsibility towards their staff, so it is always good to work through these organizations. They support and guide us in many ways. They provide us training on tube feeding assistance through Ryle's tube. We are also guided on checking blood pressure, and blood sugar, tracheotomy care, wound dressing, urinary catheter care, and many other technical procedures. Training is provided for our skill up gradations" (R57/24/N/H/U/Exp. 1 year).

George *et al.* (2017) also discussed the benefits of training offered by the agencies which enhanced their mental, emotional and physical health, a lack thereof left them stressed, undervalued, and anxious.

It was concluded that agencies play an important role in addressing the demands of care work in combination with supportive benefits like paid sick leaves, pick and drop facility, and extra payment for outstations. Agencies are also responsible for conducting training and scheduling meetings to discuss their important issues.

4.14 Job Structure of the Respondents (Nurses and General Duty Assistants)

It refers to the caregiver (nurses and general duty assistants) shift pattern. Respondents were interviewed to enquire about the job structure they were more interested in. A caregiver can choose from work shift patterns depending on their preferences.

Live-in shift refers to the job structure in which the caregiver is expected to stay round the clock with the patient for 24 hours but the working hours are limited to 8 hours per day.

Live-out shift refers to the job structure in which the caregiver is expected to stay up to 12 hours with the patient but working hours are limited to 8 hours per day. The results are indicated in Table 4.6.

Table 4.6: Job Structure of the Respondents

Job Structure		Group		Total
		Nurses	GDAs	
Live in shift - 24 hrs stay	Count	10	23	33
	% within Group	25.0%	57.5%	41.3%
Live out shift -12hrs stay	Count	20	11	31
	% within Group	50.0%	27.5%	38.8%
Both	Count	10	6	16
	% within Group	25.0%	15.0%	20.0%
Total	**Count**	**40**	**40**	**80**
	% within Group	**100.0%**	**100.0%**	**100.0%**

Note: Chi-square test value = 8.73*, among above categories with p-value = 0.01.
Source: Primary Data Collection.

It was evident from data as shown in Table 4.6 that about 50 per cent of the nurses choose the live out shift pattern as they were more comfortable working for 12-hour duty whether it is day shift or night. From in-depth interviews, it was understood that the nursing staff conducted technical procedures like wound care, and tracheostomy (an incision in the windpipe made to relieve an obstruction to breathing). Suctioning helps to remove the thick mucus and secretions from the trachea and lower airway which are not cleared by normal coughing.[1]

As in a few patients, suctioning is done when one wakes up in the morning and before going to bed in the evening. While in others, it is done after any respiratory treatment. The data reveals 50 per cent of the nurses working in home care find it very hectic to work for 24-hour shifts followed by 25 per cent who preferred to stay with the patient for 24 hours and an equal percentage choose both work shift patterns.

However, as compared to General duty assistants, 57.5 per cent of them preferred to stay with the patient for 24 hours, they reasoned that food and accommodation are provided by the patient and there are flexible work timings are depending on the need of the patient. While 27.5 per cent choose the 12-hour shift pattern followed by 15 per cent preferred both shift patterns. However, it was analyzed from in-depth interviews that women in middle age prefer to do night shifts as they tend to do their house chores in the morning and prefer to work at night.

A few of the narratives are discussed below:

> (R 29 N) said "I am generally inclined towards a 12 hours shift, as I am married. But I am comfortable doing both the shifts. I am paid Rs. 21,000 monthly for 12 hours and if I take leaves, I am paid Rs. 15,000 monthly for 12 hours" (R 29/30/N/S/U/Exp. 12 years).

> (R 19 GDA) mentioned "We are not left with many options, salaries in hospitals are very meagre, one gets good salaries in home care. I am thus working for 24 hour shift" (R19/GDA/H/U/Exp. 1 year).

Henceforth, the results analyzed were found to be significant ($p < 0.05$) as is evident from the chi-square value (8.73*). Overall, it can be evaluated that as there are two shift patterns, the respondents who want to save on their income tend to stay at patient homes for 24 hours, but a large number of nursing staff preferred working for 12 hours shift as they tend to perform technical procedures and found working for 24 hours very hectic.

4.15 Relationship with the Agency (Nurses and General Duty Assistants)

Agencies provide home nursing services and caretakers for the term depending on the underlying conditions; the care requirement may be for a few days or may last many years. They begin with creating a patient care plan. The patient care plan identifies the health and personal care activities that are to be carried out with the patient. Personal care assistants are guided on the jobs by qualified nurses who conduct home visits. The agencies have process manuals that incorporate good practices in caregiving.

Data were collected from respondents to know whether they receive respect appreciation, support or training, and effective communication in the care team.

Table 4.7 shows the relationship of caregivers (nurses/personal care assistants) with the agency. It was analyzed that overall 50 per cent of the respondents believed that they received respect from the agencies and 50 per cent of them believed that they did not receive any respect from the agency supervisors and managers.

Talking about work appreciation, 52.5 per cent of respondents (nurses/GDAs) believed that they were appreciated for their work, while 47.5 per cent of respondents believed that they did not receive any appreciation for their work.

Table 4.7: Relationship with the Agency

Relationship with the Agency			**Group**		**Total**	**p-value**	**χ^2 Test**
			Nurses	**GDAs**			
Respect	Yes	Count	23	17	40	1.80	.180
		% within Group	57.5%	42.5%	50.0%		
	No	Count	17	23	40		
		% within Group	42.5%	57.5%	50.0%		
Apprec-iation	Yes	Count	23	19	42	.802	.370
		% within Group	57.5%	47.5%	52.5%		
	No	Count	17	21	38		
		% within Group	42.5%	52.5%	47.5%		
Support (Job training and work guidance)	Yes	Count	22	26	48	.833	.361
		% within Group	55.0%	65.0%	60.0%		
	No	Count	18	14	32		
		% within Group	45.0%	35.0%	40.0%		

(*Contd.*)

Relationship with the Agency			Group		Total	p-value	χ^2 Test
			Nurses	GDAs			
Control (communication, scheduling into care team)	Yes	Count	13	13	26	.001	1.000***
		% within Group	32.5%	32.5%	32.5%		
	No	Count	27	27	54		
		% within Group	67.5%	67.5%	67.5%		

Source: Primary Data Collection.

However, on the job support, training, and work guidance, 60 per cent (nurses/GDAs) believed that they are guided on the jobs by qualified nurse managers who conducted home visits. Even GDAs are provided training on tube feeding; checking on the vital parameters. In the case of nursing staff, they are provided hands-on training on tracheotomy care, wound dressing, urinary catheter care, and tube feeding assistance through Ryle's tube. However, 40 per cent believed that they are provided no support from the agencies.

Their communication in the care team consists of three essential tasks; team coordination, communication, and shared responsibility. Effective communication is needed to facilitate coordinated care and the interactive team meetings that were scheduled to discuss patient care issues, these meetings are also important to discuss safety issues, and issues related to other behavioural, clinical, or psychological concerns in patient homes. Surprisingly, 67.5 per cent of them were not happy with the working of agencies, as they believed that they never address any of their issues whether it is related to their safety or other emotional tensions confronted at their work place. While just 32.5 per cent of the respondents felt that the agencies address their issues whenever the need arises. Henceforth, the results analyzed were found to be highly significant ($p < 0.05$) as is evident from the chi-square value (1.000***).

On the whole, it was understood that a lack of support from the agencies was identified as participants felt that their issues were not addressed. Moreover, they expressed multiple problems with in home care. It is felt that this profession lacks respect and appreciation both at the hands of agencies and families. Inexperienced staff, no paid leaves, continuously working for 6 months, lack of supervision sessions and no scheduling of meetings were some common complaints. Support and interactive meetings are very important for influencing their physical, mental, and social health. Kroposki and Alexander (2006) reported that higher patient satisfaction scores were seen in home care agencies where nurses and supervisors had good working relationships along with the opportunity for shared decision-making was present and formalization of professional guidelines existed.

4.16 Relationship with the Patients (Nurses and General Duty Assistants)

Over the world, a larger part of the long-term care recipients are seniors above 60 years of age, long term care involves a set of services designed to meet the personal and health care needs of the person. A caregiver or a certified nursing assistant can come to the elderly rescue in such a situation. A caregiver supports the elders with their activities of daily routine, toileting, grooming, bathing, eating, helping them with exercises, and also assisting them with medication.

Despite performing activities, 78.7 per cent and 71.3 per cent of caregivers (Nurses and GDAs) respectively believe that they have a cordial relationship with the patient and receive respect and appreciation for their work from the patient. While 21.3 per cent and 28.7 per cent, respectively disagreed about receiving respect and appreciation from the patients.

Talking about companionship and support, 72.5 per cent and 73.8 per cent (Nurses and GDAs) respectively act as their counterparts as companions, engage them with recreational activities, support and accompany them in many ways, take them to the park, cycling, give an ear to their life experiences, playing card games, board games, crosswords which ultimately boost their memory, increase alertness and strengthen problem-solving skills. However, 27.5 per cent and 26.3 per cent respectively believed that patients suffer from one or the other psychological disorder and so there is no point in companionship or support as they have to manage things according to the patient underlying condition. In a few cases, the patients have lost their memory and are rather very aggressive at times. However, the results analyzed were found to be insignificant ($p > 0.05$) as is evident from the chi-square value which is equal to (3.16). Home care visits are used primarily to provide long term care to patients suffering from chronic conditions. Similar results were discussed by Welch *et al.* (1996) on long-term care through home health visits. Home health aides play a larger role in providing companionship, assisting with personal hygiene or performing activities of daily living, or helping families in household chores. Such visits are the substitutes for care earlier provided by family members or friends.

Table 4.8: Relationship with the Patients

Relationship with the Patients			**Group**		**Total**	**p-value**	**χ^2 Test**
			Nurses	**GDAs**			
Respect	Yes	Count	29	34	63	.217	3.05
		% within Group	72.5%	85.0%	78.7%		
	No	Count	11	6	17		
		% within Group	27.5%	15.0%	21.3%		
Appreciation	Yes	Count	25	32	57	.084	2.99
		% within Group	62.5%	80.0%	71.3%		
	No	Count	15	8	23		
		% within Group	37.5%	20.0%	28.7%		
Companion-ship	Yes	Count	26	32	58	.133	2.25
		% within Group	65.0%	80.0%	72.5%		
	No	Count	14	8	22		
		% within Group	35.0%	20.0%	27.5%		

(*Contd.*)

Relationship with the Patients			Group		Total	p-value	χ^2 Test
			Nurses	GDAs			
Support	Yes	Count	26	33	59	.075	3.16
		% within Group	65.0%	82.5%	73.8%		
	No	Count	14	7	21		
		% within Group	35.0%	17.5%	26.3%		
Trust	Yes	Count	28	29	57	.805	.06
		% within Group	70.0%	72.5%	71.3%		
	No	Count	12	11	23		
		% within Group	30.0%	27.5%	28.5%		

Source: Primary Data Collection.

Banijamali *et al.* (2014) described in their study that home care workers provide support services to disabled people who are otherwise not able to live safely at home. Washington Home Care programme provides funds to lower-income consumers of home care so that they can hire an individual provider of their own choice. Without home care services, many people with disabilities and older adults would be cared for in more expensive and less desirable institutional settings. It was analyzed from in-depth interviews that the Indian Red Cross Society (IRCS) impart skills to young men and women from the community and render home health care to sick/elderly person and empowers youth with a skill that makes them self-reliant and employable. The staff who is employed through the Red Cross Society charges reasonable wages for their work. The relationship between home health care aides is shown in Table 4.8.

However, concerning trust, 71.3 per cent feel that they share an intimate bond with the patient which is full of respect, love, and trust. They asserted that old people are like little children who just need care, love, and trust from us. While 28.5 per cent disagreed and said rather the patient develops suspicious behaviour and will doubt us in many ways.

Overall, it can be concluded from the findings that the majority of the respondents felt that they develop good relationships with the patient and they are respected and valued for their work while few of them felt that they are rather devalued and were treated as housemaids. They asserted that they support and engage with the geriatric in many ways. The overwhelming trust, support, and companionship turn into 'attachment', which in times of separation (in sudden demise) from the patient puts the caregiver in pain for years. It is thus a fact that all the responsibilities are endowed on the shoulders of nurses and caregivers in home care.

4.17 Relationship with the Family (Nurses and General Duty Assistants)

Families play a major role in patient care as the primary caregiver is always a member of the family. The results are indicated in Table 4.9.

Despite performing activities, 72.5 per cent and 65 per cent (Nurses and GDAs) mentioned that they receive respect and appreciation for their work from the members of their family while 27.5 per cent and 35 per cent (Nurses and GDAs) believed that they did not receive any respect and appreciation for their work from the family members rather they interfere in their chores.

Table 4.9: Relationship with the Family

Relationship with the Family			Group		Total	p-value	χ^2 Test
			Nurses	GDAs			
Respect	Yes	Count	27	31	58	.317	1.003
		% within Group	67.5%	77.5%	72.5%		
	No	Count	13	9	22		
		% within Group	32.5%	22.5%	27.5%		
Appreci-ation	Yes	Count	26	26	52	1.000	.000
		% within Group	65.0%	65.0%	65.0%		
	No	Count	14	14	28		
		% within Group	35.0%	35.0%	35.0%		

Source: Primary Data Collection.

On the whole, it can be summed that home care nurses and general duty assistants experience ambiguity in their role-playing as their duties have not been clearly outlined by the agencies. Agencies must clearly discuss the roles and responsibilities of nurses and general duty assistants with the families. Domestic work is not a part of nurses' and caregivers' duties. However, by doing chores which is not related to their professional duties, they are losing their dignity and respect. Similar results were presented by Fatemi *et al.* (2019) where the home care nurses experience ambiguity in their role-playing, as their duties were not clearly defined in the government guidelines, they felt a sense of power working in a hospital but they felt it decreased when they work at patient homes.

The third objective examined the emotional well-being and challenges faced by health care staff in home health care. Respondents were asked about the job structure, the number of patients they handled, types of patients cared for, and years of experience in home care. Further questions were asked regarding problems faced concerning food, job, safety issues, and remuneration at the workplace. The questions were framed about the services performed by home care staff. Moreover, to understand their emotional well-being, questions were framed to understand the burden concerning caregiver burden scale.

4.18 Number of Patients Cared (Nurses and General Duty Assistants)

Caregivers are compassionate health care professionals, who take care of the geriatric, support them with their daily activities, and assist them with medication besides providing them companionship. The data about the number of patients that are cared for by the respondents are indicated in Table 4.10.

Data were collected to know about the number of patients handled by general duty assistants and nursing staff. It was found from Table 4.10 that the majority of them, i.e. 52.5 per cent have handled up to 20 patients, followed by 18.8 per cent of them have handled up to 40 patients. However, whether they are GDAs or nursing staff, 8.8 per cent of them have taken care of up to 60 patients. Interestingly, about 100 patients and above are handled by 18.8 per cent of the staff each respectively.

Table 4.10: Number of Patients Cared

Number of Patients Cared		Group		Total
		Nurses	GDAs	
Up to 20	Count	19	23	42
	% within Group	47.5%	57.5%	52.5%
21-40	Count	7	8	15
	% within Group	17.5%	20.0%	18.8%
41-60	Count	3	4	7
	% within Group	7.5%	10.0%	8.8%
61-80	Count	0	1	1
	% within Group	0.0%	2.5%	1.3%
81-99	Count	0	0	0
	% within Group	0.0%	0.0 %	0%
Above 100	Count	11	4	15
	% within Group	27.5%	10.0%	18.8%
Total	**Count**	**40**	**40**	**80**
	% within Group	**100.0%**	**100.0%**	**100.0%**

Note: Chi-square test value = 4.85, among above categories with p-value = .302.
Source: Primary Data Collection.

4.19 Years of Experience (Nurses and General Duty Assistants)

Respondents (Nurses and GDAs) were interviewed to analyze the years of experience of working in home health care.

Data analyzed from interviews is presented in Table 4.11. About 47.5 per cent have over 3 years of experience working in home care followed by 12.5 per cent, 8.8 per cent, and 6.3 per cent who have over 4 years, 6 years, and 7 years of work experience respectively. It was observed that 5 per cent of them have more than 9 years, 10 years, and above experience respectively in home health care.

Table 4.11: Years of Experience

Years of Experience		Group		Total
		Nurses	**GDAs**	
Up to 3 years	Count	17	21	38
	% within Group	42.5%	52.5%	47.5%
4 years	Count	5	5	10
	% within Group	12.5%	12.5%	12.5%
5 years	Count	4	3	7
	% within Group	10.0%	7.5%	8.8%
6 years	Count	6	1	7
	% within Group	15.0%	2.5%	8.8%
7 years	Count	1	4	5
	% within Group	2.5%	10.0%	6.3%
8 years	Count	0	1	1
	% within Group	0.0%	2.5%	1.3%
9 years	Count	2	2	4
	% within Group	5.0%	5.0%	5.0%
10 years	Count	2	2	4
	% within Group	5.0%	5.0%	5.0%
Above 10 years	Count	3	1	4
	% within Group	7.5%	2.5%	5.0%
Total	**Count**	**40**	**40**	**80**
	% within Group	**100.0%**	**100.0%**	**100.0%**

Note: Chi-square test value = 7.93, among above categories with p-value = .440.
Source: Primary Data Collection.

One of the nurse managers shared her experience "Earlier I have worked with Aegis home care, Max hospital, SAS Nagar, Mohali, Fortis hospital, SAS Nagar, Mohali, and now I am working with Max home health care as a nurse manager. I have over 7 years of experience in nursing, but still, my salary is equivalent to what a fresher in home care is paid" (R62/26/NM/H/U/Exp. 7 years).

> Another one shared "I have worked with many hospitals. I have over 9 years of experience in nursing and am paid Rs. 20,000 for 24 hours shift pattern"(R70/25/N/U/Exp. 9 years).

George *et al.* (2017) study explored the perception of aged care support workers and how their health was influenced by their job. In this study aides whose time spent in the home care industry ranged from six months to 28 years, as compared to the present study, where there were people ranging in experience, those who joined the industry only about 6 months ago and some (7.5%) nurses and (2.5%) GDAs who have been working for about more than 10 years in the support care industry and are continuing their profession. From in-depth interviews, it was further analyzed that the respondents who were above 45 years of age have over 20-25 years of experience and are still working as nurses and general duty assistants. As they think this is the best job they can do along with giving time to their own family, and in these few cases, the respondents especially the females preferred to work in the night shifts.

4.20 Types of Patient Handled (Nurses and General Duty Assistants)

Home care provides support in case of chronic diseases like Alzheimer's disease, Cancer, Heart failure, Chronic Obstructive Pulmonary Disease (COPD), Parkinson's disease, and Injury or fracture. When one suffers from chronic conditions which affect one's quality of life, that means home care is needed.

Data were collected regarding the type of patients handled by the nurses and caregivers and are indicated in Table 4.12. It was estimated that 83.8 per cent (neurological disease), 72.5 per cent (cancer), 92.5 per cent (diabetes), 63.5 per cent (lungs), 60 per cent (liver), 70 per cent (kidney), 80 per cent (heart disease), 82.5 per cent (hypertension), Open wounds and disease of the Muscular-Skeletal system respectively were the different kinds of patients handled.

Caregivers undertake the responsibility of cancer patient home management and organize health care services according to the changing condition of the patients. They help in activities such as physical care, symptom management, managing care devices-infusion pumps, intravenous fluid replacement, patient handling, and patient safety. They also perform domestic activities such as shopping, child care, cooking, and washing clothes (Wen and Gustafson, 2004; Stenberg *et al.*, 2010; Hazelwood *et al.*, 2012; Chang *et al.*, 2013).

Table 4.12: Types of Patients Handled

Types of Patient Handled			Group		Total	p-value	χ^2 Test
			Nurses	GDAs			
Disease of the Nervous System	Yes	Count	33	34	67	.762	.092
		% within Group	82.5%	85.0%	83.8%		
	No	Count	7	6	13		
		% within Group	17.5%	15.0%	16.3%		
Cancer	Yes	Count	30	28	58	.617	.251
		% within Group	75.0%	70.0%	72.5%		
	No	Count	10	12	22		
		% within Group	25.0%	30.0%	27.5%		
Disease of the Endocrine System (Diabetes Mellitus)	Yes	Count	34	40	74	.011	6.48**
		% within Group	85.0%	100.0%	92.5%		
	No	Count	6	0	6		
		% within Group	15.0%	0.0%	7.5%		
Lung Disease	Yes	Count	27	24	51	.485	.487
		% within Group	67.5%	60.0%	63.7%		
	No	Count	13	16	29		
		% within Group	32.5%	40.0%	36.3%		
Liver Disease	Yes	Count	26	22	48	.361	.833
		% within Group	65.0%	55.0%	60.0%		
	No	Count	14	18	32		
		% within Group	35.0%	45.0%	40.0%		

(*Contd.*)

Types of Patient Handled			Group		Total	p-value	χ^2 Test
			Nurses	GDAs			
Kidney Disease	Yes	Count	31	25	56	.143	2.14
		% within Group	77.5%	62.5%	70.0%		
	No	Count	9	15	24		
		% within Group	22.5%	37.5%	30.0%		
Hyperte-nsion	Yes	Count	35	31	66	.239	1.38
		% within Group	87.5%	77.5%	82.5%		
	No	Count	5	9	14		
		% within Group	12.5%	22.5%	17.5%		
Heart Disease	Yes	Count	34	30	64	.264	1.25
		% within Group	85.0%	75.0%	80.0%		
	No	Count	6	10	16		
		% within Group	15.0%	25.0%	20.0%		
Open Wound/ Bed Sores	Yes	Count	34	32	66	.556	.346
		% within Group	85.0%	80.0%	82.5%		
	No	Count	6	8	14		
		% within Group	15.0%	20.0%	17.5%		
Disease of the Muscular-Skeletal System	Yes	Count	34	32	66	.556	.346
		% within Group	85.0%	80.0%	82.5%		
	No	Count	6	8	14		
		% within Group	15.0%	20.0%	17.5%		

Source: Primary Data Collection.

However, with all these variables, the results analyzed are insignificant, except for diabetes, where the results were found to be moderately significant ($p < 0.05$) as is evident from the chi-square value which is equal to (6.48**).

4.21 Problems Faced with Regard to Job

Data were collected to analyze the problems faced by nurses and caregivers in home care (Table 4.13).

Table 4.13: Problems Faced with Regard to Job

Problems Faced with regard to Job			Group		Total
			Nurses	GDAs	
	Yes	Count	21	19	40
		% within Group	52.5%	47.5%	50.0%
	No	Count	19	21	40
		% within Group	47.5%	52.5%	50.0%
Total		**Count**	**40**	**40**	**80**
		% within Group	**100.0%**	**100.0%**	**100.0%**

Note: Chi-square test value = .200, among above categories with p-value = .655.
Source: Primary Data Collection.

It was found that 50 per cent of respondents faced problems related to food, salaries, respect, and the interference of families, while 50 per cent of them faced no issues.

Overall, it can be summed up that home care workers experience several challenges such as long shift hours, poor work place management, lack of peer support, feeling of being underpaid, stress, and burnout at the workplace. These workers also deal with inappropriate social status as they are more likely to be subjected to degrading reactions from family members and close relatives. Moreover, neither they are provided leaves by the agencies nor by families as the families are solely dependent upon them for caregiving. Similar studies showed sources of stress for home nurses include poor workplace, loss of peer support, unexpected events, inappropriate social status, and working time problems (Denton *et al.*, 2002; Hsu *et al.*, 2007; Carr and Kazanowski, 1994; Fatemi *et al.*, 2019; Delp *et al.*, 2010).

4.22 Problem Faced with Regard to the Food (Nurses and General Duty Assistants)

Data were collected to analyze the problems faced related to food by nurses and caregivers in home care. It was examined from the data depicted in Fig. 4.9.

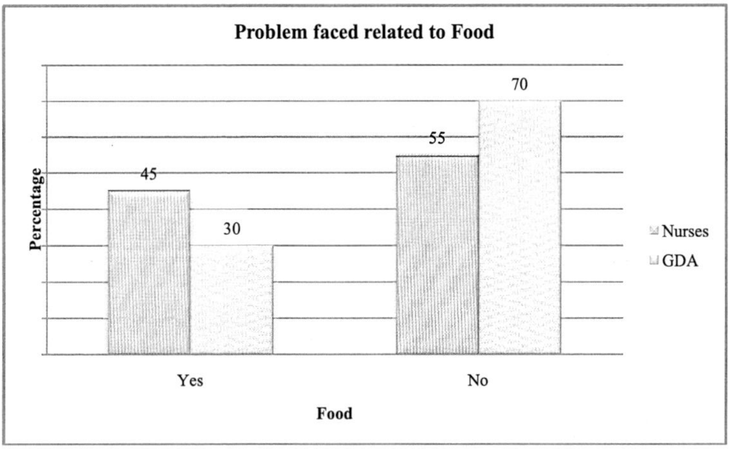

Fig. 4.9: Problem Faced with regard to Food.

Note: Chi-square test value = 1.92, among above categories with p-value = .166.
Source: Primary Data Collection.

It was investigated that 45 per cent of nurses and 30 per cent of GDAs respondents faced problems related to food while 55 per cent nurses and 70 per cent GDAs did not face any problems related to food.

> (R36 GDA) shared her experience "The last family used to scold me and tell me that you tend to eat more food and they would clearly instruct that you are not allowed to eat these things. I was given only certain foods to eat as per the family wishes, almost every time the food provided was given late" (R36/19/GDA/H/U/Exp. 1 year).

On the whole, it can be concluded that there were some families which provided good food to the health care professionals, while a number of them were just concerned about their patients and rather were not willing to provide meals even to the staff who stayed with them for 24 hours as the families consider providing meal as an extra burden.

4.23 Safety Issues at Work (Nurses and General Duty Assistants)

Respondents were interviewed regarding the safety issues at work. The results are indicated in Fig. 4.10.

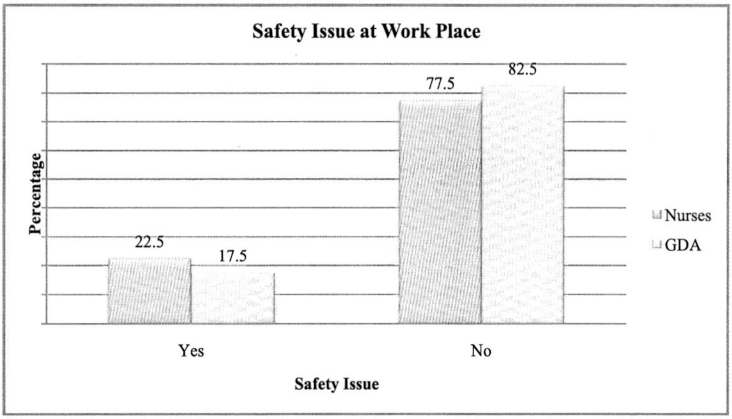

Fig. 4.10: Safety Issues at Work.

Note: Chi-square test value = .313, among above categories with p-value = .576.
Source: Primary Data Collection.

Overall, 77.5 per cent of nurses and 82.5 per cent of GDAs faced no safety issues at work while 22.5 per cent of nurses and 17.5 per cent of GDAs faced safety issues at work. Many of the respondents discussed safety issues being faced. A few of the stories are as under:

> (R34 N, Female) "Once I was coming back from duty in the late evening, it was 9 pm. Someone stole my phone, pushed me, and I was badly injured. I was very upset with the agency and had to pay more to the auto driver worrying about any mishappening further. I was furious as to why the authorities are not concerned about our safety. We receive calls if we are ten minutes late for our duty but why are we not looked after, why don't they confirm whether the staff has reached their destination safely or not" (R34/27/N/S/U/Exp. 4 years).

(R69 N, Female) narrated her story "I was taking care of a female patient who suffered a clot in the brain and was bedridden for the last 12 years. Her husband rather than taking care of her, compelled the staff to develop intimate relations with him. In anger, I once slapped her husband and warned him. He even tries to molest his daughter-in-law in the same way. Further, we are responsible for maintaining our dignity in home care, we cannot trust anyone" (R69/26/N/S/U/Exp. 3 years).

(R 34 GDA, Male) said "I faced safety issues in my last job. I was taking care of a male patient, who was not well, the wife started loving me and compelled me to be physically involved with her. She used to send pictures to me. Later, when the family members got to know about this relationship. I had to run away from their house as there was a threat to my life" (R34/22/GDA/MU/M/Exp. 6 years).

Even one of the respondents discussed about the Covid times, in grief, she shared "Even during the times of COVID-19, we were not provided kits and in many cases the patient was a suspect" (R48/31/N/S/M/Exp. 3 years).

It was concluded from the findings that providing a safe environment for the health care professional is very important and the utmost responsibility lies with the agencies and the families with they are working with.

4.24 Financial Satisfaction through this Profession

Respondents were interviewed regarding their satisfaction with the finances. The results are indicated in Fig. 4.11.

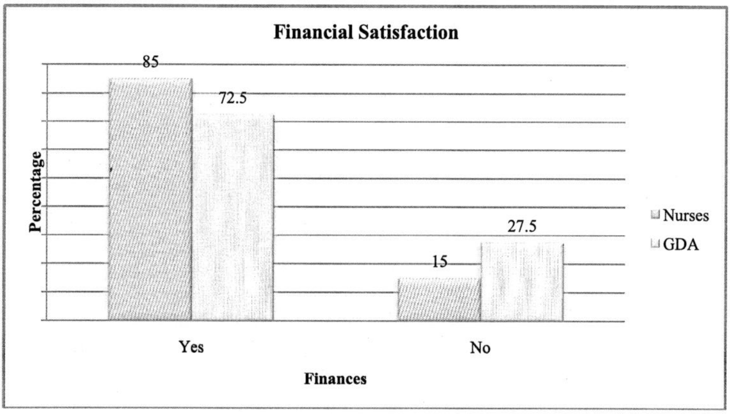

Fig. 4.11: Satisfaction with the Remuneration.

Note: Chi-square test value = 1.86, among above categories with p-value = .172. *Source:* Primary Data Collection.

It was analysed from the findings that 85 per cent of nurses and 72.5 per cent of GDAs were satisfied with the finances while 15 per cent of nurses and 27.5 per cent of GDAs were not satisfied with the finances.

> (R29 GDA) asserted "I have brought a 6-marla plot from this salary, I bought an auto rickshaw for my brother, I am saving money for my sister's wedding and purchased a bike from my salary, now I have started my business of wheatgrass juice. I go to the park early in the morning (4 am-8 am) then later I go to work from 8 am-8 pm"(R29/25/GDA/H/U/Exp.6.5 years).

Donovan (1989) study on home care workers also identified stressful working conditions, lack of benefits, low pay, lack of opportunities for promotion and powerlessness. The present study also identified stressful and hectic work environments, lack of benefits was observed but the respondents in the study elaborated that they are comparatively more eager to work in hospitals than home care, but due to meagre salaries in hospitals [Avg. salary INR

Rs. 10,000 month (134.68$)] they have to unwillingly work in home care.

It can be summarized from the findings that more respondents were satisfied with their salaries in home care whether they were nurses or GDAs. As they believed that especially in 24 hours shifts, they tend to save on food and accommodation. Very few of them believed that they are underpaid according to the workload in home care.

4.25 Nursing Services Provided to the Patients in Home Health Care Sector

Based on the initial assessment of the elderly patient's requirements, a nurse officer prepares a patient care plan that includes the mediation plan, meals plan, exercise, massage, recreation, and daily routine. The nurse officer takes the patient's vitals on his/her visits to ensure the well-being of the patient. She also addresses the issues of the family regarding the home care attendants' or nursing staff's conduct. Various procedures are handled by home care nurses in patients' homes (Fig. 4.12).

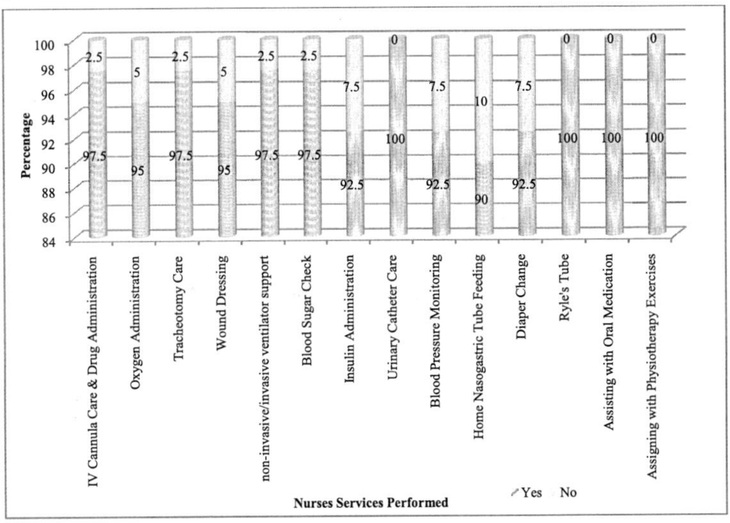

Fig. 4.12: Nursing Services Provided to the Patients.

Source: Primary Data Collection.

In the present study, 100 per cent of the nurses assisted the patient with oral medication, physiotherapy exercises, and checking vital parameters. However, 97.5 per cent of the nurses helped the patients with I.V Cannula care and drug administration. However, an equal percentage of nurses performed finger prick test for checking the blood sugar level as well as administered Insulin. Whereas 97.5 per cent of trained nurses managed patients with tracheotomy and its care by adequate suctioning, attaching non-invasive/invasive ventilator support while 95 per cent helped the patients with oxygen administration and wound dressings at home. Moreover, 92.5 per cent conducted technical procedures such as administrating the patient with Ryle's tube feeding, and urinary catheter care at home. It was analyzed from in-depth interviews that nursing staff was not comfortable changing diapers, they felt that changing diapers were not part of their duties but about 90 per cent of them had to change patient diapers in home care. Technological advances have allowed for more medical treatments to be carried out and monitored in private homes (Ward-Griffin and McKeever, 2000) such care is sometimes called "hospital at home" and is often put into practice and handled by a team of nurses delivering complex care (Temmink *et al.*, 2000).

4.26 Personal Care Services Provided to Patients in the Home Health Care Sector

The health care sector is one of the most rapidly growing sectors in India, both in terms of generating revenue and employment generation. A home health aide provides personal services to sick and bedridden patients suffering from multiple ailments in the patient's home.

It was analyzed from the data from Fig. 4.13 that 100 per cent of home health care professionals provide care services such as bathing, dressing, grooming, changing patient clothes, nail and hair care, denture care, changing diapers, assisting with commode, ambulation (assistance in walking), assisting with oral medication, assisting in physiotherapy/daily exercises and laundry services.

97.5 per cent act as their companions, carry out recreational activities, lending an ear to their life experiences, play games with them, take them for walks and listen to their stories. 95 per cent of them tend to reposition bed-bound patients to help prevent bed sores, and check their temperature and blood pressure. From In-depth interview it was analysed that initially the families are reluctant to keep staff as they are not willing to spend money on their patients, but as their condition deteriorates, the families later employed a GDA staff when almost all the patient body has bed sores. It was observed that 72.5 per cent assisted the patients with the Ryle's tube feeding and 65 per cent help them in the preparation of food and shopping for other household requirements, preparing and serving meals to the patients.

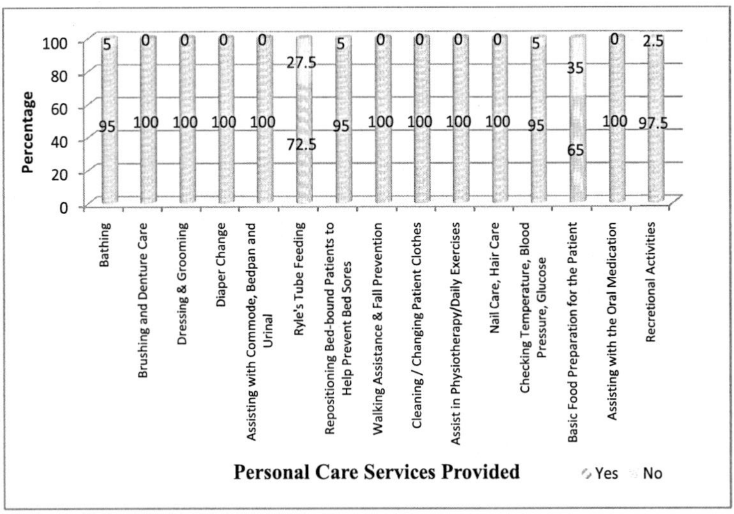

Fig. 4.13: Personal Care Services Provided to the Patients by GDAs.

Source: Primary Data Collection.

The findings are different from results conducted by Ugur *et al.* (2014) where about 54 per cent of the caregivers helped the patient in the preparation of food and looking after their nutrition, 50.36 per cent helped in assisting with the medication, 44.53 per cent helped in bathing, 26.28 per cent helped in oral hygiene,

51.82 per cent helped in changing clothes, 75.91 per cent help to shop for the patients and their house needs, 71.53 per cent acted as their companions and 48.18 per cent checked on patient body temperature. However, Hendrix and Ray (2006) emphasized that caregivers are in dire need of help with the administration of medicine management and changing patient clothes. Training programmes are important for the caregivers before and after patient discharge to reduce problems encountered by the caregivers in managing patients.

4.27 Caregiver Burden Scale

The burden experienced by family caregivers and paid caregivers is the most important caregiver-related variable in care at home in the care of a chronically-ill person. The extent of subjective burden (which is borne by the caregivers) has a significant impact on the emotional and physical well-being of the family caregivers and the paid caregivers (nurses and general duty assistants), and even influences the mortality of spouse caregivers. A comparison with a non-caregiving group shows that over 4.5 years, the risk of death of spouses burdened with caregiving was 63 per cent greater than the spouses who did not perceive home care as a burden (Schulz and Beach, 1999). In the present study, the researcher interviewed 40 nursing staff, 40 general duty assistants, and 40 family caregivers to analyze the burden they bear in lieu of their duties in caring for sick patients. It affects the way the family caregivers especially the primary caregivers, nurses, and general duty assistants deal with the care receiver and determines the time of institutionalization. In the present study, the paid caregivers tend to stay with one patient for a period of 6 months to 1 year continuously; some tend to continuously stay for 3 years also. The Burden Scale for Family Caregivers (BSFC) (Grasel, 1995) is a 28-item questionnaire that was developed to determine the burden felt by caregivers working for the patients.

Overall, it was found that 76.9 per cent of general duty assistants, 59.5 per cent of family caregivers and 40 per cent of nurses, BSFC scores ranged between 0 to 41, which means 50 per cent of the caregivers have an average extent of physical symptoms.

However, 52.5 per cent of the nursing staff, 20.5 per cent of the general duty assistants, and 12.5 per cent of the family caregivers' BSFC score range from 42 to 55, and 74 per cent of those caregivers have an above-average extent of physical symptoms. Henceforth, for 7.5 per cent of the nurses, 28 per cent of the family caregivers, and 2.6 per cent of the home aides, BSFC score ranges from 56 to 84, 90 per cent of those caregivers have an above-average extent of physical symptoms. The results analyzed were found to be highly significant ($p < 0.05$) as is evident from the chi-square value which is equal to (11.07***) showing a strong association of home health care workers who deliver the majority of home care services and shoulder the bulk of burden and responsibilities at the workplace. Burden scale was further analyzed for age, gender, marital status, religion, current residence, and social-economic status of the respondents.

Table 4.14: Interpretation of the BSFC score for Caregivers of Individuals

BSFC Score	Subjective burden categories	Risk of psycho-somatic symptoms	Family Caregivers	Nurses	G.D.As
0-41	None to mild	Not at risk[a]	59.5%	40%	76.9%
42-55	moderate	Increased risk[b]	12.5%	52.5%	20.5%
56-84	Severe to very severe	At very high risk[c]	28%	7.5%	2.6%

Note: Chi-square test value =11.07***, among above categories with p-value = .004.
Source: Primary Data Collection.

[a]If the BSFC score ranges from 0 to 41, the extent of overall physical symptoms corresponds to the expected value in the "normal population", that is, 50 per cent of those caregivers have a percentile rank (PR) of physical symptoms< 50 and the other 50 per cent a PR > 50.

[b]If the BSFC score ranges from 42 to 55, 74 per cent of those caregivers have an above average extent of physical symptoms (PR > 50).

[c]If the BSFC score ranges from 56 to 84, 90 per cent of those caregivers have an above average extent of physical symptoms (PR > 50).

Arafa *et al.* (2003) also discussed in their study about moderate to severe psychosomatic symptoms in 21.7 per cent of nurses which is an indication of mental health problems.

Piko (1999) indicated that frequency of common psychosomatic symptoms includes sleeping problems, headache and chronic fatigue is an indicator of work related stress levels.

4.27.1 Burden Scale with Regard to the Age Group of the Respondents

When the researcher tried to analyse data with respect to all the age groups of the respondents (nurses and general duty assistants). The results were indicated in Table 4.14.1.

Maximum respondents in the age group of 26-28, i.e. 66.7 per cent and 100 per cent of the nursing staff were moderately and severely burdened as compared to the other age groups. With regards to the general duty assistants, 50 per cent of the respondents in the age groups (23-25) were moderately and (17-19, 20-22) were severely burdened. The total score can range from 0-84, with a score of above 42 or more indicative of significant psychosomatic symptoms (fatigue, insomnia, aches and pains, indigestion, hypertension, headaches, and migraine). It was gathered from an in-depth interview that they tend to stay with the patient 'round the clock' which leaves behind little time for self-care and social activities for oneself and one may feel emotionally, physically, and mentally drained.

This is this age group where respondents are on the verge of getting married or are newly married and the same thoughts are shared by both the male and female respondents where they believe that this is the profession where one has to be with the patient for 12 hours or 24 hours and this occupation cannot be taken further after marriage. However, the results were found to be significant as is evident from the chi-square value which is equal to 18.9*. With regards to general duty assistants, 17- 9 years of age or 20-22 years of age means, they have just started their career and in many cases, it is due to the financial needs of the family, one has to work as a caregiver. So home care workers report a high level of burden on the job stress caring for the ill, dying, aggressive, and the disoriented.

Sansoni *et al.* (2004) have confirmed the presence of both physical and psychological illnesses among caregivers due to the stress that comes with the job. The 'round the clock' nature of caregiving for such patients leaves behind little time for oneself and one may feel emotionally, physically, and mentally drained, similar findings presented by Ferrara *et al.* (2008) confirm this assertion.

Table 4.14.1: Burden scale with Regard to the Age Group of the Respondents

Age Group of the Respondents			**Burden scale groups**			**Total**
			0-41	**42-55**	**56-84**	
Nurses						
Age	20-22	Count	0	1	0	1
		% within Burden scale groups	0.0%	4.8%	0.0%	2.5%
	23-25	Count	7	3	0	10
		% within Burden scale groups	43.8%	14.3%	0.0%	25.0%
	26-28	Count	2	14	3	19
		% within Burden scale groups	12.5%	66.7%	100.0%	47.5%
	29-31	Count	3	3	0	6
		% within Burden scale groups	18.8%	14.3%	0.0%	15.0%
	32-34	Count	1	0	0	1
		% within Burden scale groups	6.3%	0.0%	0.0%	2.5%
	35-37	Count	3	0	0	3
		% within Burden scale groups	18.8%	0.0%	0.0%	7.5%
Total		**Count**	**16**	**21**	**3**	**40**
		% within Burden scale groups	**100.0%**	**100.0%**	**100.0%**	**100.0%**
Note: Chi-square test value = 18.9*, among above categories with p-value = .041.						

(*Contd.*)

Age Group of the Respondents			**Burden scale groups**			**Total**
			0-41	**42-55**	**56-84**	
General Duty Assistants						
Age	17-19	Count	2	0	1	3
		% within Burden scale groups	6.7%	12..5%	50.0%	7.5%
	20-22	Count	9	1	1	11
		% within Burden scale groups	30.0%	0.0%	50.0%	27..5%
	23-25	Count	6	4	0	10
		% within Burden scale groups	20.0%	50.0%	0.0%	25.0%
	26-28	Count	9	1	0	10
		% within Burden scale groups	30.0%	12.5%	0.0%	25.0%
	29-31	Count	1	0	0	1
		% within Burden scale groups	3.3%	0.0%	0.0%	2.5%
	32-34	Count	0	1	0	1
		% within Burden scale groups	0.0%	12.5%	0.0%	2.5%
	35-37	Count	1	0	0	1
		% within Burden scale groups	3.3%	0.0%	0.0%	2.5%
	38-40	Count	1	0	0	1
		% within Burden scale groups	3.3%	0.0%	0.0%	2.5%
	44-46	Count	1	1	0	2
		% within Burden scale groups	3.3%	12.5%	0.0%	5.1%
Total		**Count**	**30**	**8**	**2**	**40**
		% within Burden scale groups	**100.0%**	**100.0%**	**100.0%**	**100.0%**

Note: Chi-square test value = 11.3, among above categories with p-value = .181.
Source: Primary Data Collection.

Findings of stress and pressure among caregivers are consistent across cultures (Ferrara *et al.*, 2008, Grant *et al.*, 2002 and

Lutgendorf and Laundenslager, 2009) because of the severity of the disease, a caregiver is required to do much more than just look after the patient. To name a few, getting the patient in and out of bed, feeding them, dressing them, getting them to and from the toilet, bathing them etc., are some of the many duties that a caregiver performs, along with providing necessary medical attention. This leads to consequences for the caregiver in the form of physical and psychological distress. The stress incurred is so powerful that caregivers of Alzheimer's patients have an association with poor immunity, cardiovascular issues such as higher blood pressures and decreased wound healing mechanisms, and sleep patterns overall reflecting poorly on their quality of life, well-being, and health.

4.27.2 Burden Scale with Regard to Gender of the Respondents

The researcher wishes to correlate the burden bared by nursing staff and general duty assistants at their workplace for gender. The extent of subjective burden can be visualized from Table 4.14.2.

Table 4.14.2: Burden Scale with Regard to Gender of the Respondents

Gender of the Respondents			Burden scale groups			Total
			0-41	42-55	56-84	
Nurses						
Gender	Male	Count	4	4	0	8
		% within Burden scale groups	25.0%	19.0%	0.0%	20.0%
	Female	Count	12	17	3	32
		% within Burden scale groups	75.0%	81.0%	100.0%	80.0%
Total		**Count**	**16**	**21**	**3**	**40**
		% within Burden scale groups	**100.0%**	**100.0%**	**100.0%**	**100.0%**
Note: Chi-square test value = 1.10, among above categories with p-value = .603.						

(*Contd.*)

Gender of the Respondents			Burden scale groups			Total
			0-41	42-55	56-84	
GDA						
Gender	Male	Count	17	5	0	22
		% within Burden scale groups	56.7%	62.5%	0.0%	55.0%
	Female	Count	13	3	2	18
		% within Burden scale groups	43.3%	37.5%	100.0%	45.0%
Total		**Count**	**30**	**8**	**2**	**40**
		% within Burden scale groups	**100.0%**	**100.0%**	**100.0%**	**100.0%**

Note: Chi-square test value = 2.66, among above categories with p-value = .264.
Source: Primary Data Collection.

It was found that 81 per cent and 100 per cent of the female nursing staff's BSFC scores ranged from 42 to 55 and 56 to 84. Thereby, meaning that the female staffs were at an increased risk and a very high risk of psychosomatic symptoms as compared to the male staff.

Concerning the GDAs, it was investigated that 37.5 per cent of the female staff were moderately burdened and 100 per cent of the female staff were severely burdened as compared to 62.5 per cent of the male staff who felt moderately burdened at their workplace. One of the female staff, who worked with a volatile patient for several months shared her views (R75 N) shared "There is no future in home care, as we work on one patient, less of learning as compared to learning in hospitals. Sometimes, continuously working for 24 hours makes our own life difficult. Sometimes you feel depressed and frustrated" (R75/24/N/U/Exp. 3 years). The greater the subjective burden of the caregiver, the more the caregiver's somatic symptoms (Grasel, 1998).

4.27.3 Burden Scale with Regard to Marital Status of the Respondents

The researcher further wished to analyze the burden concerning the marital status of the respondents. The results are explained in Table 4.14.3.

Table 4.14.3: Burden Scale with Regard to Marital Status of the Respondents

Marital status of the respondents			Burden scale groups			Total
			0-41	42-55	56-84	
Nurses						
Marital status	Single	Count	10	16	3	29
		% within Burden scale groups	62.5%	76.2%	100.0%	72.5%
	Married	Count	6	5	0	11
		% within Burden scale groups	37.5%	23.8%	0.0%	27.5%
Total		**Count**	**16**	**21**	**3**	**40**
		% within Burden scale groups	**100.0%**	**100.0%**	**100.0%**	**100.0%**
Note: Chi-square test value = 2.08, among above categories with p-value = .353.						
GDA						
Marital status	Single	Count	20	5	2	27
		% within Burden scale groups	66.7%	62.5%	100.0%	67.5%
	Married	Count	10	3	0	13
		% within Burden scale groups	33.3%	37.5%	0.0%	32.5%
Total		**Count**	**30**	**8**	**2**	**40**
		% within Burden scale groups	**100.0%**	**100.0%**	**100.0%**	**100.0%**

Note: Chi-square test value = 1.06, among above categories with p-value = .588.
Source: Primary Data Collection.

Interestingly, concerning the nursing staff, it was found that 76.2 per cent and 100 per cent of the unmarried respondents were moderately and severely burdened as compared to 62.5 per cent and 100 per cent of general duty assistant's unmarried respondents. It was summed from the data that the burden visualized by the unmarried respondents in the study was much more than the married respondents. As it was analyzed from in depth interviews that generally the married respondents were working during the night shifts where after completing their all-day work, they tend to sleep in the patient's room and they are very much occupied with the responsibilities of their own families too and they have no time for any further thoughts. As has been found among the few home care workers, the emotional demands workers faced on the job also affected their personal lives as many of them have sick parents at home. However, where the respondents are unmarried, they tend to stay with the patient for a longer period such as 6 months or more than a year.

Their burden was further complicated by the work environment that fails to provide them with adequate recognition and support.

Similar findings were discussed by (Arafa *et al.*, 2003) and reported psychological ill health of nurses was more encountered among unmarried nurses as compared to married nurses.

4.27.4 Burden Scale with Regard to Religion of the Respondents

The researchers further investigated the burden scale about the religion of the home health care workers. The results are depicted in Table 4.14.4.

When the researcher tried to relate the burden of respondents, concerning their religion, 33.3 per cent of the nursing staff belonging to the Hindu religion followed by 66.7 per cent of the respondents belonging to Sikh religion were severely burdened. When we talk of the burden or the visibility of psychosomatic symptoms among the general duty assistants, it was found that 100 per cent of the respondents belonging to Hindu religion were severely burdened followed by 37.5 per cent of the respondents belonging to Sikh religion were moderately burdened.

Table 4.14.4: Burden Scale about the Religion of the Respondents

Religion of the Respondents			**Burden scale groups**			**Total**
			0-41	**42-55**	**56-84**	
Nurses						
Religion	Hindu	Count	3	3	1	7
		% within Burden scale groups	18.8%	14.3%	33.3%	17.5%
	Sikh	Count	13	16	2	31
		% within Burden scale groups	81.3%	76.2%	66.7%	77.5%
	Muslim	Count	0	1	0	1
		% within Burden scale groups	0.0%	4.8%	0.0%	2.5%
	Others	Count	0	1	0	1
		% within Burden scale groups	0.0%	4.8%	0.0%	2.5%
Total		**Count**	**16**	**21**	**3**	**40**
		% within Burden scale groups	**100.0%**	**100.0%**	**100.0%**	**100.0%**
Note: Chi-square test value = 2.45, among above categories with p-value = .873.						
GDA						
Religion	Hindu	Count	19	3	2	24
		% within Burden scale groups	63.3%	37.5%	100.0%	60.0%
	Sikh	Count	8	3	0	11
		% within Burden scale groups	26.7%	37.5%	0.0%	27.5%
	Muslim	Count	2	1	0	3
		% within Burden scale groups	6.7%	12.5%	0.0%	7.5%
	Others	Count	1	1	0	2
		% within Burden scale groups	3.3%	12.5%	0.0%	5.0%
Total		**Count**	**30**	**8**	**2**	**40**
		% within Burden scale groups	**100.0%**	**100.0%**	**100.0%**	**100.0%**

Note: Chi-square test value = 3.72, among above categories with p-value = .714.
Source: Primary Data Collection.

It was also examined from in-depth interviews that almost all the patients' and their families preferred caregivers speaking the local language and most of the patients' and families' preference was care providers from Hindu and Sikh religions respectively.

4.27.5 Burden Scale with regard to Current Residence of the Respondents

The respondents were interviewed to know the burden related to their current residence of the respondents. The results are shown in Table 4.14.5.

Table 4.14.5: Burden Scale with Regard to Current Residence of the Respondents

Current residence of the respondents			Burden scale groups			Total
			0-41	42-55	56-84	
Nurses						
Current residence	Patient-owned	Count	7	10	2	19
		% within Burden scale groups	43.8%	47.6%	66.7%	47.5%
	Rented	Count	5	8	0	13
		% within Burden scale groups	31.3%	38.1%	0.0%	32.5%
	Hostel-	Count	4	3	1	8
		% within Burden scale groups	25.0%	14.3%	33.3%	20.0%
Total		Count	16	21	3	40
		% within Burden scale groups	100.0%	100.0%	100.0%	100.0%
Note: Chi-square test value = 2.27, among above categories with p-value = .686.						
GDA						
Current residence	Patient-owned	Count	18	5	2	25
		% within Burden scale groups	60.0%	62.5%	100.0%	62.5%
	Rented	Count	11	1	0	12
		% within Current residence	91.7%	8.3%	0.0%	100.0%
	Hostel-	Count	1	2	0	3
		% within Burden scale groups	3.3%	25.0%	0.0%	7.5%

(*Contd.*)

Current residence of the respondents		Burden scale groups			Total
		0-41	42-55	56-84	
Total	Count	30	8	2	40
	% within Burden scale groups	100.0%	100.0%	100.0%	100.0%

Note: Chi-square test value = 6.45, among above categories with p-value = .168. *Source:* Primary Data Collection.

As the present study showed, home health care workers are navigating a host of emotional demands on and off the jobs. It was examined from the data that whether it was nurses or general duty assistants, the respondents who stayed at the patient-owned residences were moderate to severely burden. 66.7 per cent of nurses followed by 47.6 per cent who were at increased risk for psychosomatic symptoms while 62.5 per cent followed by 100 per cent of GDAs who were staying in patient-owned residences were moderately and severely burdened. As they sense that their professional value was undermined by family members as they perceived them as housemaids.

Similar findings were studied by Franzosa *et al.* (2018) where the authors clearly described the role of a few families who asked the aides to take on an extra task that is not permitted by the agencies and perceived them as 'housekeepers'.

4.27.6 Burden Scale Regarding Socio-Economic Status of the Respondent

Respondents were interviewed to relate their socio-economic status with the burden perceived by the respondents. The results are shown in Table 4.14.6.

The analysis of the socio-economic status of respondents shows the burden felt by them at the workplace, 33.3 per cent of each of the nursing staff were severely burdened in the upper middle, upper lower, and lower segments. When asked about their job challenges, home health workers said that due to financial problems in the family they have to unwillingly work in home care. Moreover, the hospitals no longer provide jobs to ANMs and GNMs, and also the

Table 4.14.6: Burden Scale Regarding Socio-Economic Status of the Respondent

Socio-Economic Status of the Respondent			Burden scale groups			Total
			0-41	42-55	56-84	
Nurses						
SES	26-29 Upper (I)	Count	3	0	0	3
		% within Burden scale groups	18.8%	0.0%	0.0%	7.5%
	16-25 Upper Middle (II)	Count	6	4	1	11
		% within Burden scale groups	37.5%	19.0%	33.3%	27.5%
	11-15 Lower Middle (III)	Count	5	9	0	14
		% within Burden scale groups	31.3%	42.9%	0.0%	35.0%
	5-10 Upper Lower(IV)	Count	2	8	1	11
		% within Burden scale groups	12.5%	38.1%	33.3%	27.5%
	<5 Lower (V)	Count	0	0	1	1
		% within Burden scale groups	0.0%	0.0%	33.3%	2.5%
Total		**Count**	**16**	**21**	**3**	**40**
		% within Burden scale groups	**100.0%**	**100.0%**	**100.0%**	**100.0%**
Note: Chi-square test value = 21.6**, among above categories with p-value = .004.						
GDAs						
SES	16-25 Upper Middle(II)	Count	1	1	0	2
		% within Burden scale groups	3.3%	12.5%	0.0%	5.0%
	11-15 Lower Middle(III)	Count	11	2	1	14
		% within Burden scale groups	36.7%	25.0%	50.0%	35.0%
	5-10 Upper Lower(IV)	Count	18	4	1	23
		% within Burden scale groups	60.0%	50.0%	50.0%	57.5%
	<5 Lower(V)	Count	0	1	0	1
		% within Burden scale groups	0.0%	12.5%	0.0%	2.5%

(*Contd.*)

Socio-Economic Status of the Respondent		**Burden scale groups**			**Total**
		0-41	**42-55**	**56-84**	
Total	Count	30	8	2	40
	% within Burden scale groups	100.0%	100.0%	100.0%	100.0%

Note: Chi-square test value = 5.67, among above categories with p-value = .460.
Source: Primary Data Collection.

salaries provided in home care to nursing staff are pretty good. The results analyzed were found to be moderately significant ($p > 0.05$) as is evident from the chi-square value which is equal to (21.6**).

Personal duty assistants also faced job challenges and shoulder the bulk of emotional labour while caring for the geriatric population. It was found that 50 per cent of the respondents from both categories were at increased risk of psychosomatic symptoms and were from the lower middle and upper lower socio-economic groups. Ohaeri (2003) suggested existing literature on caregiving which is associated with cognitive and emotional transformations. The important predictors of burden were identified as problematic behaviour, disability, and severity of symptoms as caring for the patient requires a lot of patience and tremendous strength.

In many cases, attachment to the patient and sudden demise is one of the reasons for stress and agony for the home care providers, one of them shared:

> "One gets attached to the patient and the family. If the patient expires one feels as if their family member has gone *(itna dukh laga unke jane ke baad, apna koi mar jata ese laga mere ko)*. Further, she grieved and highlighted that families have no time for their elders and so they employ us for their care" (R15/37/N/M/Exp. 15 years).

The more greatly burdened family caregivers prefer the patient to be in a hospital rather than home care than the less burdened caregivers (Grasel, 1999; Yaffe *et al.*, 2002). As discussed through this narrative in the present study, the families due to the burden of caregiving were no longer interested in caring for the patient, and in those cases, they employ paid caregivers.

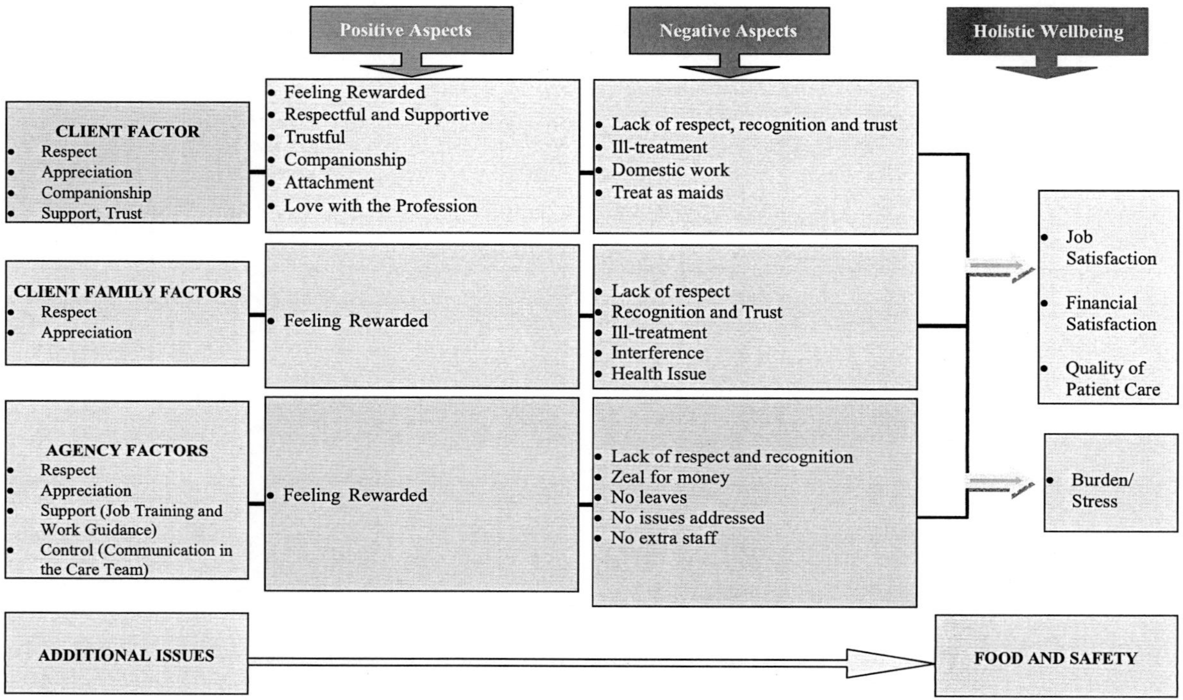

Fig. 4.14: Positive and Negative factors affecting Home Care Workers in Tricity (Chandigarh, Mohali, Panchkula).
Source: Primary Data Collection.

In the first phase of our interviews, the researcher came up with certain positive factors (feeling rewarded, respectful, supportive, trustful, companionship and attachment with the client) and simultaneous negative factors (lack of respect, recognition and support, letting them down or ill-treatment) from the patients and their families were highlighted by the nurses and general duty assistants consciously or unconsciously (Fig. 4.14). Home care workers feel rewarded, appreciated and supportive if the agencies cooperate and support them while its absence contribute to negative attitudes being formed against their duties and being associated the agencies. Additional issues related to their food and safety were also examined. On the one hand, these factors would together contribute to their holistic well-being through job satisfaction, financial satisfaction and quality of patient care or burden or stress arising out of these factors at work place.

Donaldson and Burns (1999) explored the availability of support systems, the relationship between patients, and the attitude of caregivers play a major role in determining how burdensome and stressful they find their role. Juozapavicius and Weber (2001) found that caregivers caring for Alzheimer's patients recounted many stories regarding their stress, coping strategies, barriers faced, and regrets.

All health care workers have to indulge in some kind of emotional labour or relational work required to bring trust to the patients and ensure their comfort. The majority of home care services are delivered by home care aides and personal care assistants who shoulder the bulk of the responsibility required for patients (Butler *et al.*, 2012; Rodat, 2014).

Home care workers report a high level of stress caring for ill, dying, and aggressive patients and prioritizing patients' emotional needs and happiness above their own (Arts *et al.*,1999; Hakanen *et al.*, 2008; National Institute for Occupational Safety and Health, 2010). In the present study it is reflected that the home care workers, whether they are nurses or General duty assistants, they earn more than hospital aides or nursing staff as their work is endowed with more responsibility and likely requires more judgment which is solely monitored by nurse managers. Unexpectedly, home health care workers face double the chances of illness and injuries as compared to all occupations taken together placing this job among the 30 riskiest occupations (Seavey, 2010). Similarly, aides in the present study faced health issues related to migraine, back pain, illness, and headache and in this age of the pandemic, they were even prone to infections. Still, the personal care assistants continue to work in one place for more than 2 years which have been well predicted in the study undertaken by (Kaye *et al.*, 2006), and even in the present study, the majority of the respondents had stayed with the patient for 6 months to as much as 3 years, also it is understood from the study undertaken by (Kaye *et al.*, 2006), that other low wage occupations have fewer demands and better benefits and retaining these workers could be difficult if the conditions did not improve.

Note

1. https://my.clevelandclinic.org/health/articles/4673-tracheal-suction-guidelines

5

Voices from the Field

Job Experiences of Nurses and General Duty Assistants

> Caregiving often calls us to lean into love we didn't know possible.
>
> –Tia Walker

ATLAS.ti software is software that facilitates the organization and analysis of qualitative data. This software was chosen for analyzing data as it allows the analysis to be guided by the specific objectives of the study; and the links were established keeping in mind the objectives of the study and the dominant themes emerged from the raw data. In this chapter different themes have been identified using thematic content analysis approach in the first half of the interviews, caregivers and nurses were interviewed. It was aimed to understand how the caregivers perceived their job and its impact upon their physical, mental and social health were explicitly explored. As visualized in the Ist phase of our findings as elaborated in chapter-4, there were few positive and negative factors which were highlighted by nurses and general duty assistants in home care. To gather an in-depth information, the researcher decided to collect data through focused group interviews from 15 nurses and 15 General duty assistants after the finalization of Discussion guide (Annexure-IV and V). In the first stage, the researcher through reading and re-reading interviews and transcripts made notes of ideas. Analysis of the focused group interviews were conducted following a thematic analysis approach where the content of the description of relationship formed with the patients, their family members and agencies were analysed according to common emerging themes and concepts. Further, the benefits and drawbacks of working in home care were also examined. These were classified as codes in the qualitative analysis software ATLAS.ti. Codes are short statements that can be used to index the data, grouping the main themes from each interview relating to the impact of home care. Following this, coded data from these interviews were grouped into meaningful patterns so as to generate a coding framework of the major themes, sub-themes, categories of sub-themes and sub-categories that ran through the data. An initial coding scheme was developed based on the interview guide and was operationalized using ATLAS.ti. Specifically, codes were applied to specific text within each transcript and then queried for frequencies across transcripts. The coding framework was discussed and then applied to all the 30 focused group interviews. All the data were analysed by 2 separate coders. In addition to it all data were quality checked by an experienced qualitative expert. Initially first fifteen interviews were prepared in the form of transcripts. Researchers also investigated using ATLAS.ti whether the qualitative data suggested a specific scoring algorithm of co-occurrence of themes. Researcher has produced analysis with the help of code document table that establishes relationships between codes of qualitative data.

Detailed transcripts from the audio-recorded interviews were analysed with the help of ATLAS.ti. A coding book and an item tracking matrix were developed to assure the tracking of emerging themes and concepts. Analysis of data were conducted at the participant level and then pooled together for overall analysis. A table with the codes and code frequency can be exported into Excel.

The fourth objective focused on understanding the job experiences of nurses and general duty assistants working in home health care through ATLAS.ti.

5.1 Relationship with the Patient

Among the respondents, three primary relationships were identified that affected their emotional state, patients, their family members and agency supervisors. With each relationship, participants/caregivers reported that their emotional well-being was influenced by the level to which and if they were appreciated, valued for their work and respected for their professional expertise. It was commonly reported by the caregivers that many times, they felt frustrated because of the devalued and disrespectful behaviour towards them for the duties they perform as a part of their profession in home care. Fifteen nurses working with various agencies were interviewed. A number of conceptual models have been employed to examine caregiver's (Nurses and GDAs) relationship with the client, relationship with the family and the agencies they are working with (Franzosa *et al.*, 2019). Aides and clients spend their time together building an intimacy that creates feelings of being rewarded along with the emotional demands (Delp *et al.*, 2010; Hoppe *et al.*, 2015; Franzosa *et al.*, 2019). Thus, these relationships and respondents emotional state is influenced by the patient's family members at an individual level and the role of agencies at an organizational level (Franzosa *et al.*, 2018). Banijamali *et al.* (2014) also reported that the most important reason the respondents gave for becoming home care was their commitment and obligation to care for particular clients.

Table 5.1 represents the researchers' analysis of various themes which analysed the relationship of caregivers (Nurses and GDAs) with the patients. Overall, in case of nurses, 12 themes define their relationship, namely Attachment (26.6%), Domestic work (20%), Support (46.6%), Love and enjoy (26.6%), Treat as maids (26.6%), Patient shows improvement (20%), Aggressive behaviour (26.6%), Helping outside their scope of job (20%), Plight of old parents (13.3%), Depressed and exhausted (13.3%), Trust (6.6%), and Lack of respect (13.3%). Moreover, consistent with previous research, participants (Nurses and GDAs) reported building relationship with the patient was important and they derive a sense of satisfaction by making a difference in the lives of their

Table 5.1: Nurses (Relationship with the Patient)

Sr. No.	Relationship with the Patient	D1	D2	D3	D4	D5	D6	D7	D8	D9	D10	D11	D12	D13	D14	D15	Total
	Themes																
1	Attachment	✓					✓			✓		✓					26.6
2	Domestic Work	✓						✓			✓						20
3	Support		✓	✓			✓	✓		✓		✓	✓				46.6
4	Love and Enjoy	✓								✓		✓					26.6
5	Treat as Maids			✓				✓	✓					✓			26.6
6	Shows Improvement				✓					✓						✓	20
7	Aggressive Behaviour				✓				✓		✓			✓			26.6
8	Helping Outside Scope of Job							✓				✓		✓			20
9	Plight of Old Parents					✓				✓							13.3

(Conrd.)

Sr. No.	Relationship with the Patient	D1	D2	D3	D4	D5	D6	D7	D8	D9	D10	D11	D12	D13	D14	D15	Total
	Themes																
10	Depressed and Exhausted										✓					✓	13.3
11	Trust is a Major Issue											✓					6.6
12	Lack of Respect										✓			✓			13.3

*D-Document,*N- Nurse,*GDA- General Duty Assistant, U- Unmarried, *M- Married, *S- Sikh, *H- Hindu, *C- Christianity, *MU-Muslim, *Exp. – Experience

Source: Primary Data Collection.

Table 5.1.1: General Duty Assistant (GDA) (Relationship with the Patient)

Sr. No.	Relationship with the Patient	D1	D2	D3	D4	D5	D6	D7	D8	D9	D10	D11	D12	D13	D14	D15	Total
	Themes																
1	Attachment		✓	✓			✓									✓	26.6
2	Domestic Work	✓	✓			✓			✓		✓						33.3
3	Support		✓	✓	✓	✓	✓	✓		✓		✓		✓	✓	✓	73.3
4	Love and Enjoy	✓		✓						✓		✓				✓	33.3
5	Treat as Maids	✓							✓								13.3
6	Shows Improvement				✓									✓		✓	26.6
7	Aggressive Behaviour at Times	✓				✓		✓	✓	✓	✓				✓		46.6
8	Discriminative Behaviour	✓				✓											13.3
9	Helping Outside Scope of Job		✓				✓	✓				✓	✓		✓		46.6
10	Plight of Old Parents			✓													6.6
11	Depressed and Exhausted	✓														✓	13.3

(Contd.)

Sr. No.	Relationship with the Patient	D1	D2	D3	D4	D5	D6	D7	D8	D9	D10	D11	D12	D13	D14	D15	Total
	Themes																
12	Trust is Major Issue	✓											✓				13.3
13	Lack of Respect	✓							✓						✓		20
14	Feel Good after Serving Patients		✓	✓			✓					✓				✓	33.3
15	Companionship		✓	✓	✓							✓			✓		33.3

Source: Primary Data Collection.

clients; describing spending time with the client as having fun together (Franzosa *et al.*, 2019).

With regard to general duty assistants, 15 themes define their relationship, namely Attachment (26.6%), Domestic work (33.3%), Support (73.3%), Love and enjoy (46.6%), Treat as maids (13.3%), patient shows improvement (26.6%), Aggressive behaviour (46.6%), Discriminative behaviour (13.3%), Helping outside their scope of job (40%), Plight of old parents (6.6%), Depressed and exhausted (13.3%), Trust (13.3%), Lack of respect (20%), Feel good after serving patients (33.3%) and Companionship (33.3%). For a better understanding, these themes are further explained with the help of narratives as follows:

Themes	**Narratives**
Attachment (Nurses- D1, D6, D9, D11) (26.6 %) (GDAs- D2, D3, D6, D15) (26.6%) **Love and Enjoy** (Nurses—D1, D9, D11, D15) (26.6%) (GDAs—D1, D3, D9, D11,D15) (33.3%)	D1 (28/N/S/U/Exp. 2.5 years) shared "My father is a farmer, so the family income is sparse and home care provides sufficient money, to earn more we have to unwillingly work in this sector." She also described the relationship they develop with the patient. "I **love and enjoy** being with the patient. I feel it is my responsibility to look after them and avoid any adverse events but here I have to mention the nature and behaviour of male patients is much better than female patients. I took care for a patient for around 6 months. He was 33 years old and was bed-ridden as he met with an accident, *meri bahut attachment ho gayi thi* (I was very attached to the patient). Seeing him bearing the pain, I was not able to sleep. So later, I left the job as I suffered from sleepless nights. I cried a lot when I left the patient's house and still feel that pain today." D2 (25/GDA/H/U/Exp.6.5 years) opined "The patient I was looking after was suffering from brain tumor, I stayed and cared for him for about 2 years, *Ohna da mere nal bahut pyar si* (I was very **attached** to them). I took care of the patient with full dedication, as he was like a father to me. Sometimes, in anger he used to bite my thumb. Later when he passed away, I helped the family in performing the last rites. I was deeply attached to him and it was painful for me to bear his death. *Mai tut gaya tha, mera bura hal ho gaya tha,* (I was totally shattered). It had gone to the extent that whenever I felt sleepy, It felt as if the dead body is sleeping beside me. Nonetheless, I still go there to meet aunty (Patient's wife)."

(*Contd.*)

Themes	Narratives
	D11 (26/N/S/U/Exp. 3years) elaborated "Home care sector needs properly trained staff, as we caregivers spend much of our time with the patient, we tend to develop relations with the patient and their families. One gets emotionally **attached** to the patient. I want to narrate the ordeal of a female patient. She had fallen from the first floor, her brain was declared dead by the doctors, she also suffered a fracture in the leg, she was hospitalized but later the doctors told her to take home as they could not do anymore for her. I was there with the patient for about **7 months**, the family was very nice, the children used to refer to me as '*Bua*' (father's sister). One day I had to leave for home for some urgent work and the patient passed away the next morning. Next day as I came back to the family, they said *'Bache tu na jandi ta eh vi na jande'*. (If you were there with her, they would not have left us). Talking about them she says, "Because they spend much of their time by themselves, they feel lonely and thus get very attached to us." ***Aisa isiliye hai kyuki kai families unka pura dhyan nahi karti*** (This is because families don't give proper attention and care to the patient).
Support (Nurses D2, D3, D6, D7, D9, D11, D12) (46.6%) (GDAs D2, D3, D4, D5, D6, D7, D9, D11, D13, D14, D15) (73.3%) **Companionship** (GDAs D2, D3, D4, D11, D14) (33.3%)	D2 (25/GDA/H/U/Exp.6.5 years) explained another case where he took care of the male patient. It is asserted that in cases where the patient is alone, they get very much **attached** to the caretaker. This particular patient was on oxygen administration and had a clot in the brain and was suffering from Pulmonary edema (it is the medical term for abnormal fluid collection in the extravascular space (space around the cells) of the lungs. The patient was very weak and he needed to be assisted for his daily needs and these physical activities have helped the patient's health from further deteriorating. The caregiver highlights, "**I used to take the patient for walk, assist him in exercise, eating, moving, bathing, massage the patient, changing the diaper, toileting and managing the medication.** I have worked there for 9 months and the family was non-interfering". D1 (19/GDA/H/U/ Exp. 1 year) shared "**I love and enjoy** being with the patients. I feel responsible for them and take it upon us to give them the best care possible. They always only want love and affection from us, they want us to spend time with them. Initially I felt I would not be able to do home care duties, but today I feel I am made for this work. Present family that I am working with gives me lot of **love and support**. We behave the way, the patient wants.

(*Contd.*)

Themes	Narratives
	Hum unko khush karne ke liye sab kuch karege (we try to make them happy). I have developed an understanding with the patient. I just feel good being with the patients. They always appreciate my work. We caregivers are their **companions**". D3 (25/GDA/MU/M/Exp. 6 years) "We are their **companions** as the main issue is the lack of time from the **families for their old and sick parents.** I feel that we should always remember that one point of time, we would also be old and may face the same fate." He narrated a story of the patient whose family was in Canada and his son was in Sydney (Australia) and as they could not fly back to India to look after him. "The patient stayed with his old mother and brother who were rather very old to manage things, when he passed away I along with them performed the cremation and conducted all the **last rites and condolence prayer meets**".
Domestic Work (Nurses D1, D7, D10) (20%) (GDAs D1, D2,D5,D8,D10) (33.3%) **Treat as Maids** (Nurses D3, D7, D8,D13) (26.6%) (GDAs D1, D8) (13.3%)	D1 (28/N/S/U/Exp. 2.5 years) "They expect the nurses to perform household domestic duties as well. Sometimes the families insist on doing **domestic work** like washing utensils and wiping the floor. We are treated more like **maids** than staff nurses." D3 (27/N/S/U/Exp. 4years) narrated that many times working in the home care service sector she is made to feel that she is not a professional but a **maid.** She narrated "As the patient had some personal issues, he remained irritated and told me to perform many **domestic chores** like ironing of clothes." D8 (27/N/S/U/Exp. 3 years) says, "When I was working on 24 hours duty, the patient was very rude to me, I had a very bad experience at my work place, she used to **yell on me**, '*Maine bahut sehan kara hai, majboori hai*' (I have listened to her rude talks till the time I was on duty, as I am helpless). They **treated me like 'maid'**. All the house maids and the nursing staff were given same status."

(*Contd.*)

Themes	Narratives
Aggressive Behaviour (Nurses D4, D8, D10, D13) (26.6%) (GDAs D1, D5, D7, D8, D9, D10, D14) (46.6%) **Discriminative Behaviour** (GDAs D1, D5) (13.3%) **Trust is a Major Issue** (Nurses D11) (6.6 %) (GDAs D1, D12) (13.3 %)	D4 (24/N/H/U/Exp. 7 years) deliberates upon the case of a 85 year old patient, "I looked after the patient who was suffering from psychological distress, *Dande marte the mujhe* **(he used to beat me with sticks)**, even he broke his TV. I always tolerated him thinking he is childlike. *Bachche or budhe ek hi saman hote hai* (Children and eldelrly are alike). Later when it got too much, I left the job." D1 (19/GDA/H/U/Exp. 1 year) "In the last job I did, I used to be very upset. The patient used to lie on small issues. **Trust was one major issue.** *agar hamne kuch nahi bhi kara tab bhi patient jhooth bolega ki isne mere saath ase kara,* (even if we have not committed any mistake, then also patient would complain about us). We were helpless and moreover speechless as no one would believe us. Almost all the day, I was coerced to massage patient's legs and feet. I used to feel like crying. During that time, my health was affected due to the stressful conditions at work. The patients also **discriminated** against us as once I was told to serve banana to the patient, I peeled, cut and served the banana, the patient said, that he is not ready to eat it as I have touched the fruit with my bare hands, and told me to eat it. I was so disturbed by their behaviour." D11 (26/N/S/U/Exp. 3years) shared "I think it depends upon families, if they support us, definitely the patient will **support us**. As we stay at someone else place, we need to initially gain their trust, then we have to maintain a good rapport and understanding with the patients. In some patients I have observed that the patients put all their **trust in their attendants,** so much that they tell us to be with them always."
Plight of Old Parents (Nurses D5, D9) (13.3%) (GDAs D3) (6.6%)	D3 (25/GDA/MU/M/Exp. 6 years) opined "We as caregivers tend to stay with the patient, we tend to develop good understanding with the patient and also know their likes and dislikes and we also understand their positive and negative aspects. They are totally dependent upon us as the **family doesn't give them time** and secondly, in most cases their children are settled abroad and they are left behind alone. So, we take care of them like our own parents. *Sath rehte toh aap ka bahut pyar ho jata hai patient se,* (As we stay with them, we get very attached)."

(*Contd.*)

Themes	Narratives
Patient Show Improvement (Nurses D4, D9, D15) (20%) (GDAs D4, D9, D13, D15) (26.6%)	D 9 (25/N/S/U/Exp. 1 year) asserted "One gets emotionally **attached** to the patient. They consider us like their own children. I am looking after a female who is 75 years old, she is bedridden from the last 3 years. While bathing she slipped in her washroom. I prepare the **patient care plan** that includes the bathing, grooming, massage, exercise, medication, meal plan and daily routine. I really feel bad for such patients, especially the **plight of old parents** whose children have moved away in pursuit of their lives. This particular patient was fed through the naso-gastric tube, was not able to speak properly. With the love and care provided by me and uncle (her husband) **the patient has improvised and can eat on her own now."** D4 (24/N/H/U/Exp. 7years) shared "My first patient was a lady who was 62 years old, I took care for the patient for 6 months and later when she was better, out of sheer happiness, she hosted a dinner for the owners of the agency and thanked them for the care provided by me." Another patient was suffering from brain stroke and was paralysed and had even lost her speech, even the doctors were very doubtful about her health and had told the family that the patient will not recover but in 15 days of my supervision and care, the **patient's condition improved,** her physiotherapy exercises started and she was recovering from illness. She further said, "As caregivers, we are always concerned about patient's life, and tries to have a discussion with doctors on any issues. It has never happened with me that patient's life has ever crashed in my hands, fortunately, the patient's always recovers."
Depressed and Exhausted (Nurses D10, D15) (13.3%) (GDAs D1, D15) (13.3%)	D15 (22/GDA/H/U/Exp. 3 years) narrated "Sometimes the staff commits mistake as they are **frustrated** on account of working day and night. We sometimes get depressed as night duties in winters are very cold and tough." D10 (26/N/H/U/Exp. 2 years) opined "Expectations are too much in home care. They don't consider us staff, rather we are made to work in the kitchen and clean their utensils also. Once, I took care of the female patient who was suffering from dementia. She used to bite the caregivers. She lived alone as all of her family members were settled abroad, she literally lost her memory as she stayed alone. Staying for 24 hours with such patients is a pain and sometimes we feel very **depressed and exhausted**."

(*Contd.*)

Themes	Narratives
	D15 (31/N/S/M/Exp. 12 years) said "Sometimes we feel very **irritated and frustrated** in home care and want to leave this job straightaway. There is no future in home care, as we work on one patient, there is less learning opportunities as compared to learning in hospitals. Continuously **working for 24 hours makes our own life difficult and the** quality of **life get impaired.** For a period of 6 months, I stayed at one place and served them with my utmost dedication but it was all in vain. *Kisi ka kitna bhi karlo, woh apka nahi banta* (even if you give your full support and love, even then no one will treat you like their own)."
Helping Outside their Scope of Work (Nurses D7, D11, D13) (20 %) (GDAs D2, D5, D6, D7, D11, D12, D14) (46.6 %)	D13 (30/N/MU/M/Exp. 12 years) mentioned "Sometimes we get respect and they do behave as if we are their servants, there are some families who cooperate with us. In home care we have to be loyal with our profession, even when it is not acknowledged. In case of patients, we get attached to them and want to improve his/her condition. I would like to elaborate the case of female of age 72 years. She met with an accident and had a clot in the brain, and was also suffering from hypoxia (absence of enough oxygen make it to cells and tissues. She elaborated that **the family was very loving and caring, and so she never hesitated from her job Even when it was about changing patient's diaper or cleaning her up, she would do all necessary chores required."**
Feel Good after Serving (GDAs D2, D3, D6, D11, D15) (33.3 %)	D2 (25/GDA/H/U/Exp.6.5 years) shared "One gets good salary in home care. Now-a-days, patient doesn't want to be in hospital, **They prefer home care.** We have to give lot of **personal attention to the patient and It feels really good after serving the patient."**
Lack of Respect (Nurses D10, D13) (13.3 %) (GDAs (D1, D8, D14) (20 %)	D10 (26/N/H/U/Exp. 2 years) opined "Salaries are less and there is **lot of burden** on the nursing staff, as females we have lot of **workload**, the families expect us to do **domestic chores. At times, we are not paid any respect,** not even by patient. Sometimes, It feel so **frustrated** that I want to quit the job."

Overall, it was analysed from Tables 5.1 and 5.1.1 that as the respondents continue to stay with the patient they develop attachment with them, they support the elderly in many ways and they love being with them. Participants in the study loved their job, some believe in giving free service to the client's in need. There were many who faced various issues at their work place such as workplace violence is also widespread in health care settings. Violence can be in the form of verbal abuse, aggressive behaviour, lack of respect, and humiliation. Further, they elaborated that patients are largest source of violence but they are not the only one. The patients sometimes treat them as maid, expect domestic chores. Consequently, the aggressive behaviour of the patients makes the support workers depressed and exhausted. Many a times, the respondents felt hurt as they are made to feel that there is lack of respect and recognition in this profession along with job insecurity.

5.2 Relationship of the Nurses and General Duty Assistants with Patient's Family

Relationships with the family do have a positive and negative effect on the emotional health of the respondents (Nurses and GDAs). Families play a major role in patient care as the primary caregiver is always a member from the family.

Fourteen themes define their relationship with the family. The data analysis is presented and it can be seen from the data from Tables 5.2 and 5.2.1 that 33.3 per cent nurses and 46.6 per cent GDAs believed that the families they are working with are very cooperative, while 33.3 per cent nurses and 40 per cent GDAs enjoy at their work place as the families give them lot of respect and love, while 13.3 per cent nurses and 6.6 per cent GDAs feel that building trust with the families take lot of time. Moreover, 26.6 per cent nurses and GDAs respectively spoke about families treating them like their own children, and 6.6 per cent nurses and 33.3 per cent GDAs elaborated on the support they receive from families

Table 5.2: Nurses (Relationship with the Family)

Sl. No.	Relationship with the Family	D1	D2	D3	D4	D5	D6	D7	D8	D9	D10	D11	D12	D13	D14	D15	Total
	Themes																
1	Cooperative					✓	✓			✓			✓			✓	33.3
2	Domestic Work		✓	✓				✓						✓	✓		33.3
3	Treat like their Own Children								✓	✓				✓		✓	26.6
4	Respect, Love and Enjoy				✓		✓			✓			✓			✓	33.3
5	Treat as Maids		✓	✓	✓				✓			✓					33.3
6	Interference	✓							✓		✓	✓					33.3
7	Ill-Treatment		✓	✓													26.6
8	Plight of Old Patients						✓								✓		13.3

(Contd.)

Sl. No.	Relationship with the Family	D1	D2	D3	D4	D5	D6	D7	D8	D9	D10	D11	D12	D13	D14	D15	Total
	Themes																
9	Helping Outside Scope of Job						✓								✓		13.3
10	Support					✓											6.6
11	Depressed and Exhausted						✓			✓							13.3
12	Trust								✓				✓				13.3
13	No Respect	✓	✓	✓										✓	✓		33.3
14	Not Comfortable to Carry the Duties of GDAs		✓	✓											✓		20

Source: Primary Data Collection.

at their work environment. Some even reported that families are so good and they sometimes hide their mistakes from the agency supervisors.

However, 33.3 per cent nurses and GDAs respectively complained about the domestic work which is expected by the families as a part of their job, they further explained that they are treated more like maids (33.3% nurses and 20% GDAs) than a professional. While nurses reported that in hospitals the nurses are paid lot of respect but in home care, their respect is lost, which is also reported by 33.3 per cent and 20 per cent of GDAs staff.

However, the interference of families (33.3% nurses and 13.3% GDAs) was a major issue as was reported and was reflected from data, it was analyzed from in-depth interviews that in many cases the patients were critical and at the verge of death but the families did not allow technical procedures such as suctioning at that relevant point of time. 26.6 per cent of the nurses and 20 per cent GDAs reported ill-treatment such as rude behaviour, yelling on the aides, providing stale food and not letting them have sleep. At the same time, 13.3 per cent nurses and GDAs respectively felt depressed and exhausted due to the stressful working conditions and yet were helping the families in doing chores (13.3% nurses and 33.3% GDAs) which are outside their scope of job. Further, 13.3 per cent nurses and GDAs also discussed the plight of old parents who are staying alone as their families have moved on for their livelihood abroad as they believed that now a days children are not ready to take care of their parent and so they employ staff who could look after. However, in a few cases, the families are reluctant to spend money on geriatric as mentioned by 13.3 per cent GDAs. It was also reported that 20 per cent of the nurses don't feel comfortable to carry the duties of GDAs. The themes along with the narratives describing their relationship with family are as under.

Table 5.2.1: General Duty Assistant (GDA) Relationship with the Family

Sl. No.	Relationship with the Family	D1	D2	D3	D4	D5	D6	D7	D8	D9	D10	D11	D12	D13	D14	D15	Total
	Themes																
1	Cooperative		✓	✓	✓			✓				✓		✓	✓		46.6
2	Domestic Work	✓				✓			✓		✓	✓					33.3
3	Treat like their Own Children		✓					✓	✓				✓				26.6
4	Respect, Love and Enjoy		✓	✓				✓					✓	✓	✓		40
5	Treat as Maids	✓							✓		✓						20
6	Interference								✓		✓						13.3
7	Ill-Treatment	✓				✓	✓										20

(Contd.)

Sl. No.	Relationship with the Family	D1	D2	D3	D4	D5	D6	D7	D8	D9	D10	D11	D12	D13	D14	D15	Total
	Themes																
8	Plight of Old Patients/ No Time for Parents		✓								✓						13.3
9	Helping Outside Scope of Job		✓			✓	✓						✓	✓			33.3
10	Support		✓			✓				✓			✓			✓	33.3
11	Depressed and Exhausted	✓							✓								13.3
12	Trust is a Major Issue	✓															6.6
13	Lack of Respect	✓								✓	✓						20
14	Reluctant to Spend Money on Seniors	✓									✓						13.3

Source: Primary Data Collection.

Themes	Narratives
Cooperative (Nurses D5, D6, D9, D12, D15) (33.3%) (GDAs D2, D3, D4, D7, D11, D13, D14) (46.6%)	D2 (25/GDA/H/U/Exp.6.5 years) asserted, "Few families are very interfering, but there are many who **are very cooperative**. I have built a bond with all the families I have worked with, I am still called at few places because of understanding shared with the family. Once the patient I was caring got upset with his family as he was not called upon by his son on his birthday. In aggression, he got very violent and started using abusive language. I got little upset but discussed the same with his grandson. **All the family members supported me**. *Mujhe lagta hai bache nu te bajurg nu sabhalana bhot aukha hai* (It is very difficult to handle kids and the elderly). This profession requires lot of patience. I used to stay at their place and the family gave me time for my personal activities, they looked after me and insisted me to go out and have my food at time so that I feel fresh the entire day." D4(32/GDA/S/M/Exp.13 years) opined, **"If we cooperate with families, they will cooperate with us**. We should behave well with the patient and their family members." D13 (25/GDA/C/U/Exp. 5 years) said "The patient I was caring for was suffering from **dementia who was** age 85 years and he had lost his senses and used to repeat words like (somebody has stolen my 1 lakh rupees), he also had a hump in the back, and had difficulty in walking. But overall, **I had a welcoming experience with the family as they were very friendly to me."**
Treat like their Own Children (Nurses (D8, D9, D13, D15) (26.6%) (GDAs (D2, D7, D8, D12) (26.6%)	D8 (22/GDA/MU/M/Exp. 4.5 years) opined, "Generally **all treat us as their own family**, just in few cases, some patients behave violently, such as use abusive language and in few cases they tend to find ways to trouble one like making us do home chores other than patients work." D8 (27/N/S/U/Exp. 3 years) mentioned, "Families **treat us like their own children,** in one of the families that I have worked with, they were so cooperative that **they used to hide staff mistakes** always and had a cordial relationship with all of them."

(*Contd.*)

Themes	Narratives
Respect, Love and Enjoy (Nurses D4, D6, D9, D12, D15) (33.3%) (GDAs D2, D3, D7, D12, D13, D14) (40%)	D12 (28/GDA/S/M/Exp. 7 years) shared, "The present family where she is working is very good, they pay me **lot of respect** with time, I have developed good relations with the members of family. They too consider me a part of their family and even **invite me on their occasions,** they trust me so much that they hand me locker keys and ask me to **take money on my own.**" D7 (23/GDA/S/U/Exp. 4 years) GDA opined "*Family support karti hai, hame bhi apna bachcha samajte hai,* **(They support us and treat us like their own children**). Patient's family is settled in Australia and he was suffering from liver damage, uncontrolled sugar and blood pressure. I have worked with the patient for **over 3 years.** I was there with them for 24 hours and stayed there full time and only used to just go for my exams. They gave me a lot of **love and support**. Their family always gave me leave whenever needed and allowed me to go home."
Lack of Respect (Nurses D1, D2, D3, D13, D14) (33.3%) (GDAs D1, D9, D10) (20%) **Ill-Treatment** (Nurses D1, D8, D10, D11) (26.6%) (GDAs D1, D5, D6) (20%)	D1 (19/GDA/H/U/Exp. 1 year) shared "If the families are cooperative, we get time for our studies also. The last family used to scold me on almost everything, they **never supported** me on anything. In fact, if any guest arrived, I had to work for them also. Few families are extremely **discriminating and their behaviour is unjustified, so much so that they prefer people with fair skin. If I was ever on phone,** the family used to be **suspicious** and they bluntly asked me with whom I am conversing, *Isi darr se ham apni family se bahut kam baat karte the* (I used to talk very less with my family members) We just want support from their families." D1 (28/N/S/U/Exp. 2.5 years) asserted "We are valued till the time the patient is critical and as soon as there is improvement in their condition, their families **devalue us and make us feel as we are a burden on them.** As they provide us lunch, they think that we are incurring extra charges on them. Even at the time of **paying us, their attitude changes.**"

(*Contd.*)

Themes	Narratives
Family Interference (Nurses D1, D2, D3, D8, D11) (33.3%) (GDAs D8, D10) (13.3%) **Reluctant to Spend Money on Seniors** (GDAs D1, D10) (13.3%) **Support** (Nurses D5) (6.6%) (GDAs D2, D5, D9, D12, D15) (33.3%)	D10 (23/GDA/S/U/Exp. 3 years)narrated ,"Most of the families are not able to take care of the patients *(Kayi families unka pura dhayan nahi karti).* The patient I was looking after was suffering from dementia. He used to behave like a detective. I used to work from 7 am in the morning till 7 pm in the evening. By 11 in the morning, **I used to take the patient for walk, assist him in exercise, eating, moving, bathing, massage the patient, changing the diaper, using the toilet and managing their medication.** I further helped him in activities like reading daily newspaper, he liked watching old movies, and I gave him company for that and sometimes gave an ear to their life experiences. While I felt that even though I have been taking care of the patient with full zeal, the **family interferes** in patient chores, they feel we are inefficient and to feel that we don't do anything. I worked there for 2 months later aunty told that there is no improvement in the health of patient. I **feel this could be due to the fact that families are little reluctant and they don't want to spend their money on the patient**. Later, they fired me and hired a new employee with less salary and blamed me for no reason." D8 (27/N/S/U/Exp. 3 years) "**Our personal life gets impaired in this home care,** the family I last worked. They were interfering to the extent that they did not allow us to attend our phone call during our work shift. At times families instructed us on how to handle the patient, and we are not able to work independently due to their **interference.** They try to question us and expect us to remember each and every thing. In case of hospitals, all nurses are given respect and **there are seniors and doctors for our support in hospitals."** D5 (23/GDA/S/U/Exp. 3years) asserted "Families are good, they rather **support us in many ways.** We work with them with full dedication and the patient is dependent upon us. One patient I took care was suffering from brain tumor and the **behaviour of brothers in the family was very rude with the patient,** the brothers used to push him badly as there was a family dispute going on in the family, I supported the patient to the extent possible."

(*Contd.*)

Themes	Narratives
Trust (Nurses D6, D12) (13.3%) (GDA D1) (6.6%) **Helping Outside their Scope of Work** (Nurses D6, D14) (13.3%) (GDAs D2, D5, D6, D12, D13) (33.3%)	D6 (29/N/S/M/Exp. 10 years) said, "I looked after a patient (age 84 years) who had undergone a knee replacement, I was paid Rs. 20,000 for a 12-hour shift, I was very happy and contented with the behaviour of the family as I was paid lot of respect by them. I worked there for 1 year. Another patient I serviced was 69 years old and was diabetic and hyper-intensive, I stayed there for a period of one year. The family was very **cooperative;** I used to even assist the family in **preparing meals and other household chores**. In all the families I have worked with I have spent minimum 2 months with every patient. I **think establishing trust is very difficult with the family**. I have been always treated like a daughter."
Depressed and Exhausted (Nurses D7, D10) (13.3%) (GDAs D1, D8) (13.3%)	D10 (26/N/H/U/Exp. 2 years) asserted, "One patient I cared for was a girl who had met with an accident. Her family provided me food, but took a lot of work from me, my job was very tough in the night as we as caregivers are always needed to keep our eyes on the patient but there were times when if we fell sleepy the families used to humiliate a lot, so much so that they had put cameras in the room just to keep an eye on the working staff. Once I told them, that the patient is feeling nauseous her mother started shouting at me and started aspirating the patient and in this course, she injured the patient. When I told her that you have injured the patient, her mother started yelling at me and told me that you are not able to improve the condition of the patient. I was very **depressed by the behaviour of the family."** D7 (24/N/S/U/Exp. 3 years) narrated, "For more than a year, I was there with a family, but due to a sudden death in our family, I had to leave urgently, I was shocked to know that within no time, they employed another staff as my replacement. I **felt very hurt and depressed,** as I stayed at their place for more than a year and did everything, left all my work, didn't even go for any festivals. This incident made me realize that one should always just stick to their duty and should not go out of limits to do things that are not in the scope of their job, for the sake of others. Over attachment with the family will always hurt and we should not stay at one place for more than 6 months."

(*Contd.*)

Themes	Narratives
	D7 (24/N/S/U/Exp. 3 years) mentioned, "If we are on 24 hour duty, they make us feel that we are a burden on them and even the smallest of thing such as providing us with meals will be accounted for. Even if we commit the smallest mistake, we will have to listen from them. The members of the family instruct us like doctors and also continuously interfere in our clinical procedures. In home care, our personal life is totally lost. There was a time when **they actually tortured me mentally, they questioned my qualification, and I was very depressed."**
Domestic Work (Nurses D2, D3, D7, D13, D14) (33.3%) (GDAs D1, D5, D8, D10, D11) (33.3%)	D5 (23/GDA/S/U/Exp. 3 years) said "**Sometimes the families expect us to be domestic help, they ask us to wipe the floor, wash their utensils,** but I am very upfront and refuse for such chores that are beyond the scope of my job. I would rather be fulfilling my duties, and if be, find another job but will not do the duties that are not mine to perform." D11 (26/N/S/U/Exp. 3 years) shared "Some families do **treat us like maids,** while some consider us **like their own children**. If we are at patient's home for straight 12 hours, families **interfere a lot** in our clinical procedures. We have to work at the cost of our dignity in home care."
Treat as Maids (Nurses D2, D3, D7, D11, D13) (33.3%) (GDAs D1, D8, D10)(20%) **Plight of Old Parents/No Time for Patients** (Nurses D2, D3) (13.3 %) (GDAs D2, D10) (13.3 %) **Not Comfortable to Carry the Duties of GDAs** (Nurses D2, D3, D14) (20 %)	D3 (27/N/S/U/Exp. 4 years) asserted about the behaviour of the families with the staff nurses. She narrated, "Few families pay us lot of respect while the others treat us like maids. Some families even tell us to **clean the bins. Sometimes we have to tell the families that we need a GDA for carrying out other duties of the patients like bathing, dressing, changing diapers, or assisting with the commode because some families do compel us to do all the chores which are not related to our nursing profession. If we say yes to all such odd requests, we are doing that at the cost of the dignity and respect to ourselves and our profession.** There have been many times where I am made to feel that I am not a professional but a maid. The last patient I worked with had some personal issues, he remained irritated and often told me do many of the **domestic chores like ironing his clothes**. The interference by the families is utmost a big hindrance to our work. They often through different internet sites and instruct us like doctors on many issues. I am pretty experienced in my work. I feel if the family feels we are going wrong, then only they should instruct us or otherwise let us do our jobs in peace. In few families, the patient is often alone as **some families don't have time for the patient. In such cases we are their only dependence."**

From both Tables 5.2 and 5.2.1 it can be seen that the respondents who are working as nurses and GDAs are made to work outside the scope of their jobs' work, they help the families in food preparation, cleaning the utensils, wiping the floor. It was reported that because many families give them lot of love and care and in lieu of that they tend to help them in doing all the chores. It was highlighted that this was exacerbated at the time of COVID 19 and people were reluctant to employ staff from outside so they helped the family in doing all the home chores. Appreciation received from the family was considered to have a positive influence on their social and mental health as resonant with previous literature. However, disrespectful behaviour from the families tends to bring stress at workplace. It was also found that in addition to the client's relationship, the role of client's families and agency supervisors have a strong influence on aides' emotional state. They believed that if they receive respect and are valued for their work, then their sense of confidence, ability of work is improved thus, boosting their morale. Similar findings were also reported by Franzosa *et al.* (2019) where the authors discussed that building close and trustful relationship with the client was most important for aides' emotional well-being. Wellbeing is also influenced by their relationship with the client families and agency supervisors and the level to which they felt valued for their work.

5.3 Relationship of the Nurses and General Duty Assistants with the Agencies

Participants valued the agency supervisors for their cordial behaviour and their support and appreciation boost their confidence on the work place. Tables 5.3 and 5.3.1 show the relationship of caregivers (nurses/general duty assistants) with the agencies they work for.

Twenty two themes define nurses' relationship with the agencies while 21 themes define agencies' relationship with the general duty assistants. 46.6 per cent nurses and 13.3 per cent GDAs spoke about the support, they receive from the agencies, and also mentioned that agencies are aware of their problems and in case where the help

Table 5.3: Nurses (Relationship with the Agency)

Sl. No.	Relationship with the Agency	D1	D2	D3	D4	D5	D6	D7	D8	D9	D10	D11	D12	D13	D14	D15	Total
	Themes																
1	Support	✓				✓		✓		✓		✓	✓			✓	46.6
2	Discuss Issues	✓		✓		✓	✓			✓						✓	40
3	Trainings	✓				✓	✓			✓		✓			✓	✓	46.6
4	Misbehaviour of Staff										✓		✓	✓			20
5	Not Satisfied with Salaries			✓					✓		✓		✓	✓			33.3
6	Salaries are Given Late				✓						✓		✓	✓			26.6
7	Keep Commission/ Zeal for Money		✓	✓	✓		✓	✓	✓		✓		✓	✓			60
8	Deduct Salaries										✓		✓	✓			20
9	No Leaves			✓	✓			✓	✓		✓	✓					40

(Contd.)

Sl. No.	Relationship with the Agency	D1	D2	D3	D4	D5	D6	D7	D8	D9	D10	D11	D12	D13	D14	D15	Total
	Themes																
10	No Extra Staff			✓	✓			✓	✓		✓	✓	✓		✓	✓	60
11	Inexperienced Staff				✓												6.6
12	No Appreciation							✓	✓		✓		✓	✓			33.3
13	No Career Growth							✓		✓				✓			20
14	No Support							✓			✓		✓	✓			26.6
15	Job Insecurity	✓						✓		✓			✓	✓			33.3
16	Send Employees to far off Places			✓							✓		✓		✓	✓	33.3
17	Keep our Documents		✓	✓			✓										20

(*Contd.*)

Sl. No.	Relationship with the Agency	D1	D2	D3	D4	D5	D6	D7	D8	D9	D10	D11	D12	D13	D14	D15	Total
	Themes																
18	Travel Allowances are Less												✓			✓	13.3
19	Provide Pick and Drop Facility			✓	✓			✓		✓	✓		✓	✓		✓	60
20	Sole Responsibility Lies with Agencies	✓	✓	✓						✓			✓		✓	✓	46.6
21	Don't give instructions	✓	✓	✓				✓			✓		✓	✓			46.6
22	No Commun-ication		✓								✓			✓			20

Source: Primary Data Collection.

Table 5.3.1: General Duty Assistant (GDA) (Relationship with the Agency)

Sl. No.	**Relationship with the Agency**	**D1**	**D2**	**D3**	**D4**	**D5**	**D6**	**D7**	**D8**	**D9**	**D10**	**D11**	**D12**	**D13**	**D14**	**D15**	**Total**
	Themes																
1	Support	✓										✓					13.3
2	Discuss Issues	✓						✓				✓			✓		26.6
3	Trainings	✓	✓							✓		✓					26.6
4	Misbehaviour of Staff		✓	✓						✓						✓	26.6
5	Not Satisfied with Salaries		✓		✓			✓		✓	✓	✓	✓				46.6
6	Salaries are Given Late		✓		✓	✓				✓	✓					✓	40
7	Keep Commission/Zeal for Money		✓	✓						✓	✓	✓		✓			40
8	Deduct Salaries		✓							✓				✓			20
9	No Leaves		✓	✓		✓	✓					✓	✓	✓		✓	53.3
10	No Extra Staff		✓	✓				✓			✓			✓			33.3
11	Inexperienced Staff									✓							6.6
12	No Appreciation			✓			✓						✓				20
13	No Career Growth										✓		✓				13.3

(Contd.)

Sl. No.	Relationship with the Agency	D1	D2	D3	D4	D5	D6	D7	D8	D9	D10	D11	D12	D13	D14	D15	Total
	Themes																
14	No Support										✓					✓	13.3
15	Job Insecurity						✓			✓							13.3
16	Send Employees to far off Places			✓				✓			✓						20
17	Keep our Documents			✓				✓	✓		✓		✓	✓	✓		46.6
18	Travel Allowances are Less			✓				✓		✓	✓			✓			33.3
19	Sole Responsibility lie with Agencies														✓		6.6
20	Insurance Coverage for the Employees			✓													6.6
21	No Communication			✓				✓			✓						20

Source: Primary Data Collection.

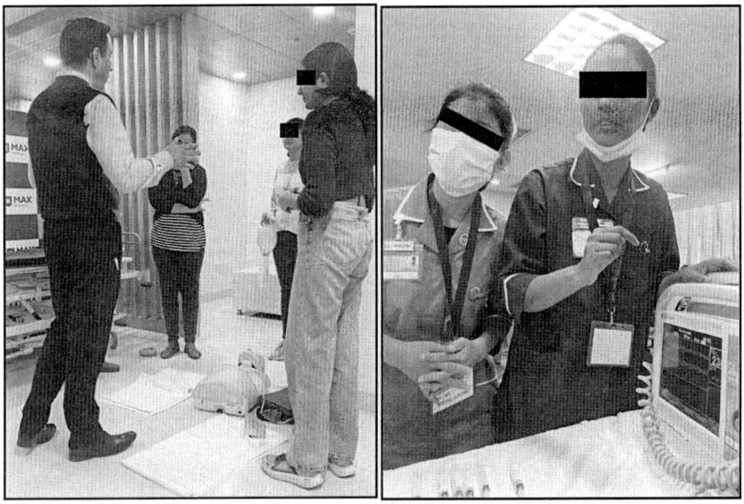

Plate 5.1: Training sessions being conducted by various agencies for training of staff

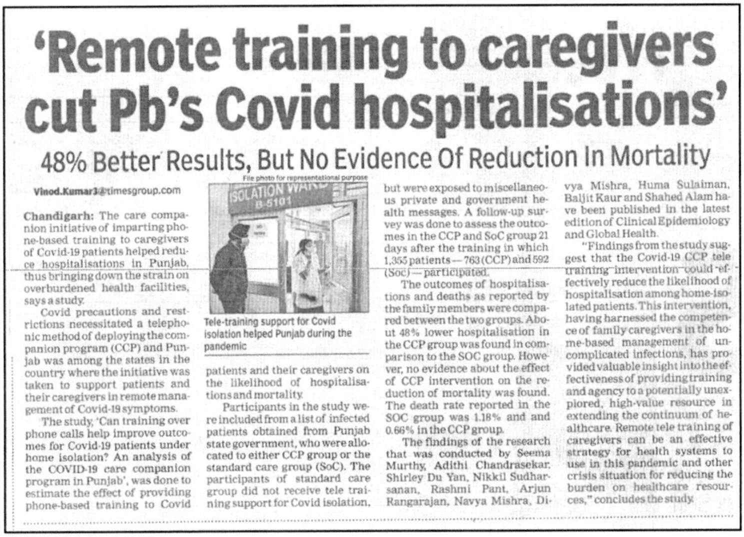

'Remote training to caregivers cut Pb's Covid hospitalisations'

48% Better Results, But No Evidence Of Reduction In Mortality

Vinod.Kumar3@timesgroup.com

Chandigarh: The care companion initiative of imparting phone-based training to caregivers of Covid-19 patients helped reduce hospitalisations in Punjab, thus bringing down the strain on overburdened health facilities, says a study.

Covid precautions and restrictions necessitated a telephonic method of deploying the companion program (CCP) and Punjab was among the states in the country where the initiative was taken to support patients and their caregivers in remote management of Covid-19 symptoms.

The study, 'Can training over phone calls help improve outcomes for Covid-19 patients under home isolation? An analysis of the COVID-19 care companion program in Punjab', was done to estimate the effect of providing phone-based training to Covid patients and their caregivers on the likelihood of hospitalisations and mortality.

File photo for representational purpose

Tele-training support for Covid isolation helped Punjab during the pandemic

Participants in the study were included from a list of infected patients obtained from Punjab state government, who were allocated to either CCP group or the standard care group (SoC). The participants of standard care group did not receive tele training support for Covid isolation, but were exposed to miscellaneous private and government health messages. A follow-up survey was done to assess the outcomes in the CCP and SoC group 21 days after the training in which 1,355 patients — 763 (CCP) and 592 (Soc) — participated.

The outcomes of hospitalisations and deaths as reported by the family members were compared between the two groups. About 48% lower hospitalisation in the CCP group was found in comparison to the SOC group. However, no evidence about the effect of CCP intervention on the reduction of mortality was found. The death rate reported in the SOC group was 1.18% and and 0.66% in the CCP group.

The findings of the research that was conducted by Seema Murthy, Adithi Chandrasekar, Shirley Du Yan, Nikkil Sudharsanan, Rashmi Pant, Arjun Rangarajan, Navya Mishra, Divya Mishra, Huma Sulaiman, Baljit Kaur and Shahed Alam have been published in the latest edition of Clinical Epidemiology and Global Health.

"Findings from the study suggest that the Covid-19 CCP tele training intervention could effectively reduce the likelihood of hospitalisation among home-isolated patients. This intervention, having harnessed the competence of family caregivers in the home-based management of uncomplicated infections, has provided valuable insight into the effectiveness of providing training and agency to a potentially unexplored, high-value resource in extending the continuum of healthcare. Remote tele training of caregivers can be an effective strategy for health systems to use in this pandemic and other crisis situation for reducing the burden on healthcare resources," concludes the study.

Plate 5.2: Remote training to caregivers helped reduce hospitalisation (Kumar, 2023)

of agencies is required their problems are heard by the agencies. While an equal number of nurses, i.e. 46.6 per cent nurses and 26.6 per cent GDAs were happy with the training sessions provided by the agencies whereas about (40% Nurses and 26.6 per cent GDAs) believed that regular meetings should be conducted to discuss their concerns regarding the safety and challenges at work place.

Kumar (2023) discussed the impact of phone-based training to Covid-19 patients and their caregivers which helped to reduce hospitalisation in Punjab thus bringing down the strain on overburdened health facilities.

Multiple issues were reported such as misbehaviour of staff (20% Nurses and 26.6 per cent GDAs), not being satisfied with salaries (33.3% Nurses and 46.6% GDAs), salaries being given late (26.6% Nurses and 40% GDAs), deduction in salaries (20% by both), keeping commission (60% Nurses and 40% GDAs), staff being inexperienced (6.6% by both), and no career growth (20% nurses and 13.3% GDAs). While most of them discussed that the home care agencies have indeed turned this noble profession caring for the sick into a business.

Some agencies solicit responsibility towards their staff as has been reported by 46.6 per cent nurses and 6.6 per cent GDAs. On the contrary, there were multiple issues faced by nurses and GDAs in home care too. 46.6 per cent nurses said that agencies don't give proper instructions to the clients and they have to carry duties outside their scope of job. However, 40 per cent nurses and 53.3 per cent GDAs elaborated that they are neither provided leaves by the family nor the agencies. This is due to the fact that agencies don't have extra staff (60% Nurses and 33.3% GDAs) at their hands so that they have to continuously work at some place for as long as 6 months straight without any work leaves. Also, 20 per cent nurses and GDAs each asserted that their concerns are unheard, and there is no communication with the agency coordinators. However, 6.6 per cent advocated the need for insurance coverage for the employees.

Similarly Andersson *et al.* (2017) also elaborated in their study about the importance of work place meetings and exchange of competencies as discussed by nurses working in home care in Sweden. Several nurses in the study also elaborated on inadequate planning, trainings and felt that it is solely up to them to participate in their competence development programmes and they were given limited opportunities to participate in development projects in home health care. A working environment that allows and encourages learning through trainings means a lot to employees. The development of their competencies adds to employees' health, well-being and personality development. These all factors leads to qualitative development in the organization.

Research studies have also shown that the higher the knowledge and competencies in caregivers reduces risks of health care damages to the patients and thus improved patient safety and quality of care (Smeds *et al.*, 2014).

The results analyzed show that 33.3 per cent nurses and 20 per cent GDAs mentioned that agencies don't appreciate their staff and at times they feel insecure about their jobs (33.3% Nurses and 13.3% GDAs). It was reported by 26.6 per cent nurses and 13.3 per cent GDAs that the agencies don't support them, and 20 per cent nurses and 46.6 per cent GDAs said their documents are taken away and kept by the agencies. Few staff members (33.3% Nurses and 20% GDAs) also reported they are sent to far off places and less travel allowances are given to them (13.3% Nurses and 33.3% GDAs). At their workplace, 60 per cent nurses advocated the need for pick and drop facility. George *et al.* (2017) also highlighted that the stress was also related with the agencies. Common issues highlighted in the study were busy coordinators, limited supervisions, concerns are not addressed, rushed communication, poor responses, lack of timely responses, last minute changes in the rosters, lack of appreciation and recognition, inadequate allocation for travel time, lack of power (as their opinions were not valued despite spending large amount of time with the clients). The themes along with the narratives describing their relationship with agencies are discussed further.

Themes	Narratives
Support (Nurses D1, D5, D7, D9, D11, D12, D15) (46.6%) (GDAs D1, D11) (13.3%)	D1 (19/GDA/H/U/Exp. 1 year) opined, "In case of any problem, we get a lot of **support from the agencies. We** are free to share our problems and can freely **discuss the same with their agency coordinators."** D7 (24/N/S/U/Exp. 3 years) shared, "Few agency coordinators **cooperat**e with us but I believe, it's always better to work through agencies. It's for the first time that since I am in this profession that the agency head has told us to feel free to discuss our problems. The agency coordinators also visit our work place to see to ensure that we are happy and content and if there are any issues at all. If need be, they even instruct the families about the nature of our jobs. **The agency also provides a pick and drop facility.** The present head guides the staff on doing all procedures, he is one of the best agency supervisors I have ever seen, and he has a very caring attitude towards his staff. He is dedicated towards his work and would never see his profit, rather he would clearly tell the patient's family about the exact condition of patient. In my career span, **this is for the first time I have observed that head of a company is visiting the patient's house to enquire about the patient's health**. Moreover, he is also concerned about his staff and will ask the staff about any issues or problems they are facing. However, the main problem is that families are not willing to give leaves to the staff, it is only the agency that **gives weekly off to the staff,** but families don't want to relieve the staff." D12 (26/NM/J/U/Exp. 8 years) asserted "I took care of a female patient who met with an electric shock, I was there with the patient for a **period of 1 year**. I have also looked after patients affected with paralysis and patients who were infected with bed sores. **As a nurse manager, my duty is to monitor the patient**, I am also responsible for finding a perfect caretaker/nursing staff according to the needs of the elderly. Part of our job is to ensure taking after the needs of the patients and their families, at times there are calls past midnight too. At the same time, I make sure to clearly instruct the client families that our staff will only do clinical work and no domestic chores will be carried by them."
Misbehaviour of Staff (Nurses D10, D12, D13) (20%) (GDAs D2, D3, D9, D15) (26.6%)	D2 (25/GDA/H/U/Exp. 6.5 years) elaborated on the working scenario of the agencies. "I was not satisfied with the behaviour of the staff and was not content with the salary received. I am the sole earner in my family so all responsibilities stay on my shoulders. Initially, I was paid Rs. 13,000 for 12 hours duty but as I have to pay for my food and room rent, it was not enough, so I did not prefer working for 12 hours. There were several other factors too. Whenever **one asks for leaves, the agency managers behave awkwardly.** After 15 days of job, I told them that I needed to go for some urgent work, but I was refused. They should understand that we too have our personal life. There are times, **salaries are given late to the employees."**

(*Contd.*)

Themes	Narratives
Salaries are given late (Nurses D4, D10, D12, D13) (26.6%) (GDAs D2, D4, D5, D9, D10, D15) (40%) **No Support** (Nurses D6, D10, D12, D13) (26.6%) (GDAs D10, D15) (13.3 %) **Agencies don't give Instructions** (Nurses D1, D2, D3, D7, D10, D12, D13) (46.6%) **No Communication** (Nurses D2, D10, D13) (20%) (GDAs D3, D10, D12) (20%) **Trainings** Nurses (D1, D5, D6, D9, D11, D14, D15) (46.6%) GDAs (D1, D2, D9, D11) (26.6%)	D10 (23/GDA/S/U/Exp. 3 years) shared "I had a poor experience with an agency. I was working with since last two and a half years. I feel the agency should realize the nature of the employee. In odd scenarios if the agency receives a complaint against the employee from any family, I think that the agency should call the employee and ask the whole situation rather than yelling on the employee. I have faced so much trouble with my agency and due to the behaviour of the agency coordinators, I would not pursue this job further. **The agencies don't value us, despite our hard work they would not increase our salary.** Even more, if we are facing any issue at our workplace, the agency coordinators **are not concerned with us. In case of any issues with the patient or family, we are blamed. These coordinators only focus on their work and they refrain from having communication with the staff. Thus, our concerns go unheard.** D 5 (23/GDA/S/U/Exp. 3 years) shared "The higher authorities don't give the staff their salaries on time, but they do take advance from the families. My salary was kept by the agency. Generally speaking, salaries in this profession are meagre, benefits are none. We were not allowed leaves, **even on my maternal uncle's death, the authorities displayed a very rude attitude and told me that duty is our first priority and family comes next."** D2 (25/GDA/H/U/Exp.6.5 years) asserted "In few cases, **agencies don't pay us on time**. As with the last agency, I had a bad experience. They were **very rude and never paid me on time."** D 10 (26/N/H/U/Exp. 2 years) said **"Agencies are just concerned with their duty**, I complained to the agency regarding the domestic chores being demanded from me but they did not change my duty nor did they reprimand the family. They do not take charge to bother to **instruct the families about the duties of staff."** D2 (25/GDA/H/U/Exp. 6.5 years) shared "I was given **one month training in** home care agency like how to handle kidney patients, how to check blood pressure. All staff members were given instructions on how to handle patients. We are also told that if the patient is in bad mood, how to handle that patient with love, how to behave with the patient, how to behave with the family etc. We are also given training on performing activities of daily living (like cleaning teeth, basic grooming and bathing). What are the things to be taken care with the patients with the wheel chair and so on. So later, when I got the job and was asked in the interview that whether I am comfortable in changing diapers then I said "*Seva karni hai man se karna hai*", (We feel good after serving others). We need lot of patience in this profession. As I progressed in this profession I prefer working for the 24 hours shift."

(*Contd.*)

Themes	Narratives
Zeal for Money/Keep Commission (Nurses D2, D3, D4, D6, D7, D8, D10, D12, D13) (60%) (GDAs D2, D3, D8, D10, D11, D13) (40%) **No Extra Staff** (Nurses D3, D4, D7, D8, D10, D11, D12, D14, D15) (60%) (GDAs D2, D3, D7, D10, D13) (33.3%) **No Leaves** (Nurses D3, D4, D7, D8, D10, D11) (40 %) (GDAs D2, D3, D5, D6, D11, D12, D13, D15) (53.3%) **Keep our Documents** (Nurses D2, D3, D6) (20%) (GDAs D3, D7, D8, D10, D12, D13, D14) (46.6%)	D3 (25/GDA/MUS/M/Exp. 6 years) opined, "Most of the money is kept by the agencies and their managers while all the work is carried by the staff who are underpaid. The staff is paid minimal salaries and there are barely any incentives. **Companies are exploiting us. Agencies don't have extra staff, we are not provided leaves, and they should provide us 4 holidays in a month and should have our replacement staff ready to go.** Companies are only concerned with their benefit; they don't cooperate with or listen to the staff. Once I received a call from the agency, a family who needed help were ready to pay Rs. 45,000 per month but the agency was demanding as high as Rs. 1,20,000 from the family. I feel we do lot of work and are paid very less as **most of the money is kept by the agencies."** D2 (23/N/S/U/Exp.4 years) said "The worse thing about the agencies is that **they charge hefty amount from the patients.** Suppose they took Rs. 30,000 from the patient, we would be paid just Rs. 22,000 rest goes in their pockets. When the amount paid by the client is more, they try to get lot of work extracted from us. There are multiple other problems in home care, we are not allowed to discuss our salary with the family. Few agencies don't give proper instructions to the patients' families and the staff has to work in miserable conditions. At times families misbehave with us, sometimes we are provided food at odd hours. I don't know whether our problems would end or not as **now this profession has become business."** D4 (24/N/H/M/Exp. 7 years) said, "One gets **no leave in home care** as the patient is totally dependent upon you and the agencies don't have experienced and **extra staff** at hands." D8 (22/GDA/MU/M/Exp. 4.5 years) shared "One of the **agencies kept the necessary documents of nursing staff like Aadhaar card** and other certificates with them."
Insurance Coverage for the Employees GDAs (D3) (6.6%)	D3 (25/GDA/MU/M/Exp.6 years) opined, "There should be **insurance coverage for the home care** staff because if something happens to the staff while he/she is on duty, his/her family can take avail the needed facility through the insurance coverage provided by the agencies."
Not Satisfied with the Salaries (Nurses D3, D8, D10, D12, D13) (33.3%) (GDAs D2, D4, D7, D9, D10, D11, D12) (46.6%) **No Appreciation** (Nurses D7, D8, D10, D12, D13) (33.3%) (GDAs D3, D6, D12) (20%)	D4 (32/GDA/S/M/Exp. 13 years) mentioned "In past, I have worked through an agency but now I am directly employed. They **used to pay me very less** and also, they **cut their share as commission. There was hardly any appreciation for the hard work."**

(*Contd.*)

Themes	Narratives
Send Employees to far off Places (Nurses D3, D10, D12, D14, D15) (33.3%) (GDAs D3, D7, D10) (20%)	D12 (26/NM/H/U/Exp. 8 years) narrated "Agencies send their **employees to far off places** like Himachal Pradesh, Haryana, Mumbai, Jhansi, although they do pay us extra for going outstation but it's a cumbersome job."
Deduct Salaries (Nurses D10, D12, D13) (20%) (GDAs D2, D9, D13) (20%) **Travel Allowances are Less** (Nurses D12, D15) (13.3%) (GDAs D3, D7, D9, D10, D13) (33.3 %)	D9 (26/GDA/H/U/Exp. 3 years) shared, **"They deducted Rs. 16,000 from my salary and do not** increase our salary. Even if I have taken a leave for a single day, the salary for the same was deducted by the agency staff." D13 (25/GDA/C/U/Exp. 5 years) said **"They actually eat out one's money. These agencies** usually **deduct our salaries** and **pay very less for the travel."**
Sole Responsibility with the Agencies (Nurses D1, D2, D3, D9, D12, D14, D15) (46.6%) (GDAs D14) (6.6%)	D14 (28/GDA/S/U/Exp. 6 years) opined, "I am comfortably working through the agency as I feel that our **sole responsibility lies with the agency** and one gets their salary on time. There is no job insecurity while working through the agency." D1 (28/N/S/U/Exp. 2.5 years) narrated "If one works directly in home care, the level of exploitation is much more, there is no one on your back to support you. Agencies are thus preferred but some agencies tell us to submit a blank cheque as they have a perception that the caregiver would enter into any direct or indirect negotiation with the client.
Discuss Issues (Nurses D1, D3, D5, D6, D9, D15) (40%) (GDAs D1, D7, D11, D14) (26.6 %) **Provide Pick and Drop Facility** (Nurses D3, D4, D7, D9, D10, D11, D12, D13, D15) (60%)	D3 (27/N/S/U/Exp. 4 years) opined "I have gained ample experience while working with Dabur. I know all the procedures. **Riders used to pick us and drop us as a safety** but these days the riders are also facing problems as they are not getting full payments for pick and drop. For this, I think the agencies should behave more responsibly. Every week, **they should conduct interviews with the staff and discuss their issues**. We should be **provided pick and drop facility.** We should get a minimum of Rs.1000 per day. Companies are taking Rs. 4000 per day from the patients but we are getting poor packages, we are not satisfied."
Inexperienced Staff (Nurses D4) (6.6%) (GDAs D9) (6.6%)	D4 (24/N/H/M/Exp. 7 years) shared "Now-a-days, the agencies don't have **any experienced staff**, sometimes the GDAs provided by them have no experience, they don't even know how to give oral medication to the patient. The staff recruited by them is rather **inexperienced."**

(*Contd.*)

Themes	Narratives
Job Insecurity (Nurses D2, D7, D10, D12, D13) (33.3%) (GDAs D6, D9) (13.3%) **No Career Growth** (Nurses D7, D9, D12, D13) (26.6%) (GDAs D10, D12) (13.3%)	D12 (26/NM/H/U/Exp. 8 years) opined, "Few agencies pay us respect and few don't. At times we feel **insecure about our jobs** as sometimes we are provided targets which seem infeasible and as now-a-days there are many home care agencies and only a few provide these services at reasonable prices so in this world of competition, sometimes we find it very difficult to find patients who can pay good amount as compensation for work in home care. At the same time, there is **no career growth** and agencies should also focus on the safety of nurses working in home care. Even as a nurse manager, I am paid only Rs. 17,000 for a month which is equal to what a fresher is paid. Moreover, there is lot of responsibility in home care, as we have no doctors to guide as at backend but nobody understands this."

Similarly, Banijamali *et al.* (2014) also highlighted the problems reported while working as home care were insufficient pay for the work done, inconvenient hours of work, no paid sick leaves, difficult to find replacement while sick or needed time off. Further the respondents wanted a less physically and emotional stressful job with better wages or benefits involving less travel time for commute. The other predominant reasons for leaving home care job was issues with the patient or the patient's family, inadequate health benefits, physical pain and long duty hours. They also advocated the need for health insurance for themselves, pick sick leaves, paid vacation time and to be extra paid for the holidays worked. The findings and problems reported were more or less similar to the findings of the present study.

Overall, from Tables 5.3 and 5.3.1 Researcher identified three primary relationships that are key successors of home care. Respondents highlighted the need for effective communication and interactive team meetings that are identified as necessary to discuss patient care issues and to discuss safety issues, and problems related to other behavioural, clinical or psychological concern in patient's homes. The respondents discussed multiple problem related to the role of agencies in home care (Lack of respect, appreciation and support) from the care team. Additionally, present study highlighted the negative aspects of working with agencies. Many issues were discussed by the aides like thirst for money, no interactive meetings from the agencies for their staff and no leaves provided. In many cases, aides are made to work at one place for more than six months. It was pointed out that majority of them were not happy with the working of agencies, as they believed that their issues go unheard whether it is related to their safety or any other emotional tension they may be facing. Additionally, from in-depth interviews, it was found that no health insurance benefits are provided by the agencies and the aides felt a need to have their health insurance covered in their jobs. Similarly, Morris (2009) also found that the health care coverage was an important factor for leavers as the newly employed were likely to have insurance coverage in their jobs.

5.4 Benefits and Drawbacks of Working in Home Care

Respondents were interviewed regarding the benefits they are availing in their jobs and the drawbacks they feel as a part of their jobs.

It is reflected from Tables 5.4 and 5.4.1 that 66.6 per cent nurses and 33.3 per cent GDAs felt that they are provided good salaries and seem content with their job. 46.6 per cent nurses and 53.3 per cent GDAs elaborated that working in a 24-hour shift is much more beneficial than other shifts, here, they tend to save upon rent and accommodation and gain much more experience and learn more (60% Nurses and 66.6% GDAs) as the sole responsibility of patient lie with them. Respondents in the study believe that home care profession requires a lot of attention and care on their end as they have to serve the patient whenever in need (26.6% Nurses and 13.3% GDAs). 73.3 per cent nurses and 66.6 per cent GDAs respectively from both categories reported about meagre salaries in hospitals and also spoke about the home care profession which is surrounded with multiple issues such as diminishing personal life (66.6% Nurses and 26.6% GDAs) as one spends much span of their time at a particular place (66.6% Nurses and 40% GDAs), longer duty hours (60% Nurses and 60% GDAs), not able to attend any personal events and gatherings (60% Nurses and 33.3% GDAs).

Table 5.4: Nurses (Benefits and Drawbacks)

Sl. No.	Benefits and Drawbacks	D1	D2	D3	D4	D5	D6	D7	D8	D9	D10	D11	D12	D13	D14	D15	Total
	Themes																
1	Good Salaries	✓		✓	✓	✓	✓	✓	✓			✓			✓	✓	66.6
2	Save upon Room Rent and Accommodation	✓	✓	✓	✓		✓	✓							✓		46.6
3	One tends to Learn a Lot	✓	✓		✓	✓		✓		✓				✓	✓	✓	60%
4	Serve the Needy								✓	✓			✓			✓	26.6
5	Handle Patients Independently		✓						✓				✓	✓			26.6
6	Salaries are Meager in Hospitals	✓	✓		✓	✓		✓	✓	✓	✓	✓	✓			✓	73.3
7	Profession is Tough	✓	✓	✓	✓		✓	✓	✓		✓	✓	✓	✓			73.3
8	Personal Life is Impaired/ Finished		✓	✓	✓		✓	✓		✓	✓	✓	✓	✓			66.6
9	Worried about Future		✓	✓		✓	✓			✓	✓	✓	✓	✓			60
10	Long Duty Hours	✓	✓	✓	✓	✓		✓	✓		✓				✓	✓	60
11	Frustrated and Depressed			✓			✓	✓		✓			✓	✓			40
12	Health Issue			✓					✓			✓					20
13	Work Load			✓				✓	✓	✓	✓	✓	✓	✓	✓		60
14	Not Attended any Family Gathering		✓	✓				✓		✓	✓	✓	✓	✓		✓	60

(*Contd.*)

Sl. No.	Benefits and Drawbacks	D1	D2	D3	D4	D5	D6	D7	D8	D9	D10	D11	D12	D13	D14	D15	Total
	Themes																
15	Stay at one place for Longer Time		✓	✓				✓	✓	✓	✓	✓	✓	✓		✓	66.6
16	Sleeping Sickness	✓	✓	✓				✓		✓	✓		✓	✓			53.3
17	Unwillingly has to Work in Home care	✓	✓	✓			✓	✓	✓	✓	✓		✓	✓		✓	73.3
18	Patient Prefer to Stay at Home		✓	✓				✓		✓	✓		✓	✓		✓	53.3

Source: Primary Data Collection.

With so many issues, 73.3 per cent nurses and 26.6 per cent GDAs felt that this profession is very tough. While 73.3 per cent nurses and 46.6 per cent GDAs are not willingly to work in home care. Incredibly, respondents face problems of sleeping sickness (53.3% Nurses and 33.3% GDAs) as reported by many of them, it is difficult for them to sleep at anyone place but they are bound as patients' needs 24 hours monitoring and care.

Similarly, Flojt *et al.* (2014) also discussed that nurses are responsible for seriously ill patient, new treatments and handling of medical equipments. Research studies indicated that heavy work load make it difficult for nurses to update themselves on new technologies, knowledge and research to improve the quality nursing care (Josefsson, 2012; Josefsson and Peltonen, 2015). Knowledge can be described as understanding the ways to handle patients or different situations (Granberg, 2014). Studies also show that nurses experience themselves as having greater responsibility towards the patients (Josefsson and Peltonen, 2015).

Health issue was also reported by 20 per cent respondents in each category and, as there is lot of work load as was reported by 60 per cent nurses and 26.6 per cent GDAs. However, despite of so many issues, they are able to handle patients independently (26.6% Nurses, and 46.6% GDAs) as they have learnt a lot working in this home care profession. Safety issue was reported by 13.3 per cent GDAs respondents. However yet, 53.3 per cent nurses and 33.3 per cent GDAs felt that patients prefer to be at their home, in the environment which is free from infections and where their near ones are always around them. Studies have indicated that home care workers have a purpose hidden in their jobs of helping people, feel good about the mission of serving the people and appreciate the variety and flexibility in their Job (Eustis *et al.*, 1993; Feldman, 1997).

Studies undertaken by Benjamin and Matthias (2004) examined various reasons on recruiting and retaining personal care assistants in home care. It is also an evident fact that wages are low, while the benefits are poor or non-existent and the hours are often long and inconsistent (Kemper *et al.*, 2008; Morris, 2009). Workers also highlighted the challenges they face in home care (low wages,

Table 5.4.1: General Duty Assistants (Benefit and Drawbacks)

Sl. No.	Benefits and Drawbacks	D1	D2	D3	D4	D5	D6	D7	D8	D9	D10	D11	D12	D13	D14	D15	Total
	Themes																
1	Good Salaries	✓		✓			✓								✓	✓	33.3
2	Save upon Room Rent and Accommodation						✓	✓	✓	✓		✓	✓	✓	✓		53.3
3	One tends to Learn a Lot	✓	✓		✓	✓	✓	✓	✓	✓		✓	✓				66.6
4	Serve the Needy		✓	✓													13.3
5	Handle Patients Independently	✓			✓				✓	✓				✓	✓	✓	46.6
6	Salaries are Meagre in Hospitals	✓	✓	✓	✓	✓			✓	✓	✓	✓		✓			66.6
7	Profession is Tough		✓	✓	✓										✓		26.6
8	Personal Life is Impaired/ Finished	✓					✓	✓				✓					26.6
9	Work Load	✓					✓				✓	✓					26.6
10	Long Duty Hours	✓	✓	✓	✓			✓			✓	✓		✓			60
11	Frustrated and Depressed			✓		✓											13.3
12	Safety Issue								✓					✓			13.3
13	Perform Nursing Procedures		✓		✓		✓		✓						✓		33.3
14	Health Issue		✓	✓	✓												20

(*Contd.*)

Sl. No.	Benefits and Drawbacks	D1	D2	D3	D4	D5	D6	D7	D8	D9	D10	D11	D12	D13	D14	D15	Total
	Themes																
15	Worried about Future	✓	✓	✓	✓					✓	✓			✓			46.6
16	Not Attended any Family Function		✓				✓	✓		✓				✓		✓	33.3
17	Stay at one place for Longer Time		✓	✓		✓	✓		✓								40
18	Sleeping Sickness		✓		✓		✓		✓	✓	✓		✓				33.3
19	Unwillingly has to Work in Home Care		✓		✓		✓	✓	✓		✓						46.6
20	Patient prefer to Stay at Home			✓	✓	✓		✓								✓	33.3

Source: Primary Data Collection.

job insecurity, lack of respect, inconsistent hours, benefits and recognition) (Ashley *et al.*, 2010). Past research had also highlighted the poor working conditions; work overload, inadequate training and lack of opportunity for advancement were also related to retention of staff (Brannon *et al.*, 2007; Jorgensen *et al.*, 2009). The respondents in the present study also identified the positive and negatives aspects of working in home health care.

Henceforth, the respondents seem worried about their future (60% Nurses and 46.6% GDAs) and feel depressed and exhausted (40% Nurses and 13.3% GDAs) due to their workload. Nevertheless, 33.3 per cent GDAs are able to perform nursing procedures. The following themes were identified and the narratives concerning them describing the benefits and drawbacks of working in home care are described further.

Themes	Narratives
Good Salaries Nurses (D1, D3, D4, D5, D6, D7, D8, D11, D14, D15) (66.6%) GDAs (D1, D3, D6, D14, D15) (33.3%) **One tends to Learn a Lot** Nurses (D1, D2, D4, D5, D7, D9, D13, D14, D15) (60%) GDAs (D1, D2, D4, D5, D6, D7, D8, D9, D11, D12) (66.6%) **Independently Handle Patients** Nurses (D2, D8, D12, D13) (26.6%) GDAs (D1, D4, D8, D9, D13, D14, D15) (46.6%) **Save upon Rent** Nurses (D1, D2, D3, D4, D6, D7, D14) (46.6%) GDAs (D6, D7, D8, D9, D11, D12, D13, D14) (53.3%)	D1 (19/GDA/H/U/Exp. 1 year) opined, "The benefit of working in home care is that we are **earning for ourselves**, we can study on our own and are earning good amount of money, along with that one tends to **save also and becomes independent**. At times, I do feel tense about my future but also feel that this profession has enriched me and I have gained **good amount of knowledge** and God forbid if in case something happens at my place, **I would be able to handle patients."** D4 (32/GDA/S/M/Exp.13 years) shared, "I have gained **lot of experience.** Till date this journey has been beautiful. I have **learned a lot and** even being a GDA, I was able to perform all nursing procedures." D14 (28/GDA/S/U/Exp. 6 years) narrated, "One gets **good salary** in home care. There are few benefits and drawbacks of working in home health care, *saare paise bachde hai, khana, peena, rehna, na koi room rent dena hota* (We tend to **save upon our money as food, accommodation** all is provided by the patient)." D8 (22/GDA/MU/M/Exp. 4.5 years) narrated, "Salaries are good in home care and I am now running my own agency, I have **learned a lot** as it is a new learning every day. I can **independently handle patients with confidence**. I am able to save **good sum.** Currently, I am earning Rs. 40,000 monthly working for a patient in a 24 hour shift."

(*Contd.*)

Themes	Narratives
	D7 (23/GDA/S/U/Exp. 4 years) opined, "We are able to save for themselves. One has the **sole responsibility of caring for the patient because they gain a lot of experience** in home care. One has a lot of work on but one has to take care of themselves."
Personal Life Impaired Nurses (D2, D3, D4, D6, D7, D9, D10, D11, D12, D13) (66.6%) GDAs (D1, D6, D7, D10) (26.6%) **Work Load** Nurses (D3, D7, D8, D9, D10, D11, D12, D13, D14) (60%) GDAs (D1, D6, D10, D11) (26.6%)	D4 24/N/H/M/Exp. 7 years) discussed, "**Our life is bound** in home care, biggest loss that we suffer is that we have stay at somebody's place for 24 hours. Some families keep us so busy that they never provide you time for yourself and we are not able to live your own life. In 24 hours shift, as one has to stay at patient's home, **one has no life of their own, eat the way they want, sleep the way as per the family's schedule.** Eventually, we have to do all chores according to the wishes of the family. It has been 8 months, since I have been home because n**o leaves are allowed."** D1026/N/S/U/Exp. 2 years) elaborated, **"One loses their personal life in home care, no privacy, no space and you cannot even talk freely**. One has to forget their own family and cannot give our view point (*Hum apna sub kuch bhool jate hai, apna view point nahi de sakte*). **There are long shift hours and no leaves.**"
Sleeping Sickness Nurses (D1, D2, D3, D7, D9, D10, D12, D13) (53.3%) GDAs (D2, D3, D5, D6, D8) (33.3%) **Worried about Future** Nurses (D2, D3, D5, D6, D9, D10, D11, D12, D13) (60%) GDAs (D1, D2, D3, D4, D5, D9, D10, D13) (46.6%) **Not Attended any Family Gathering** Nurses (D2, D3, D7, D9, D10, D11, D12, D13, D15) (60%) GDAs (D1, D2, D4, D5, D6) (33.3%)	D2 (23/N/S/U/Exp.4years) said, "The negative aspects of working in home care are firstly **we don't get sufficient sleep (*Raat ko neend nahi puri hoti*).** I would hardly get to sleep by 11pm, then would wake up at 1 am, and then again at 3 am. The patient I am taking care of is 82 years old, having psychiatric disorders. I need to reposition the patient after every 2 hours and feed them with water. Secondly, I **am not allowed any leaves**, sometimes I have to **continuously work at some place for 6 months without any leaves.** Neither we are provided leave by the agency and nor by the family, there have been times where I have not attended any family events because of my job. **Personal life gets totally impaired**, thirdly, in home care we just work on a single patient one at a time, while in the hospital we deal with multiple patients so we don't gain as much knowledge and experience but it is also a fact that we are endowed with more responsibility in home care. There is also a lot of uncertainty **about our future. The salaries**

(*Contd.*)

Themes	Narratives
Salaries in Hospitals are meagre Nurses (D1, D2, D4, D5, D7, D8, D9, D10, D11, D12, D15) (73.3%) GDAs (D1, D2, D3, D4, D5, D8, D9, D10, D11) (66.6%) **Long Duty Hours** Nurses (D1, D2, D3, D4, D5, D7, D8, D10, D14, D15) (60%) GDAs (D1, D2, D3, D4, D7, D10, D11, D13) (53.3%)	**in hospitals are meagre**, but due to low salaries in this sector we are forced to work in home care, the only good side of this profession is that the patient would always remembers us." D3 (27/N/S/U/Exp. 4 years) reasoned, "The negative aspects of working in home care are that there are **long duty hours and personal life gets impaired** in this kind of job as one has no time for themselves even on important occasions like *karwa Chauth.*" Further grieving upon; she said, "I do not get time to talk with loved ones as I am on 12 hours shift duty. We **lose our personal life in home care** as we are not allowed leaves in this job, sometimes, it gets very **irritating and frustrating.** There are thoughts sometimes to leave this job straightaway."
Serve the Needy Nurses (D8, D9, D12, D15) (26.6%) GDAs (D2, D3) (13.3 %) **Patient prefers to Stay at Home** Nurses (D2, D3,D7, D9, D10, D12, D13, D15) (53.3%) GDAs (D3, D4, D5, D7, D15) (33.3%)	D15 (31/N/S/M/Exp. 12 years) shared, "Home care is better, we tend to help the families in taking care of their family members who are suffering from so many problems but it is a certain fact that more involvement of family members, more there is demand for care. We want to **serve the needy and always pray for their good health. The patients also always prefer to stay at home with their loved ones."** D9 (25/N/S/U/Exp. 1 year) spoke, "One has the **sole responsibility of looking after the patient in home care**, one tends to learn a lot as it is a new learning every day".
Health Issue Nurses (D3, D8, D11) (20%) GDAs (D2, D3, D4) 20%	D11 (26/N/S/U/Exp. 3 years) mentioned "Few families don't pay you respect and we are ill-treated. There is hardly any time for our own family and hardly any leaves we get. **Personal life is absent and social circle diminishes**. Because we stay at one place for a longer period, we have to leave everything behind. I have not purchased clothes from the last 4 months because I think I don't get to go out, I don't want to shop. Some families are very interfering, once I **had a health issue (migraine) staying at one family's place. I have not attended any festival from the last 1 year**. In hospitals, there are fixed working hours but in home care we lose our reputation in home care, as we perform all kinds of jobs."

(*Contd.*)

Themes	Narratives
	D3 25/GDA/MU/M/Exp. 6 years) elaborated, **"Once I got mentally upset** as I used to do night duty and in the mornings. I looked after my baby because my wife had to go to work. Thus, **due to lack of sleep, I got mentally upset.** I had to consult a doctor who instructed me to have sleep for 8 hours strictly. **So now, I try to work during daytime."**
Profession is very Tough Nurses (D1, D2. D3, D4, D6, D7, D8, D10, D11, D12, D13) (73.3%) GDAs (D2, D3, D4, D14) (26.6%)	D3 (25/GDA/MUS/M/Exp. 6 years) asserted, "*Ghar walo se door ho jate hai* (In this job we get away from our family). M**y wife was working during the daytime and I used to work at night, and family time is lost because we don't get to see each other** due to our duties, so much so we don't get time to discuss even important issues of our family. Duty is important but I think family is equally important. We are earning for our family. So even our job is of no use if family life is not there." D2 (23/N/S/U/Exp. 4 years) narrated, **"This profession is very tough**. No one wants to work at someone else place but *(majboori hai, neend bhi nahi ati kisi ke ghar par)*. In compulsion and to fulfil family needs, one has to work, even **we don't get sleep at someone place."** D2 (25/GDA/H/U/Exp. 6.5 years) "The adverse effect is **we can only do this job, till we have strength in our body.** Now, I am planning to get married and cannot work for 24 hours shift as I need to give time to my family. Moreover, I would like to see my kids growing, as I would like to see my kids growing up. *(Jis bande ne apne bachae nu wade hunde nahi dekhye ohne ki dekhye)."* D4 (32/GDA/S/M/Exp. 13 years) **opined, "One has to do all the work by himself, has to prepare food for ourselves, have to wash your clothes along with the duties so there is no rest, even the 12hour shift is hectic**. Secondly, on 24 hour shift one has to stay away from their family and do not get time to take care of themselves."
Stay at one place for more than 6 Months Nurses (D2, D3, D7, D8, D9, D10, D11, D12, D13, D15) (66.6%)	D9 (25/N/S/U/Exp. 3 years) elaborated,"We get to learn more working in hospitals. **Life gets tough and time bound** '*kabhi kabhi ghumne ka maan karta hai*' **(Sometimes one feels like going out) there is lack of proper sleep.** We have to listen to the family's taunts all the time, **sometimes it gets difficult to stay with them for longer time."** D9 (26/GDA/H/U/Exp. 3 years) mentioned, "I took care of the female patient who is 95 years old with whom I have stayed for over 7 **months.** She was suffering from multiple diseases and bed

(Contd.)

Themes	Narratives
GDAs (D2, D6, D7,D9, D13, D15) (40%) **Frustrated and Depressed** Nurses (D3, D6, D7, D9, D12, D13) (40%) GDAs (D3, D5) (13.3%)	sores. I used to do dressing for the bed sores in the hip area. I even used to do suturing for the patient. The patient has recovered from her illness. Once I also took care of a patient, who had undergone buttock surgery. I **used to dress her wounds and in one month, she was able to sit."** D5 (23/GDA/S/U/Exp. 3years) said, "The negative aspects of working in home care is we have to stay away from our family, life gets tough. We can't go anywhere and have to stay at patient's home for a longer durations. We sometimes feel **depressed and exhausted."**
Safety Issue Nurses (D3) (6.6%) GDAs (D8, D13) (13.3%)	D8 (22/GDA/MU/M/Exp. 4.5 years), asserted "There are no long-term benefits in this job, one cannot pursue it **after their marriage as 24 hour shift pattern is not possible after marriage.** We have to leave our personal life behind, there is hardly any time to eat also. **Safety issue is also persistently there."**
Perform Nursing Procedures GDAs (D2, D4, D6, D8, D14) (33.3%)	D14 (28/N/U/Exp. 6 years) elaborated "One gets a handsome amount in home care as I was paid Rs. 45,000 for a 24 shift. It is also a fact that one gets to learn a lot. Even as a GDA, **I am equipped with the knowledge of all nursing procedures."**
Unwilling one has to Work in Home care Nurses (D1, D2, D3, D6, D7, D8, D9, D10, D12, D13, D15) (73.3%) GDAs (D2, D4, D6, D8, D9, D10, D12) (46.6%)	D7 (30/N/S/U/Exp. 12 years) opined, "We are paid less salaries in hospitals approximately Rs. 8,000 month. Due to lack of other options, one has to work in home care **unwillingly**. Because of working for a 24 hours shift, one has to stay continuously at patient's place, salaries are less and there is increased work load. Our life seems finished and there is no time. If one gets good salaries in hospital, **no one would want to work in home care**. This job is very tough, I am married and I have to do all the domestic chores at home too, and if in need **I take a leave then my salary gets deducted."**

Similarly, Ashley *et al.* (2010) also described the reasons given by home care workers of identifying their job as rewarding using terms such as satisfaction, gratification or pleasure. They also expressed the importance of developing relationships with the clients, valuing the time spent with the clients. Home care assistants elaborated the value of being able to help others, love for their job, helping the client out the bed, preparing meals, and being energized through their work in home care. The results found in the present study were also consistent with the study conducted by Franzosa *et al.* (2019). In the study building close relationship with the client was central to respondent's emotional well-being, which was also influenced by their relationship with the client's families and agencies. Moreover, being valued for their work tend to increase their confidence. However, aides require more communication and support from the client families and agency supervisors.

Simon-Rusinowitz *et al.* (2010) conducted a three state study and found that the workers who are directly employed through agencies were more satisfied and avail benefits such as housing, food, transportation and other benefits.

George *et al.* (2017) study explored the perception of aged care support workers and how their health was influenced by their job. It was examined that 90 per cent of them worked part-time with average 20 hours per work, with comparison to the present study, the respondents in the present study tend to work for 12 hour or 24 hour shifts with working hours limited to 8 hours per shift, so the average working hours are 40 hours per week which is double as compared to the study. Further, it was found that support work had a contradictory effect on the aides' health. On one hand, they spoke about the love they had for their work which fueled their sense of well-being while overwhelmingly, they spoke about the stress, pain and fatigue at work place impacting on their health. A similar juxtaposition which was offered by the physicality of the work as the work kept them physically fit.

In the present study too, respondents feel that this profession help them to remain physically fit and but are seemingly depressed, exhausted and stressed due to the behaviour of the patients and their families. One on hand the respondents expressed that good training and support from the agencies also boosted their morale but it was also reported by some that the lack of support from the agencies left them feel anxious, undervalued and stressed. The present study tends to understand the emotional experiences of the home care

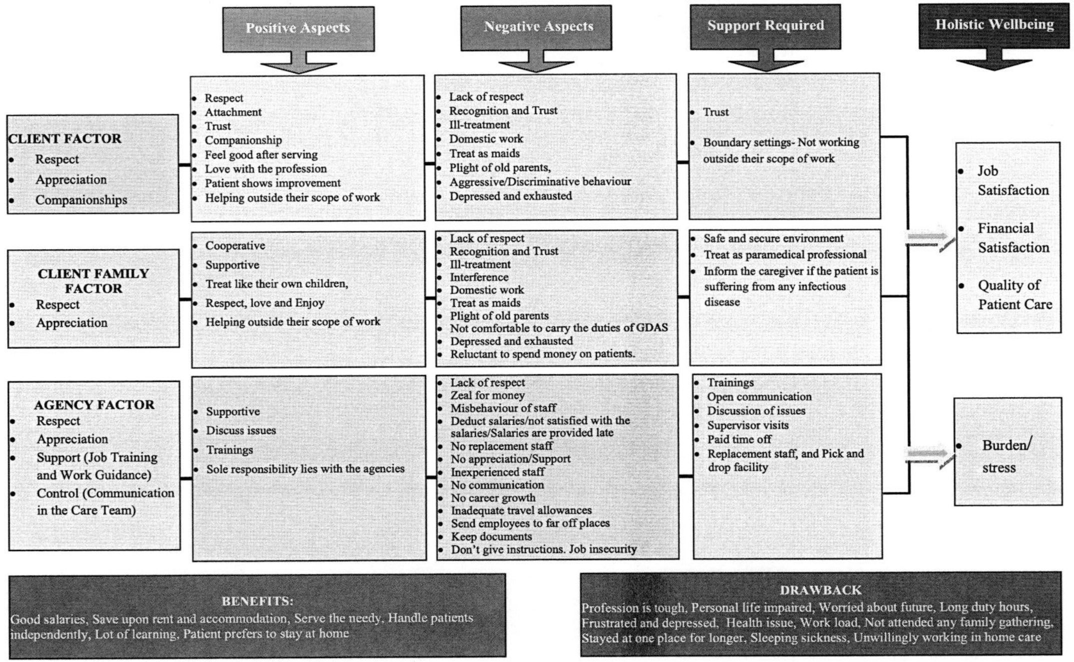

Fig. 5.1: Job Experiences and Challenges of Home Care Workers in Tricity (Chandigarh, Mohali, Panchkula)

workers and the underlying conditions under which they perform their duties and how these workers are currently managing their emotional state and what support they require from the clients, their family members and agencies.

Through an in-depth information from the respondents, the researcher came with a detailed model where in the overall factors affecting home health care workers holistic well-being was highlighted. The researcher also elaborated on the benefits and drawbacks through the analysis.

To summarize, several themes were generated such as attachment, serving the needy, families treating them like their children and so on what primarily motivated them to carry on the work, deriving a sense of satisfaction while making difference in the lives of clients, flexibility of the job, gave them valuable time to look after their own family which has a positive impact on their mental health and holistic well-being. Conversely, stress was a dominating factor which was identified among all participants. Despite of the work been officially deemed unskilled especially in case of general duty assistants, almost all the participants discussed about the exhaustive demands their job placed on them, expectations of the clients vary considerably, requiring different approaches of doing work placing additional strain on them. Further, deterioration of the client's health was distressing to the caregiver. However, majority of the participants discussed about the expectations of the client's families regarding the domestic chores which are not a part of their deal and adjustments made by the aides like working overtime and beyond what were stated in the support plan. These staff workers are also considered responsible for medications, the management pushed them to do things they are not qualified for as in many cases the general duty assistants perform nursing procedures because the client families are not willing to spend extra money on their patients and this responsibility added to the additional mental stress.

Goerge *et al.* (2017) has produced similar results where it was stated work environment contributed to stress, which affected their physical and mental health. Some clients' houses were also described as 'filthy', 'smelly' and 'unclean' that could add to this stress. Several home care aides expressed frustration due to inadequate benefits and pay by the limited ability for promotions. Lack of appreciation in home care was also highlighted. Similarly, in the same way, in the present study the results highlighted there is lack of appreciation, lack of benefits, promotions, inappropriate working schedules, long shift hours, working without leaves and multiple issues affected their mental health. They felt exhausted and depressed due to the stressful and unvalued work scenario.

Overall, it is established, the client's, their families and agencies play a major role in governing the mental, social and physical challenges faced by nurses and general duty assistants in home care. It is very important to understand their mental situations, so that they could be provided an environment which is comfortable for them to work in. The agencies should also understand their needs and the scenario where they should be provided apt leaves so there is no frustration of continuously working at one place could harm their mental health that affects their work. It is to be notably brought to light that the home care providers are going extra mile to work for the clients and thus it is the duty of the client's families and agencies to consider the needs and requirements of the caregivers and provide them a safe, healthy environment with absolutely no stress at work place.

6

Patient Demographics and their Underlying Challenges

To care for those who cared for us is one of the greatest accomplishments.

The elderly in India is a disadvantageous group as compared to the elderly from other countries. These strata of the population have special needs and peculiar health care requirements which are better dealt with home care system of caregiving. It is highlighted that at least one in seven elder lies has a functional limitation where the female elderly population is at a greater risk than the male population. Changing family landscapes have led to a change in the situation of the elderly in the country. The preference for nuclear families and the declining joint family value system have affected the elderly to the extent that they have been deprived of basic care in old age (Singh, 2017). The economic insecurity has further worsened the situation. Maples have used the term 'Silver Tsunami' to define this aging population in America.

National sample survey (2004) data on chronic profile of elderly in India is alarming. The prevalence of diseases such as whooping cough (31%), urinary problems (15%), diabetes (12%), hypertension (12%), cancer (11%), joint problems and ulcers (9%)

etc., are reflective of the state of destitution the elderly of the country are in. A home-based care approach for such geriatric patients is thus of utmost importance and need of the hour. The Ministry of Health and Family Welfare launched a national programme for the health care of the elderly (NPHCE) in 2011 to address the needs of the elderly in India, which too acknowledges that there is a lack of home-based care and no insurance for the elderly in India.

The state of geriatric care is still at a very nascent stage in India where the population out numbers the health care service providers. Although there has been an entry of home health care in both private and public sectors in India, it is still in its early years of conception and is a growing industry.

The study tends to elaborate on the in-depth data about the medical history of the patient. The researcher examined the home setting of the patient and additional information such as whether the respondent is suffering from any infectious disease (HIV/HBC/HVC/TB) was collected too. The responsibilities which were taken care by the patients and their families were further analyzed as well. Data regarding the length of engagement, i.e. the duration of time, the caregiver services were needed by the client, number of health care personnel required, and caregiver work shift pattern preferred was gathered simultaneously. Additionally, the clients were interviewed regarding the problems faced by the patients and their family members with respect to caregiving and nursing services provided at home and if there were any improvement in the condition of patients who received home care services at home.

6.1 Demographic Profile of the Patients

The primary caregivers for the patients were interviewed to know the demographic profile of the patients. Further, the families were interviewed on information such as their age, gender, marital status, and religion of the respondent.

To know the socio-economic status of the respondents. The fifth objective focused on studying the demographic profile of the patients. The family caregivers and patients were asked to provide information on the variables such as their age, address, gender, caste, marital status and religion. Further questions were asked such ascurrent residence of the patients, who is their primary caregiver, diseases they are suffering, home setting of the patient, i.e. whether the patient is staying alone or with spouse or other family members. Investigation on whether the patient is suffering from any infectious disease, and if personal protective equipment is being provided to the caregiver was also done.

6.2 Education of the Patient

The scoring is calculated on the basis for the education of the patient. Data on the education was analyzed to understand the socio-economic status of respondents. Maximum level of education attained by the respondents was considered.

With regard to the education of the patients (Fig. 6.1), it was found that the majority of the co-participants or respondents were postgraduates (27.5%), while 22.5 per cent were graduates followed by an equal number of them, i.e. 12.5 per cent were intermediates, middle school passed, and were illiterates respectively.

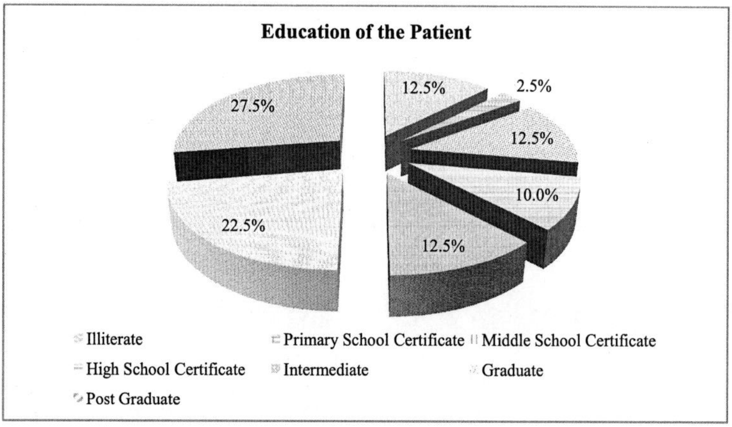

Fig. 6.1: Education of the Patient.
Source: Primary Data Collection.

6.3 Occupation of the Respondents

The occupation refers to the profession of the patient. Scoring of the occupation is from unemployed to legislators, senior officials and managers. From the Table, it can be seen that the occupation category is grouped into ten categories that are as follows.

Unemployed; elementary occupation; plant and machine operators; craft and related trade workers; skilled agriculture and fishery workers; skilled workers and shop and market sales workers; clerks; technicians and associate professionals; professional and legislators, senior officials and managers.

Table 6.1: Occupation of the Patients

Occupation of the Patients	Frequency	Per cent	Valid Per cent
Unemployed	20	50.0	50.0
Craft and Related Trade Workers	1	2.5	2.5
Clerks	1	2.5	2.5
Technical and Associate Professionals	4	10.0	10.0
Professionals	4	10.0	10.0
Legislators, Senior Officials and Managers	10	25.0	25.0
Total	**40**	**100.0**	**100.0**

Source: Primary Data Collection.

Table 6.1 presents data on the occupation of the patients. It was analyzed that majority of the respondents (50%) were unemployed, followed by 25 per cent of them who fell in the category of legislators, senior officials and managers, 10 per cent of respondents were retired professionals from various fields such as army, navy and military services and 10 per cent of them were into teaching that is considered under technical and associate professionals. It can be seen that 2.5 per cent were in the semi-skilled category job that requires some training and crafts and a few of them were into tailoring business and equal percentage of them, i.e. 2.5 per cent were into clerical jobs, they are employed as junior school teachers, junior administrators and junior medical practitioners.

6.4 Family Income per Month

Family income is the income to be assessed as total family income (per month) and not the per capita income.

Table 6.2: Family Income of the Patients

Family Income (Rs.)	Frequency	Per cent	Valid Per cent
46,129–61,662	2	5.0	5.0
61,663–1,23,321	1	2.5	2.5
≥ 1,23,322	37	92.5	92.5
Total	**40**	**100.0**	**100.0**

Source: Primary Data Collection.

As evident from Table 6.2 that for a majority of the respondents (92.5%) family income was above Rs. 1,23,322 per month, while for about 5 per cent of the respondent's family income was up to Rs. 61,662 respectively.

6.5 State-wise Distribution of the Respondents

Respondents in the present study belonged to different States of India. To see whether this variable has an effect on their socio-economic status, the respondents were asked about what states they come from.

Table 6.3: State-wise Distribution of the Patients

State-wise Distribution	Frequency	Percent	Valid Percent
Chandigarh	15	37.5	37.5
Mohali	20	50.0	50.0
Panchkula	5	12.5	12.5
Total	**40**	**100.0**	**100.0**

Source: Primary Data Collection.

Data from Table 6.3 show that 50 per cent of the respondents belonged to S.A.S. Nagar. While 37.5 per cent were residents of Chandigarh and 12.5 per cent were residents of Panchkula respectively.

6.6 Age Group of the Respondents

Data on age group was collected to further analyze the age group of the respondents.

Table 6.4: Age Group of the Respondents

Age Group	Frequency	Per cent	Valid Per cent
61-70	11	27.5	27.5
71-80	11	27.5	27.5
>80	18	45.0	45.0
Total	**40**	**100.0**	**100.0**

Source: Primary Data Collection.

Data from Table 6.4 reflect that majority of the respondents, i.e. 45 per cent of the patients were above 80 years. While 27.5 per cent of the respondents were in the age group of 71 to 80 years and 61 to 70 years respectively.

6.7 Gender of the Respondents

Gender was analyzed as to know the ratio of males and females in the present study.

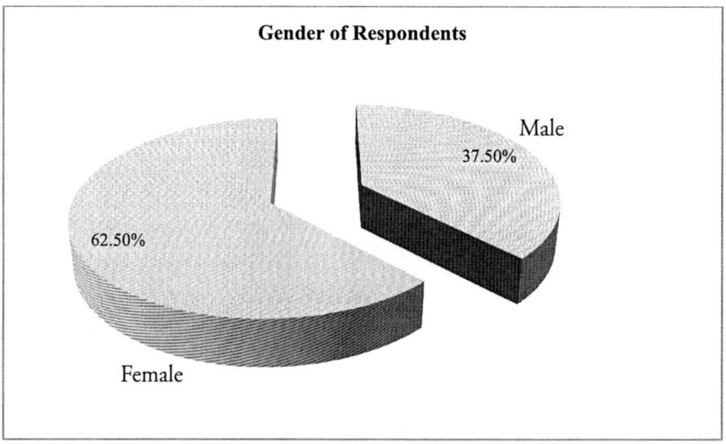

Fig. 6.2: Gender of the Respondents.

Source: Primary Data Collection.

It was interpreted from Fig. 6.2 that 62.5 per cent were female patients while 37.5 per cent were male patients.

6.8 Marital Status of the Respondents

Marital status of a person was also asked.

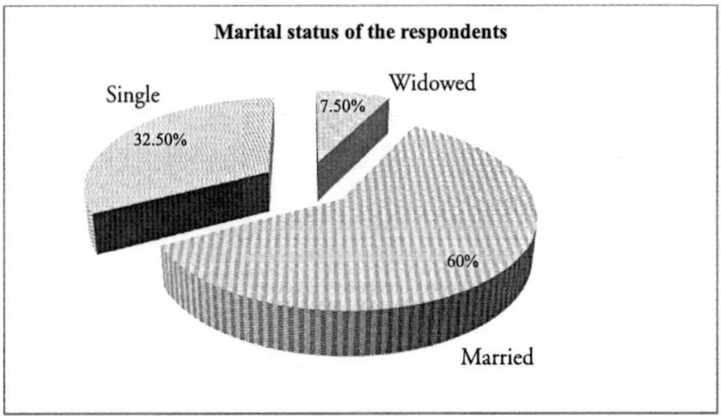

Fig. 6.3: Marital Status of the Respondents.
Source: Primary Data Collection.

From data collected, it was examined that 60 per cent the respondents were married, followed by 32.5 per cent who were widowed and 7.5 per cent were single/unmarried. The results are depicted in Fig. 6.3.

6.9 Religion of the Respondents

Data were collected regarding the religion they belong to.

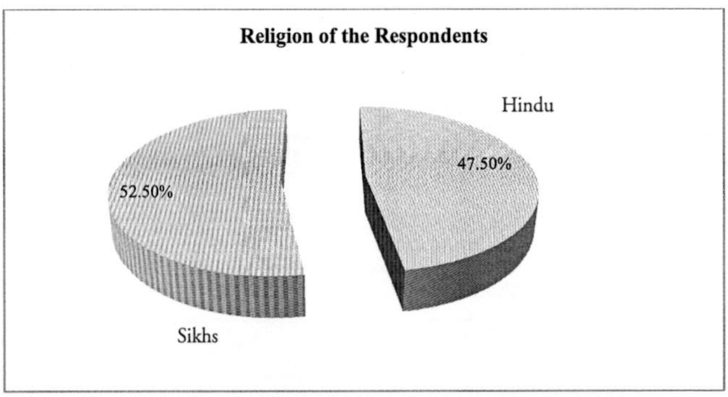

Fig. 6.4: Religion of the Respondents.
Source: Primary Data Collection.

The data collected highlight that the majority of the respondents were Sikhs (52.5%) while 47.5 per cent were Hindus. Respondents from no other religions were present in the data of the present study.

6.10 Current Residence of the Respondents

Respondents were interviewed regarding their current residence to know whether they are staying in rented accommodations and how many of the respondents had their own homes.

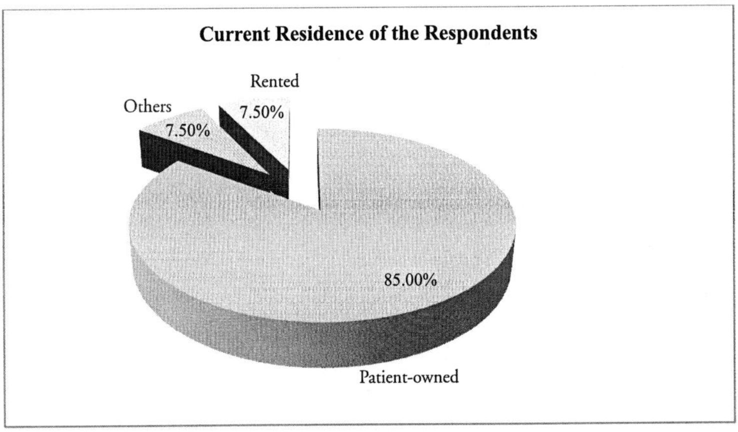

Fig. 6.5: Current Residence of the Respondents.
Source: Primary Data Collection.

From Fig. 6.5 it can be estimated that 85 per cent of the respondents lived in their own residences, while 7.5 per cent of the respondents lived in rented accommodation, and an equal percentage of them lived with their daughters as their sons have shifted abroad. This data is categorized in the 'others' section.

6.11 Primary Caregiver of the Respondents

Primary caregivers are also known as informal caregivers. They are one of the members from family, who tends to take the responsibility of looking after the patient.

Data highlight that majority of the patients (50%) were looked after by their daughters and sons while 27.5 per cent were cared for by their spouses. A significant percentage 15 per cent were looked after by their relatives (such as their sisters, daughter-in-law, brothers). A meagre percentage (7.5%) of them were nursed by their paid help as their immediate families had shifted abroad.

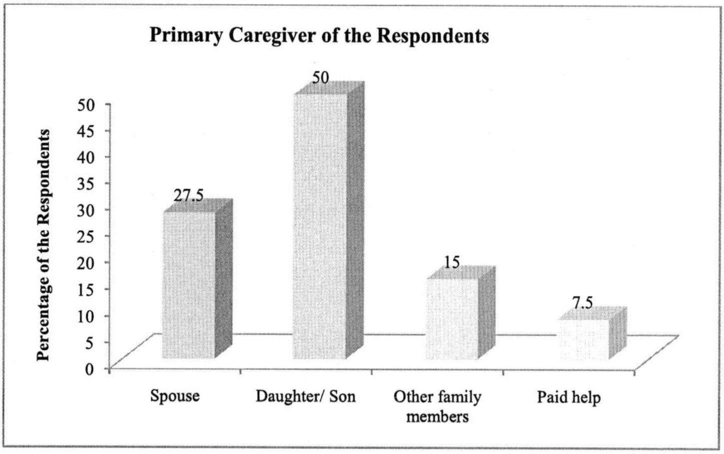

Fig. 6.6: Primary Caregiver of the Respondents.
Source: Primary Data Collection.

A somewhat similar findings were investigated by (Han *et al.*, 2013) where the authors discussed that 32 per cent of the patients were being cared by their spouses, while 27 per cent were looked after by their daughters or sons and 13 per cent were cared by other family members. A meagre percentage (4%) were nursed by their paid help.

For anyone, their family is their world and accepting that a loved one is suffering from any psychiatric disorder is challenging not only emotionally but tends to take a toll on the physical health and finances of the family too. The patient may feel more comfortable in the home environment rather than in an unfamiliar environment of the hospital and thus home care services have to be availed. Caring for a patient at home takes a tremendous toll on immediate caregiver—be it the spouse, child and the other family relatives (Sarkar and Anand, 2013).

6.12 Multiple Diseases Afflicting the Elderly

Patients were asked about if they are suffering from any disease such as disease of the respiratory system, Endocrine system (Diabetes Miletus), Muscular-skeletal system, circulatory system, Injury, open wound, skin, neoplasm, and nervous system. The patients in the study were commonly found to be suffering from hypertension.

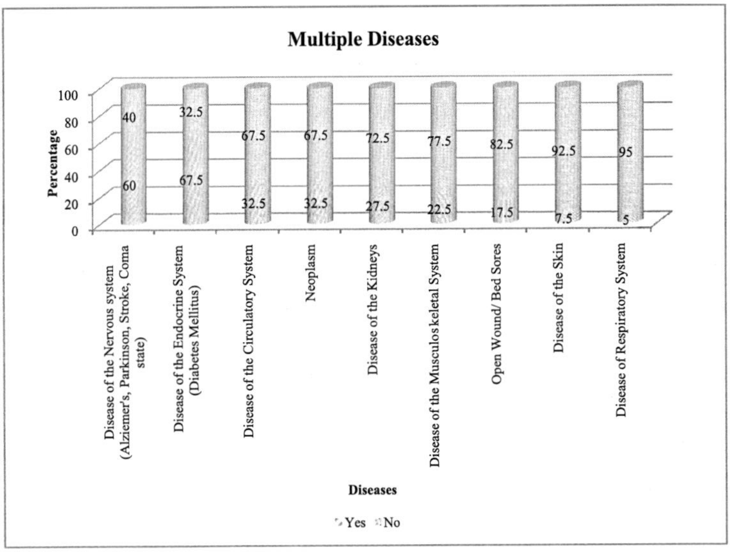

Fig. 6.7: Diseases afflicting the elderly.

Source: Primary Data Collection.

From in-depth interviews, it was found from Fig. 6.7 that majority of the respondents, i.e. 67.5 per cent were suffering from the disease of the endocrine system (Diabetes mellitus), 60 per cent were suffering from disease of the nervous system (Alzheimer, Parkinson, paralytic attack), 32.5 per cent of the respondents were living with Neoplastic diseases (means conditions that causes tumor growth) and an equal percentage (32.5%) were suffering from disease of the circulatory system (heart disease). The patients were also found to be suffering from cancer of the brain, bones, lungs, breast in females and prostate cancer in case of males. About

22.5 per cent of the respondents were suffering from Musculoskeletal diseases such as injury and fracture. There were 17.5 per cent of the respondents who had open wounds or have developed bed sores as a part of their disease. 7.5 per cent were suffering from the disease of the skin such as sclerosis (it is a rare disease that causes hardening and tightening of the skin. In patients who are suffering from this disease also incur problems in their blood vessels, digestive tract and internal organs). About 5 per cent were suffering from respiratory diseases such as asthma, lung cancer, chronic obstructive pulmonary disease (COPD). It was also examined that 55 per cent of the respondents were suffering from Hypertension in the study.

6.14 Home Settings of the Patient

Home settings of the patients here mean that whether the respondents are living alone or they live with their spouse, and their family.

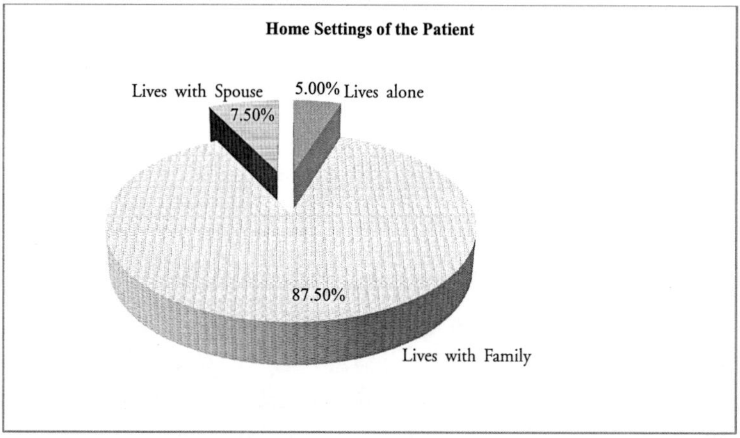

Fig. 6.8: Home Settings of the Patient.

Source: Primary Data Collection.

From Fig. 6.8, it is demonstrated that 87.50 per cent of the respondents were living with their families along with their spouses in case they were alive, while only a smaller percentage, i.e. 7.50 per cent of them were living with their spouses only and a trivial percentage 5 per cent of them were living alone. Ugur *et al.* (2014) in their study also demonstrated that 70.80 per cent of caregivers are females and 49.60 per cent are caring for their spouses. For looking after them they have employed caregivers or nurses and their immediate families have shifted abroad. There were also cases, where the patient passed away and all the last rites and related ceremonies were performed by the paid caregivers at duty. In an another study conducted by Han *et al.* (2013) where the sample was predominantly females (80%), 43 per cent lived alone, 30 per cent lived with spouse and 24.7 per cent with other family members.

6.15 Information on Patient Suffering from Infectious Disease

Family primary caregivers were interviewed regarding information on the infectious diseases the patients were suffering from (HIV/HBV/HVC/TB, HIV or AIDS). Acquired immunodeficiency syndrome is a life threatening chronic condition by human immunodeficiency virus. This disease damages the immune system. HIV also interferes with body's immune system and its ability to fight against infection and disease. It is also a sexually transmitted disease. HBV (Hepatitis B virus, which is passed from person to person through blood, semen or any body fluid). HVC (Heart and vascular or cardiovascular) diseases which include coronary heart diseases, heart attack, high blood pressure, heart defects, stroke and vascular dementia (caused by multiple strokes). TB (Tuberculosis) is an infectious disease that affects the lungs. The results are indicated in Fig. 6.9.

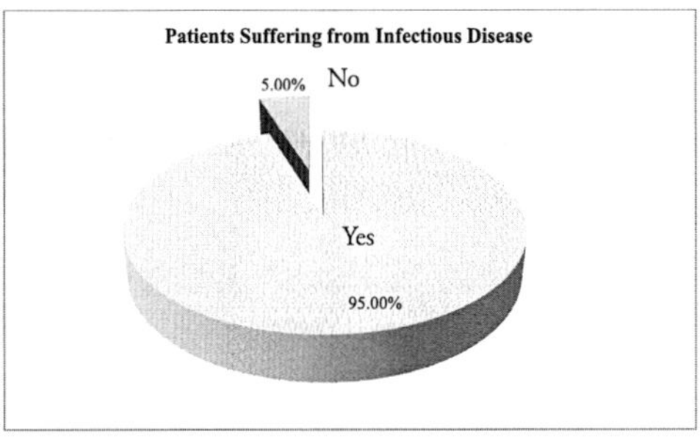

Fig. 6.9: Patient suffering from Infectious Disease.

Source: Primary Data Collection.

It was found that 95 per cent of the respondents were suffering from multiple ailments such as vascular dementia, coronary heart disease, high blood pressure, and stroke and a very small per cent (5%) of them were found to be absolutely fine, they just needed care because of their age. Caring for the patient requires tremendous strength and patience. It has been reviewed that throughout the process of caring for patients with advanced dementia, caregivers experience social, emotional, physical and financial losses, which became more significant as the disease progresses (Bullock, 2004).

6.16 Personal Protective Equipment

Primary caregivers were interviewed to find out that whether they are providing any personal protective equipment to the caregivers such as gloves, wet wipes and clean towels.

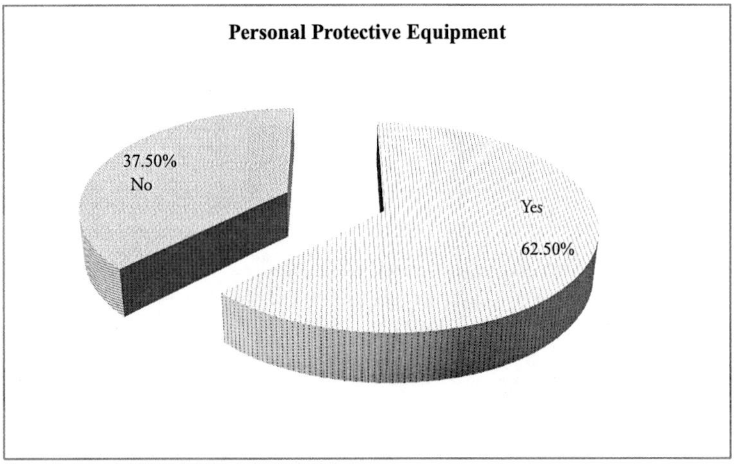

Fig. 6.10: Personal Protective Equipment.
Source: Primary Data Collection.

From the interviews, it was examined that 62.5 per cent of the respondent families provided protective equipments such as plastic gloves for cleaning patient stools. 37.5 per cent of them believed that sometimes their patient feels uncomfortable due to use of plastic gloves so they prefer cleaning the patient directly with hands. This information is represented in Fig. 6.10.

The sixth objective focused on studying the problems faced by the patients, their family members and care providers (nurses and caregivers). Questions were framed regarding the services required from the caregivers and length of engagement, preference of services required (professional caregiving or home nursing), number of health care personnel required, gender, language, and religion preferred.

Additionally, the respondents were also interviewed on caregiver's work shift pattern preferred, performance of activities of daily living depending upon the condition and severity of the disease and instrumental activities of daily living performed by them. However, whether the clients and their families were satisfied with the caregiver work and if there is an improvement in the condition of patient and the problems faced by patients and their family members with regards to caregiving and nursing services at home were studied.

6.17 Service Requirement from the Caregiver

Service requirements mean to assess that depending upon the patient's condition, whether the caregiver is required for a period of 30 days or less than 30 days.

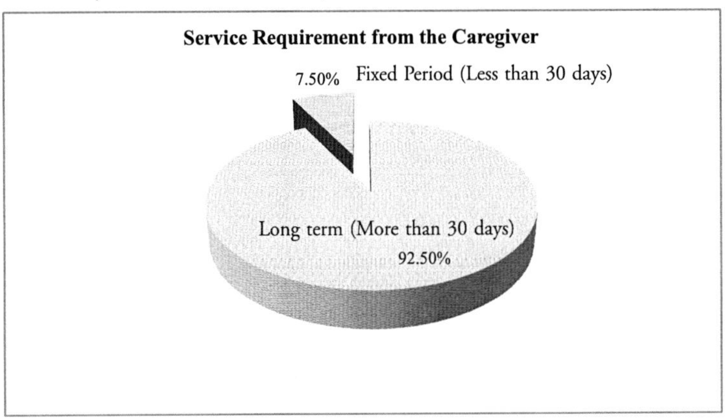

Fig. 6.11: Service Requirement from the Caregiver.
Source: Primary Data Collection.

It is visibly evident from Fig. 6.11 that 92.5 per cent of the patients engaged paid caregivers for a longer term, i.e. more than 30 days. Only 7.5 per cent of the patients required caregivers for smaller period of time, i.e. less than a month because some of them were found to be suffering from curable diseases and they required the caregiver's help for performing their activities of daily living. As their condition improved, they were found to be able in managing their things on their own and no longer require caregiver services. Welch *et al.* (1996) also discussed that home care visits are often a part of long term intervention. Almost 61 per cent of the patients in the study received six or more months of home health care while 4 per cent of the patients received such care for a period of one month.

6.18 Professional Caregiving Services and Nursing Services

Professional caregiver services include bathing, dressing, grooming nail and hair care, denture care, changing diapers, assisting with commode, ambulation (assistance in walking), assisting with oral medication, assisting in physiotherapy/daily exercises and laundry services. There are various nursing procedures which are handled by home care nurses in patient's home, which is directly dependent upon the underlying condition of the patients.

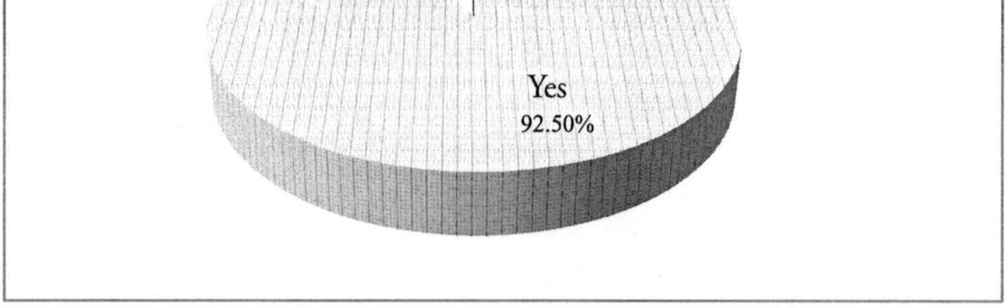

Fig. 6.12: Professional Caregiving Services.

Source: Primary Data Collection.

The data from the study reflects that about 92.5 per cent of the patients have employed formal caregivers whether they were nursing or general duty assistants (Fig. 6.12) depending upon the needs of the patients while 7.5 per cent of the patients were being looked after and being cared by their family caregivers.

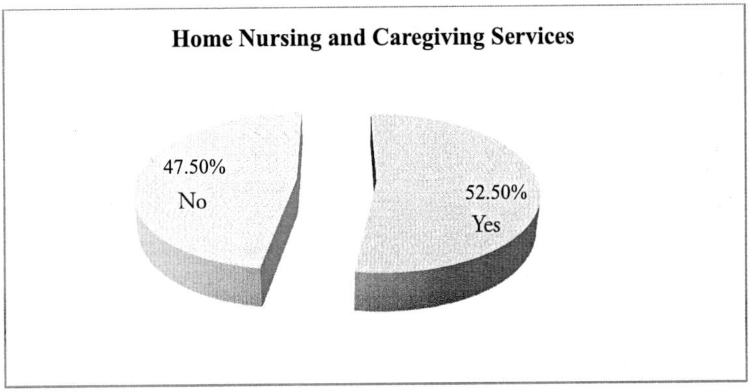

Fig. 6.12.1: Nursing and Caregiving Services.

Source: Primary Data Collection.

However, depending upon their illness, 52.5 per cent of the patients availed the nursing services at home, while 47.5 per cent of the patients were being cared for by the professional caregivers and also their family primary caregivers, which is shown in Fig. 6.12.1.

Martens and Mellor (1997) study found that patients with heart failure, who received home care nursing services following discharge from hospital had significantly fewer hospital readmissions after 90 days of their hospital discharge.

6.19 Home Health Care Personnel

Patients and their family members were interviewed regarding the number of health care personnel employed by them for patient care. Additionally, they were also inquired about gender of the personnel they prefer, along with religion and preference for language. The results on this data are shown in Fig. 6.13.

It is demonstrated that 60 per cent of patients have employed one caregiver or one nursing staff for looking after them which depends on the condition the patient is suffering from. 40 per cent of the family members said that they have employed one caregiver and one nursing staff, or more than 2 staffs as the patients are suffering from chronic illness such as dementia, cancer, Parkinson's disease, stroke, heart attack and require technical procedures to be performed by the nursing staff. Moreover, 37.5 per cent of the patients employed male staff, while 62.5 per cent of the clients have employed female staff for their care. There was an evident inclination towards female staff. 87.5 per cent of the clients felt comfortable if the caregiver's language is Hindi or Punjabi that is spoken by them too. Thomas (2017) in the study discussed about the importance of language that through multilingual and effective communication the health care providers can establish a supportive relationship with the patient and win patient's trust and confidence. Health care professionals should, therefore, make serious attempt to learn local language and should speak language preferred by the patient. Furthermore, just 10 per cent of them showed preference for religion, while 90 per cent of the respondents were only concerned with having efficient and good staff and religion was no bar for them.

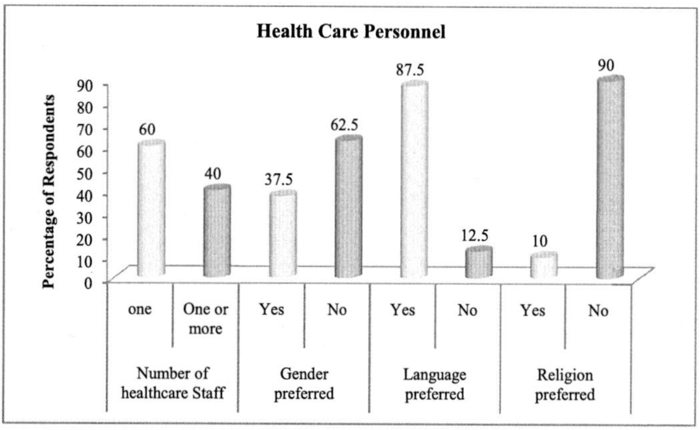

Fig. 6.13: Home Health Care Personnel.

Source: Primary Data Collection.

6.20 Shift Pattern

It refers to the caregiver (nurses and general duty assistant) shift pattern followed by them in their job. A live in shift refers to the job structure in which the caregiver is expected to stay round the clock with the patient for 24 hours but the working hours are limited to 8 hours per day. A live out shift refers to the job structure in which the caregiver is expected to stay up to 12 hours with the patient but working hours are limited to 8 hours per day.

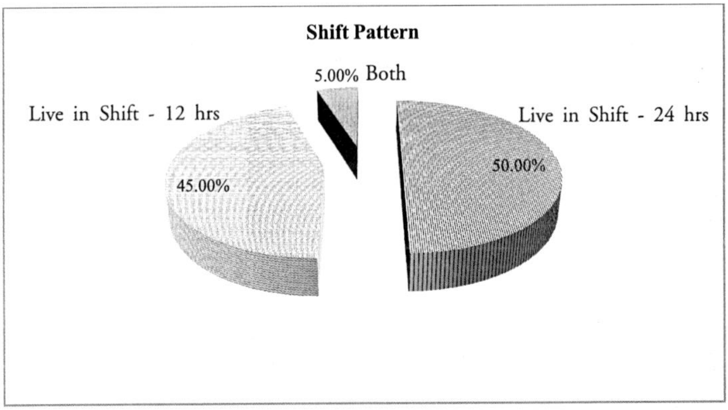

Fig. 6.14: Shift Pattern of the Caregivers.

Source: Primary Data Collection.

Overall, it was found that 50 per cent of the clients employed caregiver services for 24 hours, while 45 per cent of the clients employed caregivers for 12 hours shift (Fig. 6.14). Only 5 per cent of the clients were comfortable with both the shifts and they have recruited more than two staffs. As one of them is there with the patient for 24 hours and other one works for 12 hours.

6.21 Performance of Activities of Daily Living (ADL) and Instrumental Activities of Daily Living (IADL)

Performance of daily activities includes bathing, dressing, grooming, brushing teeth, denture care, changing diapers assisting with the commode, oral and tube feeding, repositioning bed bound patients, walking assistance and fall prevention. Instrumental activities of daily living include basic food preparation for the patient, washing patient clothes, transportation, housekeeping and shopping.

ADL represents health status as well as ability for performing activities for independent living. IADL represents the level of instrumental independence (Han *et al.*, 2013).

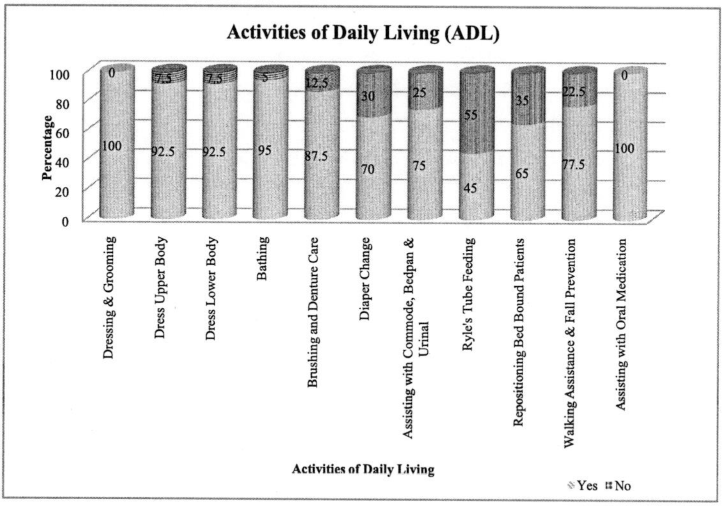

Fig. 6.15: Performance of Activities of Daily Living.
Source: Primary Data Collection.

It is evident from Fig. 6.15 that 100 per cent of the patients received care services such as assisting with the oral medications, dressing and grooming, bathing (95%), brushing and denture care (87.5%), dressing upper and lower body (92.5%), changing diapers (70%), assisting with commode, bedpan and urinal (75%), repositioning bed bound patients (65%) to prevent bed sores and ambulation (assistance in walking and fall prevention) (77.5%) from the staff recruited. 45 per cent patients were helped by the caregivers for Ryle's tube feeding assistance.

Ory and Cox (1994) investigated that seven million Americans aged more than 65 years depend on others for help for performance of activities of daily living. Keepnews *et al.* (2004) reported improvement of ADL and IADL in 78 per cent of patients who received home health care for less than 60 days. Hadley *et al.* (2000) examined functional status of the patients who were discharged from the hospitals and 6 months later. The authors found that functional status of patients who received home care showed improvement than the non users of home care service.

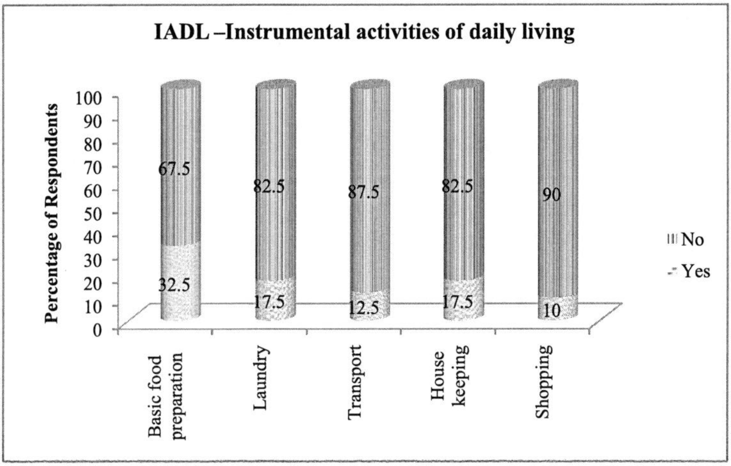

Fig. 6.15.1: Performance of Instrumental Activities of Daily Living.
Source: Primary Data Collection.

About 32.5 per cent caregivers also assisted by the helping staff in basic food preparation (Fig. 6.15.1), and were serving meals to the patients as well. 12.5 per cent of them helped them bringing in the patient to the hospital and elsewhere, 17.5 per cent were even found to be helping the patients and their families in domestic chores and laundry. 10 per cent caregivers helped them in shopping for food and other household requirements.

A study conducted by (Ugur *et al.*, 2014) also demonstrated that 54.01 per cent of caregivers helped in patient's nutritional needs, i.e. helping the patient in food preparation and nutritional needs, 50.36 per cent helped in administration of medicinal use, 26.28 per cent helped in maintaining oral hygiene, 26.28 per cent help to meet urinary needs, 51.82 per cent were helping in dressing and changing patient clothes, 38.69 per cent helping the patient to communicate with their environment and 71.53 per cent help to bring the patient to hospital or outside.

Another study was conducted by HelpAge India, they reported that with ageing, there are numerous changes taking place in the body which affect the ADL such as reduction in eyesight, heard of hearing, difficulty in walking thus reducing an individual to have a independent living for which one needs help and assistance from others. Further they elaborated that about 53.8 per cent of the elderly needed help from others to carry out their activities of daily living. However, an overwhelming percentage of the elderly needed support in IADL (97.8%), the activities involving travelling to hospital or somewhere else, difficulty in managing money, shopping, and commuting to unfamiliar places. However, the female population (57%) outnumbered the male population in need for help. The results of the study indicates that majority of the elderly population requires assistance from other. The study also revealed that the beneficiaries (immobile and bed bound patients) preferred family members and someone familiar to them to deliver the care.[1]

When these data is compared to that of the present study, the activities performed by the caregivers are found to be more or less the same depending up on the requirements of the patient and majority of the elderly population requires assistance from other to carry out their ADL and IADL activities.

6.22 Problems Faced by Patients and their Family Members

It was analyzed from the data that the patients and families were happy with the services provided by the caregivers. While many of the families were dissatisfied with the caregiver work. The results are shown in Fig. 6.16.

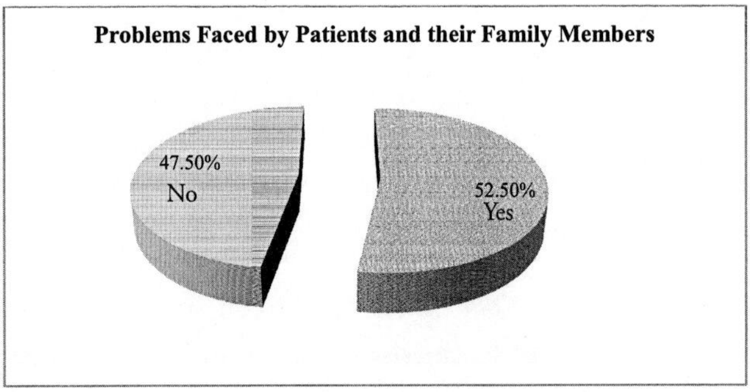

Fig. 6.16: Problems Faced by Patients and their Family Members.

Source: Primary Data Collection.

It was found (Fig. 6.16) that 52.5 per cent of the patient faced problems with the services given by the caregiver. The information obtained from in-depth interviews points to the fact that few of the caregivers used to talk on phone all the time, they were not ready to wash patient's clothes or change their diapers and some of the nurses were not ready to even clean their own bed, they refused to change the patient's diapers as they believed that this is the work of home care aides. Some of the home health care aides were inexperienced and untrained, which has led to adverse problems with the patients.

Blais *et al.* (2013) in their study also corroborated the fact that caregivers contribute to 20.4 per cent of adverse events and health care personnel contribute to 46.2 per cent of the same for the patients. Moreover, few families said that that they have to rather work for the caregiving staff such as by providing them meals and setting their beds.

6.23 Improvement in Health Condition of Patients

Patients' families were interviewed to know the improvement in the condition of patients after receiving caregiver services at home.

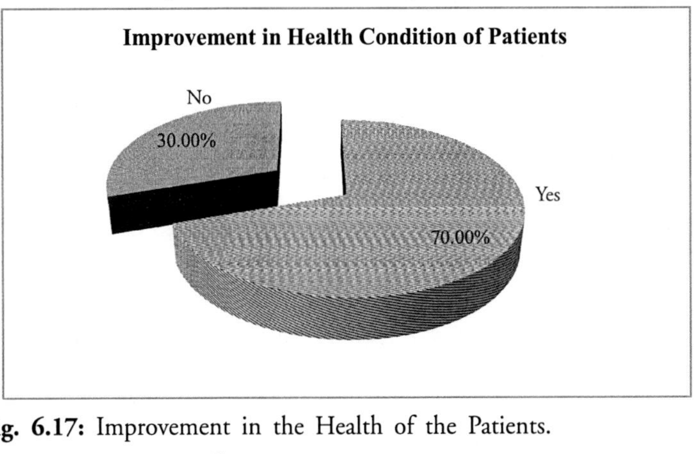

Fig. 6.17: Improvement in the Health of the Patients.
Source: Primary Data Collection.

It is set forth from the findings that 70 per cent of the respondents reported that there was improvement in the condition of patients, they stringently believed that the patient has lived longer due to the help and care provided by the caregivers. While 30 per cent of them asserted that there was little or no improvement in the condition of patients as in few cases, the discharge summaries were not clear or were lost as a result the aftercare was not clear. This data is demonstrated in Fig. 6.17. In a few cases it was also noted that the staffs provided by the agencies were not trained according to the patient requirements.

Fagermoen *et al.* (2006) was of the view that discharge summaries are always given to the patients after hospitalization, but this paperwork might get lost or discarded as a result it is difficult to understand about the primary discharge diagnosis thus providing inappropriate information about the patients comorbidities. Van *et al.* (2011) was also of the view that the caregivers often do not provide appropriate information due to poor memory, miscommunication and misunderstanding.

6.24 Zarit Burden Interview Scale

Past and recent researches showed that family caregiving is a stressful job. However, it has not been well established that at what point these stressors contribute to real risk for decreased mental health. The purpose of the present research work was also to determine a statistically valid cut-off score for the Zarit Burden Interview (ZBI) in order to identify family caregivers at risk for depression and in need of further assessment and intervention.

The ZBI was administered to the populations of family caregivers (n=40) of older adults. Findings suggested that a cut-off score ranging 0-20 predicts little or no burden, 21-40 shows mild to moderate burden, 41-60 shows moderate to severe burden, and 61-88 shows severe burden identifying caregivers at risk for depression.

Considering the combined physical and emotional stress, burden can be significantly expressed as state of experiencing fatigue, sleep disorders, pain in muscles, disorientation, impatience, anxiety, depression, tension and irritability (Gratao *et al.*, 2012; Bianchi *et al.*, 2016).

Table 6.5: Zarit Burden Interview Scale

Zarit Burden Interview scale	Frequency	Per cent	Valid Per cent
0-20	10	25.0	25.0
21-40	13	32.5	32.5
41-60	14	35.0	35.0
61-88	3	7.5	7.5
Total	**40**	**100.0**	**100.0**

Source: Primary Data Collection.

The results were enumerated through 24 questions of ZBI in caregivers of patients with cancer, dementia, Parkinson, brain disorders and injuries. Data in Table 6.5 show that 7.5 per cent of the family caregivers were severely burdened followed by 35 per cent who were moderately to severely burdened followed by 32.5 per cent who were mildly to moderately burdened.

Reportedly, caregivers with a lower degree of burden are more likely to show positive results related to well-being, better perceived health, fewer depressive symptoms and lower levels of stress (Buyck *et al.*, 2011; Adelman *et al.*, 2014).

Previously, it has also been demonstrated that caregivers experience challenges due to following factors such as patient nutrition, administration of medicines, oral and body hygiene, stomach tube feeding, concern of dropping the patient, feeling incompetency in managing fever and body temperature, fatigue, and lack of personal time (Ugur *et al.*, 2014).

6.24.1 Burden Scale with Regard to Socio-Economic Status of the Respondent

Respondents were interviewed to analyze the correlation between the socio-economic status with respect to the burden on the respondents. The results from the data are tabulated in Table 6.5.1.

Table 6.5.1: Burden scale with regard to Socio-economic Status of the Respondent

Socio-economic Status of the Respondent		**Patient burden felt by family caregiver**				**Total**
		0-20	**21-40**	**41-60**	**61-88**	
26-29 Upper(I)	Count	4	2	2	0	8
	% within patients burden	40.0%	15.4%	14.3%	0.0%	20.0%
16-25 Upper Middle(II)	Count	6	11	12	2	31
	% within patients burden	60.0%	84.6%	85.7%	66.7%	77.5%
11-15 Lower Middle(III)	Count	0	0	0	1	1
	% within patients burden	0.0%	0.0%	0.0%	33.3%	2.5%
Total	**Count**	**10**	**13**	**14**	**3**	**40**
	% within patients burden	**100.0%**	**100.0%**	**100.0%**	**100.0%**	**100.0%**

Note: Chi-square test value = 15.9*, among above categories with p-value = .014.
Source: Primary Data Collection.

With regard to the socio-economic status of respondents and the burden felt by them as on staying with the patients. 66.7 per cent of the family caregivers were severely burdened in the upper middle-class category followed by 33.3 per cent who were severely burdened in the lower middle segments. The results were found to be significant as is evident from Chi-square value which is equal to (15.9*) showing association of socio-economic class with the burden perceived by the family caregivers.

Sarkar and Anand (2013) also discussed that there is a direct relationship with the socio-economic status and average burden beared by the family. The treatment process for the patients accounts for substantial costs. It has been observed that the financial strain was experienced by 52.5 per cent of caregivers which ranged from moderate to severe.

6.24.2 Burden Scale with Regard to Gender of the Respondents

The researcher wishes to correlate the burden beared by family caregivers with respect to gender. The extent of subjective burden was visualized from Table 6.5.2.

Table 6.5.2: Burden Scale with Regard to Gender of the Respondents

Gender of the respondents		**Patient burden felt by family caregiver**				**Total**
		0-20	**21-40**	**41-60**	**61-88**	
Male	Count	5	2	8	0	15
	% within patients burden	50.0%	15.4%	57.1%	0.0%	37.5%
Female	Count	5	11	6	3	25
	% within patients burden	50.0%	84.6%	42.9%	100.0%	62.5%
Total	**Count**	**10**	**13**	**14**	**3**	**40**
	% within patients burden	**100.0%**	**100.0%**	**100.0%**	**100.0%**	**100.0%**

Note: Chi-square test value = 7.48*, among above categories with p-value = .05.

Source: Primary Data Collection.

It was found that 100 per cent of the female family caregivers were severely burdened as is visualized from the scores (61-88). Thereby meaning that the female family caregivers were at an increased risk and at a very high risk of depression as compared to male family caregivers. The results were found to be significant as is evident from chi-square value which is equal to 7.48* showing strong association of gender with the burden perceived.

Previous literature has also emphasized that caregiving is influenced by cultural structures (Robison *et al.*, 2009) and that caregiving is a responsibility traditionally fulfilled by female members of the family (Todd *et al.*, 2002; Adams *et al.*, 2009; Serfelova, 2012).

6.24.3 Burden Scale with Regard to the Age group of the Respondents

The burden with respect to the age group of the respondents was also analyzed. The results are indicated in Table 6.5.3.

Table 6.5.3: Burden scale with regard to the Age Group of the Respondents

Age Group of the Respondents		**Patient Burden Felt by Family Caregiver**				**Total**
		0-20	21-40	41-60	61-88	
61-70	Count	2	5	3	1	11
	% within patients burden	20.0%	38.5%	21.4%	33.3%	17.5%
71-80	Count	5	3	2	1	11
	% within patients burden	50.0%	23.1%	14.3%	33.3%	27.5%
>80	Count	3	5	9	1	18
	% within patients burden	30.0%	38.5%	64.3%	33.3%	45.0%
Total	**Count**	**10**	**13**	**14**	**3**	**40**
	% within patients burden	**100.0%**	**100.0%**	**100.0%**	**100.0%**	**100.0%**

Note: Chi-square test value = 14.6, among above categories with p-value = .264.
Source: Primary Data Collection.

With regard to the age of the respondents, it was found that 64.3 per cent of the family caregivers whose patients were in the age group of above 80 years fell in the category of moderately to severely burdened followed by 33.3 per cent of the family caregivers who were severely burdened.

6.24.4 Burden Scale with Regard to Primary Caregiver

Primary caregivers were interviewed. Their burden was analyzed with regard to their relation with the patient. The results are indicated in Table 6.5.4.

Table 6.5.4: Burden Scale with regard to the Primary Caregiver of the Respondents

Primary Caregiver		**Patient Burden Felt by Family Caregiver**				**Total**
		0-20	**21-40**	**41-60**	**61-88**	
Spouse	Count	5	3	1	2	11
	% within patients burden	50.0%	23.1%	7.1%	66.7%	27.5%
Daughter/ Son	Count	3	5	11	1	20
	% within patients burden	30.0%	38.5%	78.6%	33.3%	50.0%
Other Family Members	Count	0	4	2	0	6
	% within patients burden	0.0%	30.8%	14.3%	0.0%	15.0%
Paid Help	Count	2	1	0	0	3
	% within patients burden	20.0%	7.7%	0.0%	0.0%	7.5%
Total	**Count**	**10**	**13**	**14**	**3**	**40**
	% within patients burden	**100.0%**	**100.0%**	**100.0%**	**100.0%**	**100.0%**

Note: Chi-square test value = 16.7*, among above categories with p-value = .05.
Source: Primary Data Collection.

It was analyzed, as is reflected from the data in Table 6.5.4 that with respect to relation with the patient, in cases where the patient is cared for by the spouse, 66.7 per cent were severely burdened.

78.6 per cent were looked after by their sons or daughters and were moderately to severely burdened. In cases where the patient is looked after by other family members such as daughter or son-in-law, the burden perceived is much lower as compared to the burden perceived by the spouse or their son or daughter. However, the results were found to be significant as is evident from chi-square value which is equal to 16.7* showing strong association of their relation with the burden perceived by the primary caregivers.

Family caregiving has been recognized as a relative challenging issue in the existing scenario of health in India. Literature indicates that the stress associated with care giving results in a long-term health effects for the family caregivers (Sarkar and Anand, 2013).

Overall, it can be concluded that majority of the patients were taken care of by their families at homes by their sons, daughters, spouses, other relatives and paid help. Elderly population in India is at a disadvantageous position as compared to other countries in terms of geriatric specialist, health care and insurance benefits. However, it is important for every country to reassess and redesign its health care system to cope with the challenges put forward by demographic and financial variables.

In the present study, the patients also engaged the nursing staff and caregivers for performance of activities of daily living and instrumental activities of daily living.

Study undertaken by home health care in Korea also found that home health care helps to improve activities of daily living (ADLS) and Instrumental activities of daily living in patients suffering from chronic illnesses (Han *et al.*, 2013). Further it was found that the patients and their families were facing problems with regard to nursing and caregiver services. Finding assimilated through the Zarit Burden Scale found that female family caregivers were at an increased high risk of depression as compared to male family caregivers and the caregivers were severely burdened in case of patients whose spouses were responsible for looking after them. The medical history of the patients and challenges faced by the patients and the family caregivers are discussed in detail in the chapter that follows.

Note

1. Home care-Report.pdf (helpageindia.org)

7

Understanding the Lifestyle Adopted by Patients and their Care Providers to Cope up with the Disease

Too often we underestimate the power of a touch, a smile, a kind word, a listening ear, an honest compliment, or the smallest act of caring all of which have the potential to turn a life around.

–Leo Buscaglia

The health care industry altogether is an integration of various sectors within the economic system, that provides goods and services to the chronically ill and bed ridden patients. With ageing, one tends to suffer from multiple diseases, in few cases, some diseases are curable, while the others need persistent monitoring and care.

Grunfeld (1997) examined the preference for home-based care over institutional care. In home-based care the expectation is such that family caregivers are always available at home to support patients. The tradition of family caregiving is recognised as fundamental to our society and family caregivers are deeply motivated towards their commitments to the patients. The demographic trends have placed elderly population in double jeopardy, suggesting that there is need for formal caregivers, as the family members are not always available for care when needed.

The number of people affected by dementia in India are set to triple reaching six million by 2040 (Ferri *et al.*, 2005). The awareness for this diseases among the health care professionals and in the community is limited and there are few services available for elderly with dementia and their caregivers (Patel and Prince, 2001). Caring for an elderly person with dementia creates a situation of chronic stress, that adversely affect caregiver's health (emotionally and mentally) (Morris *et al.*,1988, Schulz *et al.*, 1990, Chappell and Penning, 1996). Many studies report that there are increased symptoms of depression and anxiety among family caregivers (Canadian Study of Health and Aging Working Group, 1994; Schulz *et al.*, 1990; Livingston *et al.*, 1996; Baumgarten *et al.*, 1992; Baumgarten *et al.*, 1994; Cohen and Eisdorfer, 1988; Gallagher *et al.*, 1989). Further it has also been suggested that spouses providing care are more affected than children, while men and women family caregivers are affected differently depending upon the condition of the patient (Morris *et al.*, 1988; and Baumgarten *et al.*, 1992).

Chappell (1992) advised that if formal care support is not provided, informal family caregiver will burn out. Canadian study of Health and Aging Working Group (1994) suggested that when the patients suffering from dementia are matched for their disability, they received fewer caregiving support services than those suffering from other ailments. There can be various reasons—support may be expensive, the caregiver may sometimes deny receiving support, personally, the caregiver may have conflicts abandoning his caregiver role and utmost, caregiver may be embarrassed about needing any help or assistance. It is also a possibility that the caregiver may be stigmatised that changing caregivers will disrupt the condition of patient. Townsend *et al.* (1990) reported that people who are suffering from multiple illnesses prefer to die at home until and unless, 24 hours care at home is available, the involvement of a family caregiver is very essential for palliative care for patients in need (Townsend *et al.*, 1990; Dunlop *et al.*, 1989; McWhinney *et al.*,1995; Zimmer *et al.*, 1985; Sherbourne and Stewart, 1991; Bly and Kissick, 1994).

With this background, the present chapter tries to understand the journey of the patients as narrated by their primary caregivers and how this formal caregiving has helped them through the years, as the responsibilities of family caregivers extend beyond personal care and involves sophisticated forms of treatment which are handled by trained nurses and caregivers. The elderly home care training by qualified nurses constantly supports caregivers on their job and ensures that they follow the personalised care plan (PCP), which includes, bathing, dressing, grooming, changing diapers, helping the patient with the commode, repositioning patients to prevent bed sores, tube feeding assistance, walking assistance and fall prevention. In many cases, personal care assistants work along with physiotherapist, nursing staff and nurse manager to follow an exercise plan for the patient.

The seventh objective focused on understanding lifestyle adopted by the patients and their care providers to cope up with the disease. 40 family caregivers were approached to understand the condition of the patients. 70 per cent of the family caregivers freely discussed their challenges, and 28 case studies were generated with the help of in-depth interviews from the client and their families. 24.5 per cent of them refused to discuss about the patient stating that they did not feel like discussing about the condition of the patient further while some of them did not want to hold a conversation on this matter as the patient was no more with them, they felt discussing about them is hurting their near ones. One of the respondents asserted "My mother is no more; she suffered a great deal while she lived and was in acute pain due to cancer, I don't think it's possible for me to be discussing about her anymore." A small percentage, i.e. 5.5 per cent of people did not respond to any message or call.

7.1 CASE 1

7.1.1 Disease of the Musculoskeletal System—Rheumatoid Arthritis, Injury (Fracture); Diabetes; Disease of the Cardiovascular System—Heart Disease

A daughter-in-law (age 55) of the patient (age 80) narrated her mother-in-law's experience after her fracture. She elaborated;

> "My mother-in-law is a very intelligent lady. She holds a degree in Hindi literature and was a teacher by profession. She has always been obese, weighed around 130 kg. An interesting fact about her is that she was also a 'self-styled doctor', and used to run a clinic. After an accident, she broke her femur bone and was left fractured, she incurred a phobia after this, that if she would stand, she would fall down as she also suffered from arthritis. This scared her to such an extent that she did not take bath for continuous 7 years."

7.1.2 Involvement in Daily Routine Activities by the Caregivers

She expressed, all responsibility of her mother-in-law's caregiving was on her shoulders as she is also a working individual, thus it is not possible for her to take long leaves and stay at home for looking after her. Thus, she has employed two caregivers who also helped to prepare food for her and the family. The caregivers start the duty by giving the patient a sponge bath in the morning and a fixed sum of Rs. 200 was given to the caregiver whenever they changed her diapers. She elaborated that it was a tedious task to change her diaper due to her weight. They had to use sellotapes after putting her diaper to make sure the diaper stuck in its place. She doesn't not allow anyone to use plastic or gloves for cleaning her stool either. She had to wear diapers 24×7. Later, her body is cleaned with Dettol and water, antiseptic cream and anti-fungal powder helped her to prevent bedsores in the hip area. Further she mentioned, her mother-in-law has a habit of spreading about 6-7 bedsheets over her bed, which has made changing her diapers and overall bedding a painstakingly complicated and exhausting process that oftentimes take more than an hour.

> *"Raat wali caregiver is very nice, usne bhot zyada seva ki hai, mai bhi nahi kar sakti."*

(The caregiver who used to come in the night was very helpful, nice and courteous, the extent to which she served my mother-in-law, I am doubtful I would ever be able to do as much).

My mother-in-law also suffers from diabetes, and had a heart attack few years back but I would call her a brave heart, despite her illness, she gathers the courage to get up and sit down on her own and help in chores.

She goes on saying that one of the caregivers was working in the factory during the day. She comes for duty by 5pm and leave by 9 am in the morning. She prepared meals for our family too. She leaves on Saturday and comes back by Monday morning. During this time, she (my mother-in-law) faced a lot of difficulty and stress even for freshening up in the morning. With the caregiver's help it usually takes her about 3 hours for her to bathe and get freshen up, she is very efficient and never compromised on anything. She ensures her attendants are happy and satisfied. The caregivers take care of the most basic needs of my mother-in-law and helps us immensely be it preparing meals for the family or washing clothes or utensils.

7.1.3 Difficulties Faced with the Staff from Agencies

She elaborated that we cannot adjust with the staff from the agencies, as they will not help us with any domestic work and they charge more. She informed that she is also a working individual and the mother-in-law stays home alone from 9am in the morning till 1pm in the afternoon. In between these hours, if needed, she rings a bell to call her son but mostly she would prefer sleeping at this very time. She also goes on to saying, "My mother-in-law is a very strong lady, even if she is bedridden since the last 7 years, she helps with chores such as cutting vegetables, folding clothes, and organise all the activities in the Gurdwara Sahib from home but all of these she does from her bed. She doesn't blame anyone for her illness but the problem is that *woh kabhi bed se nahi uterte the* (only the problem is that she does not get up from her bed because of the phobia of falling).

7.1.4 Having the Formal Caregivers with us is like a Blessing

The daughter-in-law continues to say, "Caregivers assist the patient with all the activities of daily living like—grooming, dressing up, bathing, denture care, changing diapers, assisting with the commode, bedpan and urinal, repositioning patients, walking assistance and fall prevention. The caregiver is also indulged in buying food for patient, doing their laundry, washing utensils and shop for things requested and needed by the patients. This has been great help through these years otherwise it was not possible for me to continue working."

Altun (1998) also reported that primary daily activities performed by the caregiver are accompanying the patient to hospital, taking the patient for a walk (90.15%), shopping for the patient and household needs, assisting with oral medications (66.67%), and cleaning the environment where patient lives (66.66%).

7.2 CASE 2

7.2.1 Disease of the Nervous System—Depression; Disease of the Musculoskeletal System—Fracture

A daughter (age 69) shared the story of her 91-year old father who was alright through his life but because of his age, he was suffering from depression. He suffered a fracture after an incident. She (The daughter) found it difficult to assist him in moving around because of his newly developed fear of falling. "He holds my hands very firmly while walking," she explains.

7.2.2 The Caregiver Really Helped him to Uplift his Spirits

The caregiver (age 26) employed to look after him used to insist him in walking, she encouraged and boost his confidence by telling him "I am a trained caregiver, I will not let you fall". This helped my father immensely, and he was convinced to be more active. They follow a basic exercise schedule twice a day. With the support from the caregiver, he also started to go out for evening walks. With her dedication and optimism, over time, his balance, strength and flexibility massively improved. Now he can walk through the corridor without support. They both share a beautiful bond. She is like a family to us. She followed the patient care plan provided to her.

7.3 CASE 3

7.3.1 Disease of the Respiratory System—Pulmonary Embolism; Disease of the Musculoskeletal System—Injury (Fracture)

A professional doctor (age 52) narrated the help his father (age 79) received from the caregiver. "My father was infected with COVID. He suffered a spinal fracture as he slipped from stairs. Later, he was also detected with pulmonary embolism (a condition in which one or more arteries in the lungs become blocked by blood clot). The personal care assistant we employed was provided with all necessary requirements and he willingly assumed responsibility; in desperate times he even cleaned soiled bed.

> *"Usne ta kabi vi nahi veham kita, usne patient ko nahalaya."*

(He never acted suspiciously, rather he used to perform all activities of daily living such as bathing, grooming and dressing.)

7.3.2 Catering to the Needs of the Caregiver

We share a special bond with the caregiver, after leaving us, he still meets us. If we will behave awkwardly, they will not take care of your family. By the time he left us, we were really attached to him, we never treated him differently, we used to give him same food as we had and even now if there are any family functions or gatherings, he is always invited. *Asi ohnu apne family members di tarah rakhiya,* (We always treated him like our family member).

Franzosa *et al.* (2019) discussed that aides perform off-plan work when they felt that it was important for client or when a family member was nice.

7.4 CASE 4

7.4.1 Disease of the Nervous System

The son (age 62) explained the condition of his mother (age 89). He elaborated that due to disturbance of the gray matter, she has been bedridden in a comatose state for a long time with non-functional senses but her vital organs are functioning normally.

7.4.2 Paid Help since Last 6 Years

The caregiver (age 25) has been very helpful, she is to our liking. Although the patient has not been in a position to express herself, but in our opinion, we did not face any problem with the caregiver. It is to be understood that due to the severity and gravity of the disease and the age of the patient, there was not much improvement in the health of the patient. However, as far as patient care was concerned, proper hygiene conditions were maintained and efforts were put in by the paid help.

> *"Bahot dhiyan rakhti thi, bed sores na ho, woh sab maintain huya tha kabhi smell nahi ayi. Hum logo ne bhi dhyan diya."*

(The caregiver took very good care of her, she ensured that proper hygiene is maintained and it never happened that the patient developed bed-sores or emitted any pungent smell in the room. We as a family have also been cognizant of her needs, we have taken good care of all her needs and ensured daily chores and activities of daily living such as bathing, dressing, grooming, denture care, repositioning the patient and assisting the patient in giving medicines have been happening with utmost care and needed attention.)

7.5 CASE 5

7.5.1 Neoplasm—Carcinoma; Blood Pressure; Disease of the Endocrine System Diabetes

A daughter-in-law (age 52) narrated the story of her brave mother-in-law (age 74) whom she defines as a very strong and active lady, she describes that her mother-in-law has been suffering from cancer of the stomach for 7 years and has undergone three surgeries. She is in serious pain but likes to take delight even during her illness, she makes the most of her time she loves to travel, has gone on world tour thrice. *Jab wo Europe gaye the toh urine bag laga hua tha.* (When she went to see Europe, her foleys catheter was in place). She puts forth, "My father-in-law is very supportive. We employed one nurse and one GDA for her care, at the same time we always have guests at home as mummy felt very happy having her near and dear ones besides her."

7.5.2 Care given by the Caregivers and Nurses

> "*Hum do bar massage jaroor karvaate the* (Twice in a day, we ensure they massaged her body). We actually feel that just due to the money we paid them, nurses took good care of them, *shayad unhi ki wajah se woh itne saal nikal gaye. Hum sab ne unki bahut care ki hai.*"

(I give all the credit to our home care staff members, I believe my mother-in-law has lived all through these years only because of their care). It would not be wrong to say that all family members have also taken very good care of her. My husband was very concerned for his mother as he was the one who used to take her mother to Gurgaon for her chemotherapy and later, while she was undergoing treatment from Max Hospital, SAS Nagar, Mohali, he ensured all amenities for her.

McCorkle (2000) also elaborated on the newly diagnosed cancer patients for a solid malignancy who were randomised to the specialised home care survived 7 months longer than the usual group. The group receiving specialised home care was significant among the late-stage patients, where the patients in the intervention group have 2 years survival rates twice than the usual care group.

7.6 CASE 6

7.6.1 Disease of the Nervous System—Alzheimers; Blood Pressure; Disease of the Endocrine System—Diabetes; Hearing Loss

A housewife (age 58) shared story of her mother-in-law (age 85) who is suffering from Alzheimer from the last 9 years. Back in the 1980s, we used to stay in Mumbai and my mother-in-law ran a boutique with 6-7 tailors. She was physically very fit even till the age of 70. All through her life she had her mind made-up to the fact that she always wanted to remain financially independent and she was able to be so, she always helped her sister and brother with monetary help, whenever needed. The problem started when she started to forget her work, in her job her work included cutting the fabric but the things which she did for years started fading away from her mind. *Woh cutting bhulne lagi thi* (She used to wrongly cut the fabric). She was not able to recognise which shirt will go with the salwar. She was not able to match the outfits according to their colour coordinates.

7.6.2 Difficult Behaviour of Patients Suffering from Alzheimer

She further elaborated that, Alzheimer is a strange disease, the patients suffering will talk to everyone with utmost love and later could ask 'who was that lady, I don't remember her'. Once she was in shock as she was not able to get visa for Australia, the doctor who was enquiring about her health got to know that she was suffering from some psychological disorder, as she remembered her Mumbai address, but did not remember her current address. She goes on to saying, we need lot of patience to handle such patients, we used to have numerous arguments with each other, *mummy bhot roti thi* (mummy used to cry a lot). *woh mere se nafrat karne lag gaye the* (she started hating me). She used to take out money from her son's purse and put it in her purse, and tells all that this is my house, you all please leave my home and let me stay alone, we had to forcibly assert and vehemently tell her that this is your home, how will you stay here alone. Due to her disease, our life totally changed.

She narrated an incident, "One day the cook was making Dosa, I told her to serve the Dosa first to mummy, she got very suspicious, she used to think we might poison her. In suspicion and anger, she struck hard at the maid's back and told her to serve others first then her." Yaffe *et al.* (2002) also analysed the baseline characteristics in dementia patients showing difficult behaviours such as psychotic symptoms (hallucinations, suspiciousness), anger, aggressiveness, dangerous to self and others (wandering) and wakes caregiver up at night.

The narrator further discussed, "For taking medicine, she used to take 10 minutes to chew a single tablet, and even then, when left unobserved she would throw the medicines without anybody knowing. Then, we started to give her medicines in the juices or aerated drinks. All these duties and tasks were assigned to us and none of the relatives ever helped us. Dias *et al.* (2008) in their study discussed similar findings where 86 per cent of the principal caregivers who lived with the person with dementia, the majority (58%) having no help from any relative for the caregiving.

In another incident she narrates, "Once we left her at her brother's house, she felt so insecure as she felt we are planning to shift her from our house to her brother's place, she got so violent that she ran towards the gate of the house." In agony, she corroborates the fact that the people suffering from this disease would be more suspicious towards their primary caregiver. She said that my mother-in-law only had issues with myself. We (all the family members) used to feel very scared, *hum ne apas me baat karna band kar diya tha* (we had actually stopped talking to each other in front of her as my mother-in-law became so suspicious and no relative came to our help. Sometimes, her deteriorating condition has turned the family environment very stressful. Even the economic burden of caregiving is very traumatic. Dias *et al.* (2008) found that caregiving is associated with worsening mental health, high burden on the caregiver and greater out of pocket health care cost, which is also due to home care visits by the private doctors.

Further, she emphasized on the need of trainings for caregivers, she asserts, "I think there should be special training (formal and informal) to be organised by the neuro departments for handling such patients."

The study conducted by Alzheimer's Society (2009) identified that working with people who are suffering from dementia is very exigent particularly in patients with behavioural problems (getting upset and angry, depressed and no more interested in anything, hitting other people, hiding things and believing that others are hiding). Further, the study elaborated that in India there is no separate facility available in emergency departments either for older patients or for the patients with specific problems such as dementia. Health care attendants, nurses and even treating physicians are not trained to deal with dementia patients. Yaffe *et al.* (2002) examined that caregiver burden is associated with increased risk of nursing home placements for patients with dementia as by doing this, caregiver stress and depression can be averted. A comprehensive counselling intervention for the caregivers helps to teach the caregiver behavioural management techniques to condense difficult patient behaviour. The researchers also underlined the need for training caregivers, who would be able to handle difficult patients. Unfortunately, physicians fail to notice the caregiver stress and depression and the services are not always within reach. Lower rate of nursing home use by some caregivers is also associated with economic hardships. And thus, the demands and cost associated with caregiving will always become a matter of concern.

She tribulates, "People should cooperate and relatives should spend time with the patients, rather than doing mere formalities. Patients suffering from this disease are very difficult to handle, *Subah subah uthi, woh gir rahi thi, unko koi attack ah raha tha,* (once she woke up in the morning, she had a stroke), immediately we took her to hospital. The stroke was major, and her left hand was paralysed. *Baad me unki speech chali gayi thi* (she also lost her speech because of her suffering).In aggression she used to attack the maid at times. I often covered up for her and had to tell them *tumne kuch galat kiya isliye unhone galat kiya tumare saath* (you might have committed some mistake, that is why she is angry). In 2015, we met one doctor, after taking his medicines she had to calm down. I had noticed that she had the habit of doing hemming on the clothes because of her business, her hands were always moving into some kind of an involuntary movement with the help of pencil. From her facial expressions, we would decipher that she is suffering from some psychological issues. Upon consulting with doctors, we were told that because she has been doing strenuous work all her life such as working on the machine, so it can be possibly one of the reasons that she is suffering from this disease."

7.6.3 Caregiver Work Duties

The daughter-in-law in distress further elaborates, "She was bedridden for about 6 months, I used to monitor her day and night, most of the time, I instructed the caregiver to ensure she had a quilt at night. Sometimes, I had to check her body by using torch light to see if she had any bedsores over her body. In her case, there was also a problem of bed wetting." Additionally, she continues, *Bar bar tange wash karni padti* (we have to wash her legs in case she soils herself in bed). My home care staff used to tell me '*Madam aap bhot dhiyan rakhte ho*' (Madam, you are actually very concerned about her health). She has become very childlike, at times, she took more than an hour for eating food, sometimes she used to play with the spoon. *Raat ko uth ke chal padti thi* (she used to walk in her sleep), and so we got very scared. Once during night time, she got up from her bed and starting walking, she then fell down due to knocking herself over with the dressing table in her room. She started bleeding profusely and we had to immediately take her to the doctor and later we removed all furniture and left only a bed in her room. Day by day, her condition has deteriorated for instance there was a lot of bed wetting, she had no idea about the day of the hour, she walked in the night, she was not able to identify time by looking at clock. For looking after her, we employed two lady caregivers, one used to come in the night for 12 hours and another used to come in the day. My mother-in-law was like a child to me, I used to give her lot of love and affection and she reverted it back, she used to hold my hand and *mere upar haath pherti thi* (used to pat my head with love). In the past 8 to 10 years, I have changed at least 10 caregivers because there have been instances, *woh gadbad karte hai kai bar* (they creates mess many times). Once my daughter caught the caregiver slapping her, I clearly instructed her not to behave aggressively with the patient. Grafstrom *et al.* (1993) discussed that the more greatly burdened caregivers are more aggressive in their behaviour towards the person they are caring for than the less burdened caregivers.

7.6.4 Having Caregiver is a Great Help

Having someone to help you and share your burden makes you feel little independent. We have changed many home care assistants including the nursing staff, one stayed at our place for 3 years, another is with us from the last 6 years, she is very nice and is trustworthy. At least it's a great help, one feels independent.

7.6.5 Suggestions Given by the Family Caregiver

One has to monitor the caregiver, installing cameras to keep an active eye on them is a good option. Our caregiver in order to avoid dealing with the patient sometimes used to throw her food away and to showed us that she had eaten the food. So, I always sit with mummy while she ate. One cannot show blind adherence towards the caregiver. Their job is such that they have to be awake at night, but they tend to sleep, sometimes we understand that one needs sleep for 2- 3 hours, but we expect them to stay awake rest of the time.

7.7 CASE 7

7.7.1 Disease of the Nervous system—Alzheimer; Blood Pressure; Disease of the Endocrine System—Diabetes Mellitus; Hearing Problem; Neoplasm—Prostate Cancer

A daughter (age 70) narrated the story of her father who is suffering from Alzheimer's disease, prostate cancer at the age of 93 years.

She narrates, "My father was into textile business, in 2013, I brought him to my house as my husband shares a strong bond with him and takes very good care of him. With declining age, he is suffering from multiple issues like prostate cancer and due to this issue, he has had a urinary catheter in place."

7.7.2 Difficult Behaviour Accompanied with Alzheimer

Now as due to his old age, he is not keeping well. There is a bed wetting issue due to prostate problem. Last winters, due to frequent urination we had installed Foleys catheter in place to help him ease himself. Now, he wears diapers, yet sometimes I don't understand why he tends to take out his diaper himself and throw his used diapers around. This could be due to Alzheimer's disease. His dietary preferences have also changed. He doesn't like to eat vegetables now so we give him eggs as a replacement. He speaks in English but now has a problem in hearing. So, he rarely engages in any kind of conversation.

7.7.3 Caregiver Duties

Regarding the home care staff, she elaborated that the caregiver (age 27) is very nice. He is more like an extended family member to us. I believe that although all responsibilities are taken upon by the primary caregiver, yet one has to be very vigilant. The staff can perform all activities such as bathing, grooming, cleaning the patient and, changing their diapers. The patient is able to get extra affection and care in their presence.

She simultaneously narrated the story of her mother who was also suffering from Alzheimer's disease and was also looked after by a caregiver. The staff cooked for the patient and in our presence, she performed her duties very efficiently but, in our absence, she would ignore my mother and would not listen to her. We got to know about this when we installed cameras in the house and so, I believe that monitoring of the patient by one or the other family member is very important. We should not leave our elders solely dependent upon these caregivers. There have to be a means of monitoring the impact of these health services on society as a whole or on the health services indeed. These mechanisms help to monitor the quality of care provided by a family caregiver or a professional (Fast *et al.*, 1997; Coyte and Young, 1997).

7.8 CASE 8

7.8.1 Disease of the Nervous System—Alzheimer; Neoplasm—Carcinoma; Bedsores; Blood Pressure; Disease of the Endocrine System—Diabetes

A wife (age 72) narrated the story of her husband (age 76), who was suffering from cancer of the stomach (Carcinoma). She goes on to saying, "I have taken lot care of my husband, I have employed physiotherapist for his exercises and other than this I help him personally, for instance, at the time he has to relieve himself, I have taken the responsibility of helping him and cleaning him after he is done."

7.8.2 Problems Faced due to Caregivers

The caregivers used to charge a fixed sum of Rs. 15,000 for 12 hours a day and Rs. 20,000 for 24 hours a day per month. I am an ardent believer of the fact that we need to ourselves look after our patient. When I was looking after him and took responsibility of repositioning him after every two hours, he never ever had bed sores. *Ohna nu mai koi taklif nahi hon diti, mai 'Sai Baba ji' di vibhuti lagadi si ohna de* (I tried my best that he never felt the pain ever, so I bought a charismatic *vibhuti* from Sai temple). With time, his health deteriorated and he even starting missing on and calling out his old friends who passed away a long time ago.

I was not satisfied with the job done by caregiver. He was reluctant in cleaning him and was not willing to wash his clothes. He behaved so awkwardly that at times, he was not even ready to put the used diaper in the dustbin. Moreover, the caregiver's presence felt like an additional task for me, as I had to prepare breakfast, lunch and dinner for him. It was not possible to afford the caregiver as rather than him working for us, I had to work for the caregiver. I would rather spend that time to my husband. With time, his condition is further deteriorating and he has started suffering from dementia. At times, he does things which are incomprehensible for me or others to understand. He insists on not wearing diapers and in extreme situations he would undo his diaper and put his faeces on his body. I was the one who used to change bedsheets at least three times a day. *Har koi seva nahi kar sakde, khana vi khud hi khilana hai* (Wife has to look after and take care of her husband, I always cook food and make him eat myself). I would never employ caregiving staff from any agency as they extract lot of money from the patient's and their families.

Similar results were explored by Vyasamoorthy (2014) through case studies where the author elaborated on the neglect/abuse of the elderly by caregiver in residential settings. Formal caregivers who tend to stay with the patient had to take care of physical needs and provide company to the patient. He discussed the general problems faced with the home-based caregivers. Issues highlighted with the caregiver were the absenting from the work with or without notice, adjustability with the patient and family members, problem in providing food to the caregiver and language of communication. As hiring caregivers were generally through agencies, the age of the caregivers ranged from 19 years to middle aged women and majority of the staff employed were women. Moreover, the caregivers hired gave lot of trouble one after another.

7.9 CASE 9

7.9.1 Disease of the Musculoskeletal System—Cord Compression; Blood Pressure, Disease of the Endocrine System—Diabetes Mellitus

A daughter (age 62) explained the reason of her mother (age 85) who is not able to walk due to cord compression in the spine. "*Backbone dabi huyi hai* (Her backbone is compressed). When this problem happened, she was with me and she needed immediate surgery. The surgery went well but she still has issues in walking, lower part of her body is almost dead."

7.9.2 Care Provided by the Caregiver

Further she elaborated, "My mother has been looked after by a caretaker from the last 15 years. He was just 7-year-old, when he came to our house now his son is 21 years old, he holds a special place in our house and family, once when he was in need my mother gave him 10 lakhs for his sister's surgery. She even purchased a house for him as she is not able to walk, the caregiver helps her in bathing, grooming and dressing. She always says *Sadde wich naukar maalik wala sambandh nahi hai. jina mai kar sakdi ha mai kardi ha. Ohna nu sadi lodh nahi, sanu ohna di lodh hai* (She always says that we have a beautiful bond, there is nothing like owner and slave, how much ever I can do for him and his family I do, moreover we need them and not they need us)."

Corroborating on the importance of their caregiver in their life, the patient asserted "All my family resides in the United States. My caregiver who is more like a son to me is taking care of my house and me from the last 15 years and I think now I can think of living without my family but cannot think of staying away from my caregiver. My whole house is in his hands, from bringing vegetables to buying small or big things, it is all his responsibility." Banijamali

(2014) also indicated that home care workers job satisfaction, which is also influenced by extrinsic rewards (wages, fringe benefits etc.), training and career development. Because home care workers in the study were primarily working for clients who were alone in their homes, and considered the client as their family.

7.10 CASE 10

7.10.1 Disease of the Nervous system—Depression, Parkinson Disease; Blood Pressure, Disease of the Endocrine System—Diabetes Mellitus; Disease of the Kidneys

A husband (age 85) narrated the condition of his wife (age 82) who is diabetic from the last 20 years along with that, now she is living her life with Parkinson's disease from the last 2 years. To add on he says, my wife is suffering from depression from the last 20 years. I think the reason for her depression is she has no son and has four daughters. Due to depression, now there is very little movement in the body and day by day her condition is getting worse. Now, she cannot walk without the help of walker.

7.10.2 Help provided by Caregiver

Jad to caretaker aah gayi hai, hun sare kam chad dite hai (As we have kept caregiver for her care, now she has totally stopped doing all the work). She is also dealing with increased creatinine, urinary tract infection and bed wetting. *Bimar pe gai si, jad ethe aye si, actually himmat nahi, kam karan di habit khatam ho gayi hai* (She fell sick as we shifted here, actually she has stopped doing all the work). We have no issue with any caretaker, we cannot discriminate on any basis as they are extremely helpful to us. We are paying Rs. 1500 per day to them for their services.

7.10.3 Satisfaction with the Staff from Agency

Initially, the caregiver we employed had ran away. Now, we have waged staff (age 36 years) from the agency, and we are very satisfied with their work. She (caregiver) is also contented with the salary provided, she does her job with utmost professionalism and feels satisfied with her job. *Sari kitchen us de hawale hai* (all the work in the kitchen is also handled by her). We don't interfere with her work at any cost. There is improvement in my wife's condition, the main problem was earlier was that she felt lonely earlier in Bareilly but now since we have shifted to Chandigarh on rent, things have eased up, our daughter lives very nearby, her presence is a great motivation for her, she does everything for us. Despite of her very busy schedule, she manages everything.

Thoda left hand kambda hai, thoda chalde huye body disbalance ho jadi hai (Her left hand trembles due to Parkinson disease, she loses her balance, rest she is fine. I consider these home care staffs as a boon for sick and old people. Now, since the caregivers are with us from the last 1 year and we are totally dependent upon them and I would say, in every aspect my life has become very easier.

7.11 CASE 11

7.11.1 Disease of the Nervous System

A mother (age 84) narrated the story of her 61-year-old daughter who has been bedridden since she was 9 months old.

The mother narrates her ordeal saying, "Initially for the first few years, I tried everything that I could possibly do that was feasible or not so feasible to help improve her health. Born as a completely healthy child, I was hopeful that one day she will walk, she will talk, she will sit and with this hope I would spend my entire day working towards her health, grooming and taking her to physiotherapist 60km away everyday in the morning, giving home therapies with the tutor in the evening, giving her medicines after every two hours, being very regular with her sitting standing schedules with all her equipment. However, nothing changed, in fact with time her health worsened. Five years into it, I went into severe depression, it took a great toll on my life and health too. I didn't know when the day started and when the day ended. I had forgotten the meaning of the words "family life" or "social life" or "peaceful sleep", even in my sleep I would keep murmuring the timings of her medicines."

I had to send my other two daughters to the hostel, so that I could devote more time towards her. There came a time I was put on sleeping pills for several months and my doctor strictly advised me to maintain distance with her, he said that if I continued living that way, I would have gone mad. Though, I always had help from beginning but there was some sort of hesitance, it is only with time I learnt to trust them and to rely on them. Gradually, with my daughter's growth, even the basic tasks have become very difficult as she cannot even control her neck, with age, her weight and height have increased, she started getting periods, and things just got worse. The journey so far has been very painful, as a mother to see my child just lay on the bed helpless.

7.11.2 Caregiving was a Blessing to me

I am so thankful to the staff that takes care of her, because I know what they are doing for her, with my age and physique even I cannot do for her. It's because of the caretakers I am able to now lead my life normally. Rest of my two daughters are already married.

The staff that takes care of her is also like family to us, we now and we live, laugh, cry, celebrate together. I cannot thank enough to them for taking care of my daughter. They have been always been there for me, as well as her, they stuck by when times got tougher. Many times, when she has gotten really sick and it felt like there is no coming back, they gave her the best care. They cry or get sad as much as I do, their dedication in their work is paramount, I have never seen them feel disgusted by her or while doing personal chores for her such as changing her diapers. Sometimes, they had to also put their family behind like miss their family functions or occasional holidays for her sake. I love them like my family and try my best to also help them in their hard times as much as I can. There are no words to thank the caretakers, it's because of them we can live and move on with our lives carefree. My own children could have never helped me the way they have.

7.11.3 Message for the Families who have Employed Caregivers

I would just like to tell the loved ones of such patients that we should not forget that these caregivers are also humans, they also have a family. We should understand and realise that if we were ever put in their place, we wouldn't be able to handle the patient and come to their aid with so much efficiency, we should give them a leeway at times and understand that mistakes are bound to happen by anyone. Irrespective of whatever we are paying them, we should always be thankful to them for taking care of the patient like their own family.

7.12 CASE 12

7.12.1 Disease of the Nervous system—Alzheimer, Depression, and Disease of the Musculoskeletal System—Osteoporosis

A daughter (age 59) narrated the story of her mother (age 88) who is suffering from Alzheimer. In 2015, we lost our father, before his death she did everything for him. She stays upset, she feels very lonely and is also suffering from Gastritis and bowel incontinence. Yaffe *et al.* (2002) study explored the baseline characteristics of Dementia patients along with anger, aggressiveness, and psychotic symptoms, about 49 per cent of the patients were also suffering from bladder or bowel incontinence.

Continuing her ordeal the daughter says, "She is now getting disoriented *maine bolna ap bhul rahe ho* (I told her that you tend to forget things). Her condition is deteriorating. The prevalence of anxiety symptoms are also observed, she has been feeling restless. She is very attached to my brother and used to tell him, "I don't want to stay with your sister here, you take me home (*Tere sath ayi hu, tere sath hi jaugi)*, as she is now getting older, she is also suffering from osteoporosis."

7.12.2 Difficult Behaviour Accompanied with Alzheimer

She get aggressive at times (*Gusa to kam hi hota hai, naraz ho jati hai)* and tells us that I am not wrong, I don't forget anything. Sometimes, she feels like she has lost interest in everything. Recently, she has now been forgetting things, old memories are still fresh in her mind, but recent moments she forgets that she had breakfast in the morning. She doesn't remember the name of simple fruits. Sometimes, she claims to meet people she has not met from very long time. She gets anxious all the time and has lost interest in almost everything. From sometime, she doesn't express her interest to eat anything. We have noticed this problem from the last 2 years but I think now it has aggravated.

Her memory is in a jinx these days, she tends to mix the days of months with days of week. We used to tell her, "Mom, you have started to forget everything", in reply she always insisted that this is due to old age and did not accept that this is possibly due to her condition. My brother feels that she stays worried all the time and tells us that 'I don't want to stay alone' and after sometimes it's as if nothing happened, she does not remember anything. This I believe is due to the mood swings which people suffering from dementia go through. Muller-Spahn (2003) explored behavioural disturbances in demented patients. Psychological symptoms and behavioural abnormalities are common characteristics of dementia. These symptoms include depression, memory loss, anxiety, loss of interest/apathy, delusions, irritability, dis-inhibition, wandering, psychosis, aggressiveness, urinary incontinence and sleep disturbances.

7.12.3 Caregiver is like a Blessing to the Family

The narrator continues to tell, "Due to her ailing condition, we have waged a caregiver who is there with us for 24 hours as this disease requires 24 hours monitoring as the behaviour of person changes and much of the time, the person behave suspiciously. They go so extreme in their mind that wild thoughts such as that their near ones are now willing to disown her are common to them. I believe a caregiver is like a blessing to family, as she is very concerned about our patient and luckily, we are a finding an improvement in her condition."

Grunfeld *et al.* (1997) discussed about caring for dementia patient is one of the most difficult challenges that are faced by caregivers. In Alzheimer's disease, the cognitive deterioration progresses steadily with no possibility of remission. The cognitive problems impair their social skills of the person and would lead to disruptive or difficult behaviour and also changes appear in their personality, and they generally suffer from physical disability as well. So, the patients with advanced dementia requires 24 hours surveillance.

7.13 CASE 13

7.13.1 Neoplasm—Bone Cancer; Blood Pressure; Disease of the Endocrine System—Diabetes Mellitus

The daughter-in-law (age 43) of the patient (age 67) elaborated on the sufferings of her father-in-law who was suffering from cancer of bones. She recounts, "Our house is on the 2nd floor and we needed to call the ambulance after every two days. It was a miserable time, so, we thought of renting the room at ground floor. It started gradually, one day he was not able to walk. *Waist toh niche wala portion almost dead ho gaya si* (Body below the waist is almost dead). Once, he went to pick his granddaughter and he fell down. He complained he feels pain in bones. As we got his PET scan done, we got to know he is in his 3rd stage of Cancer. He used to feel pain in knees and used to depend on painkillers very frequently. By this time, he was in the last stages of his suffering. Doctors clearly told us that he has just 6 months to live and this was in December 2021. He later passed away in May 2022."

7.13.2 Problem Faced with Caregiver

When he lived, we had a really tough time finding caregivers for my father-in-law. My husband used to help in the evenings and mornings but else there was a great problem as we were only able to find male caregivers for his care and we found that female staffs were reluctant to work for a male patient. We paid Rs. 500 daily for 12 hours a day and later we employed two caregivers as my mother-in-law was not ready to do anything for my father-in-law. She did not help with any of his chores. Once when the caregiver was not present, my father-in-law had peed in his diapers and my mother-in-law straightaway refused to clean him. He lied in that wet diaper for long until my husband came home and cleaned him.

7.13.3 Dissatisfaction Regarding Caregiving Services

I used to feel bad about my father-in-law's condition. I was not satisfied with the caregivers as they were not responsible, sometimes they used to be late and sometimes they were reluctant to clean his stool. Initially, his condition improved till he was hospitalised. After 3 sessions of chemotherapy, there was rather no improvement. He was later admitted in ICU (Intensive care unit), his blood pressure was being on the higher side and later due to multi- organ failure, he passed away. With regard to the home care services, we were not satisfied with the caregivers, we changed many caregivers, but overall, just two of them who we had employed at the end of his journey were good. Similar results were discussed by Vyasamoorthy (2014) where the series of caregivers hired gave lot of trouble one after another. Only one among the eight were nice, cooperative and helpful.

7.14 CASE 14

7.14.1 Neoplasm—Breast Cancer; Blood Pressure

A daughter-in-law narrated the condition of her mother-in-law who was suffering from breast Cancer. She elaborated, "My mother-in-law felt a cyst in her breast which was excruciatingly painful for her, as we got her PET scan done, she was in her second stage of cancer. After 2 days of detection, she underwent through a surgery and the doctors removed the breast. Later, after her surgery, there was vomiting, dizziness, weight loss, and hair loss. Initially, she had very long hairs till knees but due to chemotherapy, all her hairs were lost. Her breasts were removed during the surgery and she had lost her zeal to live, she no longer wanted to do basic things such as dress up or colour her hair anymore."

7.14.2 The Home care Staff was a Great Help

For period of one month the caregiver used to help her in bathing, grooming and dressing, massage her body and took her for a walk. Moreover, she also provided oral medications and meals at proper timings. The care my mother-in-law received helped her to restart her life and she is perfectly fine now.

7.15 CASE 15

7.15.1 Disease of the Nervous System—Paralytic Disease; Blood Pressure

A daughter (age 55) elaborated on the condition of her father (age 89), who suffered a paralytic attack. She mentioned her father prior to the attack was a self-sufficient man who owned a cloth shop and fend for himself. Later, after his condition worsened, he was unable to talk, unable to walk and was even not able to hold his plate by himself. He had lost the ability to talk and used to converse through gestures.

7.15.2 Duties Performed by the Caregivers

We employed two home care staffs to look after him, each for him worked towards his care for a 12-hour shift. We paid them 12,000 monthly for working 12 hours a day. The caregivers supported him with their activities of daily routine, helping him with the toilet, grooming, bathing, eating, helping them with exercises, used to take him to the park on wheel chair and also assisted him with medication. While the experience with most of the staff employed were very good on the contrary, some boys were reluctant to change diapers and spent long hours on talking on their phones or consuming content over the internet.

7.16 CASE 16

7.16.1 Neoplasm—Rectal Cancer; Bedsores; Disease of the Endocrine System—Diabetes Mellitus

The daughter-in law (age 50) narrated the sufferings of her mother-in-law (age 78) who was suffering from rectal cancer. Her cancer was detected on 28th January, 2021. She had few symptoms of rectal cancer. There were changes in bowel movements such as constipation, diarrhoea and there were more frequent bowel movements. Grievingly, her daughter-in-law asserted that her mother-in-law has been in pain, her health has been on the downside, there was unexplained weight loss, abdominal pain, feeling that you haven't completely relieved yourself. Frequently, there was blood in stool. Talking about her mother-in-law's strength and resilience she says, "One thing I would always remember that despite of having so much pain, she remained very calm and content all the time."

7.16.2 Being in the Shoes as a Primary Caregiver

For a period of about 3 months, we did not put her on using diapers. I used to help her with everything. I used to clean her up, prepare meals for her and help and support her in performing activities of daily living. There was no help from other relatives. Given *et al.* (2001) reported that caregiver experience challenges in caring for cancer patients in pain management, activities of daily living, patient mobilization, and communication with the health personnel, medicinal management, and the management of emotional reactions of the patient and often feel helpless due to uncontrolled patient pains.

7.16.3 Problems Faced by the Staff from Agencies

Emphasizing on her stance, she says "I employed two lady caregivers for my mother-in-law, but I feel we have to remind them for many things. I had to keep an eye on them. They were never helpful in the kitchen, I prepared meals for my mother-in-law and they only helped her in having her meals. Many a times, the agencies used to change staff on their own and it wasn't always a smooth journey with everyone. Some were unwilling to clean her up, they were also not ready to wash her dirty and soiled clothes." She extrapolates that the presence of primary caregiver is very important, however, if the family is not keeping an eye on the staff, they will sometimes fool us in some way or the other. She continues, "I felt that the caregivers are not paid adequate amount by the agencies. The amount charged by the agencies was Rs. 18,000 per shift (per month) from us and the caregivers too feel that with the salary they are not able to cover for their expenses and they are not able to save up. Vyasamoorthy (2014) also discussed the causes of caregiver behaviour such as caregiver is stressed, lack of empathy towards the senior citizens, lack of cooperation from senior citizen, abusing behaviour of the patients, low salary, lack of trainings, anger/dissatisfaction with the hiring agency, long working hours, demanding employers and other reasons.

7.17 CASE 17

7.17.1 Multiple Ailments—Hearing Loss, Vision Problem

A daughter (age 62) elaborated on the changes which she is visualizing in her mother (age 89). She elaborated that we feel that she tends to forget things, sometimes repeat little things. We have employed two trained personal care assistants for her care. She is suffering from multiple problems such as weakness, difficulty in walking, with age she has become hard of hearing and also her vision is also very weak. The caregivers employed for her in performing activities of daily living such as bathing, dressing and assist in walking and fall prevention.

7.17.2 Patient and Caregiver Share Beautiful Bond

Anita (age 25) and Reshma (age 21), the caregivers are also content with their job. They have been working in the said household from the last one year. They told, that they come from far away and that their home is around 10 km away, to reach here they take an auto. They insisted that they always maintain a cheerful demeanor and feel at home with the patient.

The daughter further shares, "Earlier, my mother was rejecting all the caregivers, but now she feels happier and much relaxed when these caregivers are besides her. It is their warmth, behaviour and personality that has endeared them to the family and the patient. Now my mother has a new fondness for life as she is getting better, she likes to put on her traditional outfits as whenever she goes out and likes to do activities she desires."

7.18 CASE 18

7.18.1 Blood Pressure; Bedsores; Disease of the Endocrine System—Diabetes Mellitus; Disease of the Kidneys—Kidney Failure; Disease of the Musculoskeletal—Hip Fracture

The patient (mother-in-law, age 65) was battling many challenges with her health. Despite that, the family is closely knit who continue to manage to keep a smile on their faces, they are brave hearts and have taken their troubles in stride.

The daughter-in-law (age 46) narrates, "For a long time, my mother-in-law (age 65), a person with diabetes, hypertension, hip fracture managed her medications on her own and with the help of the family members. However, things took a turn when her kidneys were infected. The family felt it risky to let things be. She was undergoing infusion therapy (to balance body electrolytes and levels, it is a long-term treatment that can help minimise the need of kidney dialysis or kidney transplant). Later, there was an electrolyte imbalance in the body and water retention in the whole body which led to severe swelling. The conditions worsened, there were a slew of problems such as heart was working 15 per cent, electrolyte imbalance, water imbalance and kidney issue which was accompanied by weight loss, swollen ankles, blood in urine. Unfortunately, there was a multi-organ failure and she could not be revived."

7.18.2 Help Provided by the Caregivers

We employed caregivers to manage her numerous medicines, the home attendant was delegated with the task of helping the patient with her activities of daily living, keeping her engaged with light exercises, personal grooming, relieving her stress with various modes of entertainment among other things. Her job also includes regularly monitoring her BP and blood sugar levels and most importantly administer her insulin. I think they have been a great help. She is compassionate and extremely sensitive to the patient needs especially their mental health issues.

7.19 CASE 19

7.19.1 Disease of the Musculoskeletal system—Arthritis, Disease of the Endocrine System—Diabetes Mellitus; Disease of the Cardiovascular System—Heart disease, Hypertension, Macular Degeneration, Disease of the Skin—Sclerosis

A daughter (age 68) explained the condition of her mother (age 92) who is suffering from Sclerosis (it is accompanied with the outgrowth of interstitial tissues).

She illuminated about her mother's condition, "In these cases, the geriatrics have to undergo surgery to address long-standing problems and, if they do not recover well, their mobility will get compromised. As a result, elder assistance in the form of professional post-operative care becomes essential. A good idea is to seek elder assistance in the form of an established home nursing care provider. My mother has been availing caregiver services for the last four years now. She suffers from heart disease, hypertension and macular degeneration (It happens when the small central portion of the retina which is called macula wears down, it is often age-related macular degeneration, this usually does not cause blindness but might cause severe vision problems). Doctors explained that the blood vessels underneath her macula and these vessels leak blood and fluid into retina. She underwent surgery for macular degeneration at the same time. Because of this, she was in need of post-operative care and her condition warranted 24-hour monitoring and professional elder assistance. Also, owing to the progression of arthritis, the onset of the disease affected her ability to coordinate the movement of her limbs. Therefore, she cannot balance herself. Earlier, she was able to perform all her activities of daily living."

7.19.2 Having Home Care Attendants has Become Part of our Family

It is a wonderful relationship that the home attendants share with us, they have all bonded well with the family. This bond is mutual even we treat them like our own children. Now, we have one caregiver (age 27) who stays round the clock with my mother to attend to her needs like toilet care, food and medication.

These workers are called support worker who are employed and paid to provide assistance with a variety of activities, including personal care and activities of daily living (Access Community Health, 2012; Careers, 2014).

7.20. CASE 20

7.20.1 Disease of the Nervous System—Paralytic Disease; Blood Pressure; Disease of the Endocrine System—Diabetes Mellitus

A daughter (age 58) describes the condition of her mother (age 83), who is suffering from paralytic disease and is wheelchair-bound. She gives an account of her mother's case, "It was in 2009, when my mother had a stroke (a stroke is the common underlying condition that trigger partial or complete paralysis in patients. In partial paralysis, the patient has still partial control over the affected muscles and in complete paralysis, the patient has no control over the affected muscles). She suffered from partial paralysis. At that time, she stayed in Haridwar and the medical facilities were not up to the mark in the city as the specialist doctors were unavailable. Keeping in mind her underlying condition, we shifted her to Chandigarh in 2013. We then employed two nursing staff for her care, the first caregiver used to work from 7am to 7pm and the other worked after this till morning.

7.20.2 Help Provided by the Nurses and Personal Duty Assistants

We have seen a total of 15-18 home attendants come and go. Presently, we have a nursing manager (NM) who visits the household every month. The NM monitors her health condition. In addition to that, the NM evaluates the home attendant's performance and offers guidance. Owing to her health constraints, she spends long hours in bed, her condition is called Hemiplegia (it is a type of paralysis where a person loses control over one side of the body). With passing years, she has lost her will power. The caregivers indulge with her and keep her engaged with light exercises, performing personal grooming, relieving her stress with various modes of entertainment among other things. They also regularly monitor her blood pressure and blood sugar levels. Due to her condition, she is being fed through the Ryle's tube. It has been years now, since 2009 she is in the same condition.

7.20.3 The Caregivers I believe were a Great Help

Although it is a fact that caregivers have put in consistent efforts but my mother never felt comfortable with them. Now, she doesn't put any efforts for her own as it has been so many years. She has lost all hope of getting back on her feet and getting better. She highlights the importance of caregiver training on aspects concerning mental health.

Several care workers in the study also acknowledged the benefits of training and stated that they have learnt a large amount of their work by simply being on the job. This included efficient techniques needed to help the patient in showering, hand hygiene, dressing and drying the patient, lifting, manoeuvering, medications, common health conditions, client safety and their own safety (George *et al.*, 2017).

7.21. CASE 21

7.21.1 Disease of the Musculoskeletal System—Injury; Disease of the Endocrine System—Diabetes Mellitus; Disease of the Cardiovascular System—Heart Disease

A daughter (age 55) elaborated the condition of her father (age 88). "He met with an accident 35 years back. He does not have a knee joint, so his leg is straight. He is able to do all his work except if he falls down, he cannot stand on his own. Once he fell down, now he is not able to move his right shoulder. Along with that few years back, he underwent a bypass surgery, leading to which there were a few complications in the surgery, and his water vein was clipped, and for circulation of water, we used a machine, we also had to make him wear the socks which are used in varicose veins, otherwise there would be swelling in the whole leg. Additionally, he is also a diabetic patient. It was a family decision and friend's suggestion to opt for a caregiver for him because it was becoming difficult to move him around as he was too heavy."

7.21.2 Help Provided by the Caregiver

The daughter enlightened how this decision helped them immensely and the family members were able to find some time for themselves. They felt they got much-needed respite. In addition, caregiver's (age 31) cordial attitude helped the patient feel much better. He helped the client in performing activities of daily living, bathing, dressing, grooming and also engaged him in physiotherapy exercises, so that he could move his right shoulder along with that, he engaged in conversations with him every now and then which made him feel happy.

7.21.3 Happy with the Home Care Given to Senior

The patient's daughter and family members are content and happy with the quality of home care he received. She discussed that she could not ever point any negligence in their dedication towards their work and was satisfied with their service. The caregiver remains with the family and is serving them from last two years.

7.22. CASE 22

7.22.1 Disease of the Nervous System—Parkinson's Disease, Dementia

Sometimes, home care becomes inevitable. A daughter (age 57) discusses, "My mother's (age 86) life has not been the same ever since she was diagnosed with Parkinson's disease, initially, she used to complain about back pain in the spinal area. Over the last year, she had two falling incidents, although she escaped unhurt, she has developed a fear of falling which led her to cut down on her physical activities. As a result of this, there is slowness of movement and she is experiencing difficulty in walking. This disease is accompanied with degenerative disorder of the nervous system that has mainly affected the motor system. She adds on, I am visualising the cognitive and behavioural problems such as depression, anxiety, irresponsiveness in my mother from a span of 10 weeks. She has started experiencing weakness. And she could not muster the courage to get back to her normal activities. When a senior citizen who has always led a very active life suddenly became lethargic and their confidence level drops. Cognitively, she is not any better, she cannot move independently, she doesn't recognise me. She is now suffering from Parkinson's disease and dementia as there is a huge memory loss, by now she is in the advance stages of the disease."

7.22.2 Training Needs required for Formal Caregivers

The caregiver (age 26) was an enthusiastic and confident professional home care giver who came to offer elderly assistance. She offered her mobility assistance. She has been there with us for 4 months now. She is versed with how to engage the patient. She also helped her with activities of daily living and managed her medication as well.

Presently, at this movement, we have somebody else but I am not satisfied with their nursing services. She is quite happy to change her diapers but I have to remind her about so many other things, she is not trained according to the patient's requirements. The last caregiver was very trained who understood that falling down again and again can affect the quality of a senior's life adversely. She also was aware on how such falls could be prevented to a large extent. Therefore, she paid extra attention towards very basic but little things such as keeping her bathroom dry was always a high priority for her. Also, when she notices any kind of risks that may lead to a fall, she was quick to take precautions. She made a relationship with my mother and our family and she understood her needs and how to deliver them. One has to understand the Parkinson's disease takes years to develop. Definitely, my mother is improving. At one point she could not even recognise me which has gotten better now. It is all due to the personal care that matters a lot. I believe home care team needs more training as the home care staff has the sole responsibility of looking after the patient and they should be well trained according to the underlying condition of the patient.

Agencies should identify patient characteristics associated with hospitalization as high-risk patients require specialized intervention beyond the traditional home care services provided (Ellenbecker *et al.*, 2008).

7.23. CASE 23

7.23.1 Neoplasm—Cancer of the Lungs

A daughter (age 40) narrated the story of her mother. She explained that her mother was diagnosed with lung cancer at the age of 60. By the time it was identified it was already in an advanced stage. Her doctors told that she has very less time to live yet she survived 4 years and she passed away very recently in 2022, this was when she was 64 years old.

7.23.2 Her Journey during Cancer was not easy

She faced many problems including financial troubles. It was totally a private treatment so it costs much more as compared to government hospitals-based treatment. During her chemotherapy she faced many health issues including social stigma due to hair loss. Many of our close relatives who came to visit her often asked her many questions regarding her baldness. Being a female, it was really a very tough phase to accept all these harsh and painful remarks on her looks. On the other hand, her medicines had so many side effects including dry itchy skin, loss of calcium and low hemoglobin. The most important factor in a cancer patient's life is the emotional struggle they go through. They are also well aware with the harsh reality that they may not be left with much time and yet they have to fight on and try to live keeping up a brave face and maintaining their inner strength to fight against the dreadful disease. The economic burden faced by family caregivers is significant as they report financial losses, getting out of their pocket expenses, lost wages due to time taken for caregiving (Addington *et al.*, 1992; Covinsky *et al.*, 1994; Stommel *et al.*, 1993).

7.23.3 Help Provided by the Home care Staff

The caregiver *Samita* was extremely helpful, she helped my mother in performing all activities of daily living and was there with my mother for 24 hours. They would sit and talk, she used to feel happy when *Samita* was around her. As me and my sister were busy in our lives, she would spend and dedicate much of her time with our mother. The caregiver kept her cheerful and engaged in her, she even helped my mother in the kitchen. We truly believe, it is the home care staff who is responsible for all their work.

Tsigaroppoulos *et al.* (2009) examined the problems faced by relatives caring for cancer patients at home. The most frequent problems reported were anxiety (61.8%) regarding what will happen in the future to the patient, 54 per cent felt pain due to the patient condition, increased economic burden and financial burden was felt by (51.3%) primary caregivers. Additional problems faced were problems with patient feeding (54%), depression (48.7%), emotionally upset (47.4%), worsening of patient behaviour and personality (38.2%), difficulty in establishing a positive attitude towards their underlying condition (34.2%) and assistance from wider family circle (25%). Similar problems were faced by family members suffering from cancer in the present study.

7.24. CASE 24

7.24.1 Neoplasm—Bone Cancer; Blood Pressure; Disease of the Endocrine System—Diabetes Mellitus; Disease of the Cardiovascular System—Heart Disease; Disease of the Respiratory System

A daughter-in-law (age 61) narrated the story of her mother-in-law (age 88) who is suffering from bone cancer. She orates, "I meet and interact with the nursing staffs to understand various aspects of geriatric care. Initially many years back, she (mother-in-law) underwent through bypass surgery. She was suffering from a slew of problems and was bedridden from the last 1 year. In addition to this, she was battling illnesses in the form of faecal incontinence (uncontrolled bowel movements, causing stool (faeces) to leak unexpectedly from the rectum). Later, the diagnosis revealed she also had Stage III bone cancer. By the end, she was bedridden and needed help with all activities of daily living. She would have food through Ryle's tube. As she was quite heavy, moving her on a bed and off was a tough task."

7.24.2 Adjustment made from the Families towards Nursing Staff

The family then decided to keep one nursing staff and one general duty assistant to look after the ailing patient. Talking about the experience with them they say, the caregiver (age 32) helped in giving medication to the patient, washed and ironed her clothes and massaged her body throughout the day but the nursing staff (age 31) was very fussy, she was not ready to clean the bed where the patient slept but overall, she was well trained and was good at her job. The family maid used to wash her clothes. We paid her Rs. 25000 per month for working 12 hours a day. The whole family cared for her. During her last days, the doctors clearly told us that there is no scope of any surgery but she was a lady with strong will power, and she wanted to spend time and stay at home with her family. By this time, she was on oxygen support as she also suffered from issues of breathing from a long time and the illness has aggravated this condition. Her death was not natural, as the oxygen machine was on inverter support and there was some issue with electricity. At some point the machine stopped working and it was due to lack of oxygen that she passed away.

Studies have reflected that developing countries are facing several technological and social challenges, which affect the supply and demand for home care services (Beer *et al.*, 2014; Megaritis *et al.*, 2018).

7.25. CASE 25

7.25.1 Disease of the Nervous System—Dementia; Disease of the Musculoskeletal System—Fracture

A son (age 52) narrated the story of his mother (age 89) who had started developing_dementia around two years ago. Sadly, the disease has slowly progressed since then. She tends to forget things, for instance she would forget where the washroom is. If there is a change of room, she would feel as if she is not at home and is somewhere else. She forgets to take her medicines, and instead of taking one medicine, she takes the same blood pressure medicine thrice. Whenever, she talks on phone, she only recalls her old memories. She would not remember recent events as in what she had for breakfast in a particular day she will not remember. Sometimes, she behaves aggressively, but she always feels and insists that she remembers everything. In December 2020, she accidentally fell at night and broke her femur bone. As a result of the accident, she is bedridden now and needs help with activities of daily living.

It is suggested that falls are the leading cause of injury related death for the geriatric population. Centres for Medicare & Medicaid Services (2006) suggested that emergency care for injury caused by accidents or falls is one of the adverse events occurring for patients receiving care at home. 30 per cent of the people (age 65) fall each year and one in every five patients requires medical attention (Gillespie *et al.*, 2003).

7.25.2 Training covered by the Home Care Staff

The son continues, "We decided to avail professional care from a home nursing care provider. Keeping our mother as comfortable as possible in the given situation was our goal. We believe post-hospitalisation, the care is very important. This training covers basic physiotherapy exercises for geriatric. It also focuses on the importance of fall prevention and aspects of mobility assistance for seniors with different underlying conditions. I am hopeful that my mother is improving as caregivers work round the clock and follow a patient care plan."

7.26. CASE 26

7.26.1 Disease of the Nervous System—Alzheimer; Blood Pressure

Sharing her agonizing experience, A female shares, "I was born as an illegitimate child as my father left my mother while I was still in the womb. My mother though gave birth to me but she never really was a mother to me, she wanted to love me but she was so caught up in her misery and loneliness that her soul and heart were just not only capable of giving the warmth that I deserved. With time her sadness turned into loneliness and then into madness and instability. I was just 12 years when she tried to kill me by forcing me to drink poison it was then that I was sent to an orphanage and my mother to a mental hospital. I spent my entire childhood in the confusion and dilemma alternating between the questions as to what was better that I am an orphan and have none to love and call family or that my only family "my mother" is the sole reason for me being called an orphan. I was 24 years old, doing good for myself, had a decent job, was earning enough to have a decent life and then I received a phone call that shook my so called "self-made life". It was from the hospital, that my mother wasn't a danger to anyone anymore though they made it clear that she could still have her episodes of depression and is also suffering from Alzheimer's disease. Anyhow, I took the decision to get her home the same way that she had made a call years ago to give birth to me with a heavy heart and no understanding of what future holds for her.

She was there right in front of me, and all the time, it was frustrating to even look at her, I was infuriated to have her in my surroundings, she was the same women, the women I hated the most yet the only women I could ever call my family. Life had given me one chance that I neither wanted nor wanted to miss upon. My heart wept when I had to be the mother to her that she never was to me. It was fine till I had to cook for her, or even spend on her medicines etc. I was earning good and I didn't mind taking care of her expenses but suddenly I had company while I was used to living alone as I had spent my entire life yearning for the love and affection of a family and that killed me from inside. However, there were times when she had her episodes of panic and dementia and she would zone out and would be unable to physically to do anything for herself and I had to feed her and even give her a bath. I just couldn't do that; I didn't have the strength mentally to do that. I would often wonder what life had thrown at me, what on earth I had done to relive the misery. However, on the other hand, that period made me realize that god had put me in her shoes. It felt exactly the same, once she had blamed me for her misery, now I blamed her for mine. This is when I understood why it was so hard for her to love me and give me the warmth that I needed.

We were both stuck in this viscous cycle and both of our lives were so tangled but I had no one to turn to or ask for help. It felt like I was turning into her, for my sanity it became very necessary that I hire a help, a third party who would save both of us from drowning. That was a changing point, the less I was around her in her misery, the more quality time I was able to spend with her. Initially, I didn't care much if the help did the needful, but with time it mattered, if everything was on time and done in a proper way. We have had the same lady caregiver from the beginning and she has been the witness of our life in a major way. I am married now and my mother (age 65) and caregiver (age 50) lives with us. Things are better, though we both still have our episodes of sadness but there are also times when we are happy and content. I would say that if I didn't hire help that time, I would have drowned with my mother and she saved us both."

7.26.2 Caregiver is more than a Family

Sometimes, I feel she (caregiver) played the much-needed role of the mother in my life. She was ears to both of us, we both would talk about each other to her (caregiver) and vent our hearts out but she was always a mediator, it felt she was a mother to her two children. I can never thank her enough for helping us mould our lives and move on. There was a time I was called an orphan and now I have two mothers, a loving husband and two very beautiful children.

Due to dementia, sometimes, my mother still utters the same sentences that she used on me when I was a child. "Why were you born, how can I kill you?" She sometimes gets confused and behave suspiciously but I know it's the dementia talking. Now as her age has progressed, there is huge memory loss, she does not speak properly. Day by day, her condition is deteriorating. But still once again I give the entire credit to the caregiver to fill the void in our lives and be our guardian angel. Life would have passed anyhow but now at least I have a family now.

7.27 CASE 27

7.27.1 Disease of the Nervous System—Alzheimer

Another son (age 55 years) shared the story of his mother (age 89 years), "After my father's retirement, my mother and father used to live in village. We are five brothers and after my father passed away, my mother preferred to stay with my elder brother. It was tragic that as his son got married, they shifted our mother to the drawing room. From that day on, she started feeling annoyed and disturbed. Even she used to get aggressive with her grandsons and daughter. She felt she has been shifted out of her room. There were changes in her behaviour. Around the same time she suffered a clot in her brain.

Due to her ailing condition, I bought her at our place in Chandigarh. Now as she was staying with us, there was little improvement in her condition. All brothers decided to keep mother for three months. In agony, she once grieved and said you all tend to send me here and there *(mere ko idhar-udhar bhejte ho).* After having her breakfast, she used to cry a lot, take her clothes out and throw in the bag, she threw her blanket in the bag and it seemed that she is waiting for someone to go somewhere. One day, she was looking confused and disoriented. After seeing her condition, we all got little alert by her behaviour

Now in the mornings, we take her for a walk, but she started getting aggressive day by day. It felt like she has really lost her memory. Doctor prescribed medicines for memory enhancement for a period of 6 months. She was showing uncharacteristic jealousy, sometimes screams loudly, bangs on the doors, takes off all her clothes, forgets to wash her hand after using toilet and spills her food and tea. One day while walking in the park, she slipped and broke her hip joint bone. It was the time of COVID-19 when she had the surgery. I was surprised by the attitude of my brother at that time who told us to send mother to him only after getting a COVID test done.

By this time, we needed a caregiver for her care. Initially, she used to get annoyed with her caregiver who used to take to her to the park, massage her body, and wash her clothes, she adjusted with her with time and mother used to give her blessings. *Kabhi Kabhi bachpan ki bate karte hai, unke apne maike jana hai* (She talks about her old memories and the will to visit her parents' house). She used to wake up at night and walk around and she once hit her head into the shelf but she is better now. I think the main problem is that she is not able to stay at one place for a longer period as no one wants to really keep her. She always insists that she wants to go to her native village. Sometimes, she sits and stares at me and tells me that I am trying to cement your face into my memory.

Because no one was actually ready to take her responsibility, having a caregiver with us was a blessing. Doctors clearly told that she will have more memory loss with time. Once without informing anyone, she went to out of home too, upon asking she told that she was going to the railway station without knowing the reason why.

7.27.2 Caregiver was like a Family to us

Mother ki pension hum rakhege. Jitna kharcha aata hai, mother ki pension se use karege (We will keep her pension now, and will carry all her expenses out of those).We have now employed two caregivers, one who comes in the morning and another who does the night shift. *Even medicine lene me problem, khane me panga karte hai, khana kum khaya tab mujhe tension, toilet nahi kari tab mujhe tension* (She is not ready to take her medicines, don't want to take her food and I feel tense if she don't have her food or get constipated. All my family members worry for me they feel I might get sick caring for her. I am attached to my mother, but no other children are attached to her. I value my mother while others don't value her. *Joint families khatam ho gayi hai* (There are no more joint families now), when I get busy with some work, mother will throw tantrums such as she would throw her food here and there. When she is outside, she would tell all neighbours that they don't want to keep me at home and do not provide me food. She forgets that she has had her breakfast. Sometimes, I feel as helpless as my mother too feels that we all don't understand her. Therefore, I feel having home care staff is a blessing for all of us, as now-a-days, nobody has really time for their parents and nor anyone is interested to spend money on their parents.

7.28. CASE 28

7.28.1 Disease of the Nervous System—Alzheimer; Disease of the Endocrine System—Diabetes Mellitus; Neoplasm—Prostate Cancer

The son-in-law (age 56) described about the condition of his father-in-law who is aged 88 years and is living his life with Dementia. He recalls his old memories but could not recall recent memories as to what he had in the morning. He lives alone in his own home as he only has one daughter who is now married but he likes to stay at his own home. We always try to spend weekends at his place, sometimes, insist him to stay with us but he is reluctant to leave his house. So, we have employed one caregiver to look after him.

7.28.2 Caregiver and the Patient share a Beautiful Bond

The caregiver (age 29) possesses good handling skills. They help us with all simple activities like peeling vegetables. They share a beautiful bond like daughter and father. He is also suffering from prostate cancer. So we have also waged one male nursing staff (age 32) to monitor his daily vitals. "He remembers a lot about the good olden days and has many stories to share" remarks the caregiver. "He is occupied and active and that is all we want, we are happy. We enjoy spending time dancing and singing, this creates an environment of happiness and cheerfulness."

By far it is established that home care services are very important to support people who are caring for senior population in the advanced stages of diseases (Philp *et al.*, 1995; Howarth and Willison, 1995; Istjanson, 1989). It is very important that family caregiver must be present in the home for caring for patient with dementia or other terminal illness. Management of dementia involves care for the behavioural, functional, cognitive and emotional changes that occur as a part of illness. As the stress of caring for a family member has adverse effects on the health of primary caregivers. They tend to develop depression and anxiety symptoms in the process of their caring. The absence of an able and willing caregiver has been identified as an obstacle in providing palliative care services at home (Lubin,1992; Ley,1989; Bruera *et al.*,1990). However, most of the caregivers interviewed in the present study found caring for their sick member burdensome with effect of illness on the family finances, disruption of normal family routine, sleep sickness, separation anxiety and the production of stress symptoms in both the caregivers and patients. The physical dependency of the patient reduces their interaction with other family members, relatives and also curtail their participation in social activities. Research also focuses on how the tradition of caregiving has taken a dramatic emotional, physical and financial tool on the primary caregivers (Sarkar and Anand, 2013). Having a home care staff is a blessing, as families don't have time for their loved ones and most importantly, home care is often the preferred option for many patients and their families though the physical, monetary and emotional cost of providing care at home can be a burden to patients, their families and caregivers and home care enables people to age in place and keeps families in tact.

Through all these findings, the researcher came up with the few points that can help to understand the insight of working with the caregiver. Furthermore, the researcher also discussed the responsibilities of clients and the benefits of home health care to geriatrics.

7.29 Insights of Working with the Caregiver

- Care giving is a tough job and mental fatigue is common. The ability to give the caregiver a sense of purpose and advancement determines whether she continues to stay on or quit after a brief inning of work.
- One should not assume that caregivers would immediately understand the senior, their illness, and their needs. There are certain specificities about the patient/senior that only one can know and tell as family members. For example, have a list that one would talk about in the first few days

to the caregiver, or that the mother-in-law likes slightly warm water for bathing- it should not be too warm. The expectations should be discussed for example- the bathroom should not smell foul or the bathroom should be dry at all times.

- The caregiver must be informed about the challenges and the ways of dealing with seniors suffering from conditions like Alzheimer's disease and dementia. One should never assume the caregiver would be familiar with all the behavioural manifestations of the disease. Talk with them about it on the first day itself.
- Any tips that one may have, must be shared with the caregiver. Making a list and sharing it with the caregiver on their first day will boost the confidence of the caregiver. It will help them feel more confident about handling the senior. For example, one may discuss that sometimes, my mother-in-law does not understand how to swallow liquids and food. She can hold food in her mouth for a very long time without swallowing it. If one prompts her to speak something, she is likely to swallow her food first. Another trick is offering her yet another morsel of food or water. This also reminds her to swallow the previous morsel.
- One should be specific about how much water they want the senior/patient to drink in a day and how much food they want them to eat. If the patient refuses to eat, let the caregiver know what alternative supplements or drinks can be given.
- It is deemed helpful to print a medicine chart and paste it on the wall or cupboard in the patient's room. The medicine chart should list the medicine name, the dosage to be administered, and the time of the day. If caregivers can't read the medicine names well, use of colour codes may be helpful.
- One must ensure to prepare a timetable for the caregivers to follow. For the first 2-3 days, let them know that the

timetable is to be followed strictly. Ensure they stick to the time as much as possible. One must allow caregivers sufficient rest also if they are performing a live-in shift (24 hrs).

- One must print all important phone numbers that caregivers can refer to in case of an emergency. Stick this information next to the medical chart and timetable.
- One must spend the first 1 or 2 days supervising the caregiver and setting expectations. If the first two days are managed well, sailing through the remaining days is rather smooth.
- All seniors should be engaged in meaningful activities of their choice and caregivers can shoulder this responsibility, including specific activities in the daily timetable and ensuring that caregivers adhere to them as much as possible.
- There must be dedicated time everyday for exercise. All seniors irrespective of their condition should exercise in some way or the other. Bedridden seniors benefit from passive movement exercises suggested by a physiotherapist. Massage can also help. All expectations must be on the first day. Video record the exercise regime so that the new caregivers in the future can use this recording.
- In the case of a senior who uses wheelchair or walker, one must ensure that the caregiver knows how to use it too. If not, they should be explained or demonstrated about their use.

7.30 Responsibility of Clients

- It is the responsibility of the client's to provide a safe and secure environment to the caregiver. The patient/client shall take full responsibility and care to ensure that there is no verbal, mental, or physical harassment or abuse of the caregiver at the patient's location including, not exposing them to any hazardous and infectious work environment.

- Treat the caregiver as a paramedical professional and not utilize him/her for jobs outside the scope of work.
- To provide caregivers tools and equipment to carry out his/her job including "Personal Protective Equipment" like disposable gloves, masks, aprons etc. to care for the patients.
- To inform the caregiver if the patient is suffering from any infectious disease like TB, HIV/AIDS, or Hepatitis which can adversely affect the health of the caregiver.
- To provide immediate medical attention to the caregiver in case of any sickness or accident without any delay.
- To not keep the caregiver against her/his wishes. Retaining the caregiver against her/his wishes construes illegal detention and only the client will be responsible for arising from the behaviour of the client or any harm done to the caregiver.
- To provide food and accommodation to live in for the caregiver.

7.31 Benefits of Home Health Care to Seniors

- With home care, the patient is not one among many patients as in a hospital, he/she is the only patient in home care. The personalized approach helps in building a trustful relationship between the patients and care providers and ensures collabourative effort for recovery.
- Seniors are more comfortable in their homes in their familiar surroundings and the attachments they share with their families. Receiving treatment at home is known to have a positive effect on the patient bringing about a better recovery.
- In-home care settings, the relationship between the general duty assistant/nursing staff and the seniors can be customized and supervised by a family member. With support from the family and the comfort of the home, the patients inherently recover faster.

- Even in cases of advanced dementia, where the patient lacks communication, the presence of loved ones makes a lot of difference.
- Home care reduces hazards that are induced in hospitals (infections and stressors) as well as medical errors.
- Seniors can remain active and independent as they would have activities to perform that they are familiar with.
- Several engagements like card games, crosswords, board games etc. can boost memory and concentration, increase alertness and strengthen problem-solving skills thus slowing down cognitive decline.
- Activities like cycling, and walking in the park can keep the seniors relaxed besides improving their mobility, balance, flexibility, strength, coordination, and agility.
- All types of physical, social, and mental benefits reduce stress, increase their self-confidence and result in a better quality of life for seniors.

8

Summary and Conclusions

We can't help everyone, but everyone can help someone.

– Ronald Reagan

The market size of home health care in India is valued at USD 7.4 billion in 2021 and is expected to grow at a compound annual growth rate (CAGR) of 19.27 per cent from 2022 to 2030. The rising disposable income, the shift of trend from communicable to lifestyle diseases, advancement in technologies, need for better quality post-operative, primary care and the increasing availability of improved home care services with the technology-enabled platform are expected to drive the market growth.

As the growing geriatric population and dependency ratio in India is expected to drive the demand for home health care. According to the Economic and Social Commission for Asia and the Pacific, the aging population of India is expected to reach 298 million by 2051, accounting for 17 per cent of the national population. With the introduction of advanced home health care services in the country, high-quality health care can now be delivered in the comfort of one's own home.[1]

8.1 Home Health Care—Adjustment Between the Patients, their Family Members, Caregivers and Role of Agencies

The present study focused on studying the demographic profile of the patients, nurse managers, nursing staff and general duty assistants. The study also focused on studying the adjustment between the patients, their family members, caregivers and agencies. Further the study examined the emotional well-being and challenges faced by health care staff in home health care. Case studies were generated to understand the life styles borne/adopted by the patients and their care providers to cope up with the disease.

8.1.1 Challenges Faced by Home Care Nurses and General Duty Assistants

The study focused on exploring the perceptions of nurses and general duty assistants on how their work impacted their overall emotional state, the challenges faced by them and the support they expected from the client families and agencies. The researchers identified three primary relationships as the key to the success of home care workers. Majority (78.7%) of the participants believed that they have a cordial relationship with the patient. Appreciation received from the client was considered to have a positive influence on their social and mental health (as has been reasonably emphasized in earlier literature). Studies have shown that home care workers have the hidden purpose of constantly helping people, feeling good about the mission of serving the people and appreciating variety and flexibility in their job (Eustis *et al.*, 1993; Feldman, 1997).

However, the disrespectful behaviour from some of the clients tends to cause stress at workplace. One of the respondents asserted,

> "We are valued till the time the patient is critical. As soon as there is improvement in their patients, condition, the families of the patient devalue us and make us feel as if we are a burden on them."

Donovan's (1989) study on home care workers also identified stressful working conditions, lack of benefits, low pay, lack of opportunities for promotion and powerlessness. The present study also identified a stressful and hectic work environment and examined the lack of benefits and reasons why some respondents in the study were more willing to work in hospitals than home care.

According to Elwer *et al.* (2010) support workers feel exhausted with the stress arising from the excessive demand of clients organisational instability and limited recognition of overall efforts, all of which were borne out by the current study as well. However, respondents also discussed about the overwhelming trust, support, and companionship that turns into 'attachment', which in times of separation (in sudden demise) from the patient puts the caregiver in pain for years. It is thus a fact that all the responsibilities are endowed on the shoulders of nurses and caregivers in home care.

In addition to the client's direct relationship, the role of the client's (Patient) families and agency supervisors exerted a strong influence on the emotional well-being of the caregivers. Several of them (78.7%) believed that they received respect and were valued for their work. This improved their sense of confidence, ability to work and boosted their morale. Ashley *et al.* (2010) described the reasons given by home care workers for identifying their job as rewarding by using terms like satisfaction, gratification or pleasure. The results showed that the present study was consistent with the study conducted by Franzosa *et al.* (2019) which highlighted that building close relationships with the clients was central to the respondent's emotional well-being. It also influenced their relationship with the client's families and agencies. The caregivers require greater communication and support from the client's families as well as agency supervisors. One of the respondents mentioned,

> "Home care agencies have turned this noble cause of caring for the sick into a lucrative business. The worse thing about such agencies is that they charge a hefty amount from the patients but give a pittance to the

> actual worker. When the amount paid by the client is more obviously they try to get a lot of work extracted from the staff."

In the present study, the caregivers have highlighted the need for effective communication and interactive team meetings as a necessary step for discussing patient care issues. Such meetings are also important to discuss safety and other issues related to various behavioural, clinical or psychological concerns in patient homes. The in-depth interviews highlighted another fact which is that no health insurance benefits were being provided by the agencies. The caregivers felt a need to have health insurance coverage in their job. Morris (2009) also found that the health care coverage was an important factor for those who leave their jobs because the newly employed were more likely to have insurance coverage.

For decades, wages and benefits have been stagnated at low levels for home care personal assistance workers, from in-depth interviews it was clear that for a fresher in home care, the average remuneration for a 24 hrs shift and 12 hrs shift for GDAs was Rs. 600 and Rs. 500 per day respectively. The average daily earnings for the nurses for the 24 hrs shift and 12 hrs shift is Rs. 1,600 and Rs. 800 respectively. The average age of the home care worker is 31 years in the present study. This ranges from a younger segment of about 17 years to an older one of about 46 years all of whom are working as home care staff.

The researcher observed that the home care workers, whether nurses or GDAs, earn more than hospital aides or nursing staff as their work is endowed with more responsibility and requires greater judgement which is solely monitored by nurse managers. The home health care workers face double the chances of illness and injuries as compared to all other occupations taken together. This placed home care to be among the 30 riskiest occupations (Seavey, 2010). In the present study several respondents reportedly faced health issues related to migraine, back pain, illness, headache and during times of the pandemic, they were all the more prone to infections. Craven *et al.* (2012) identified the safety concerns of the support

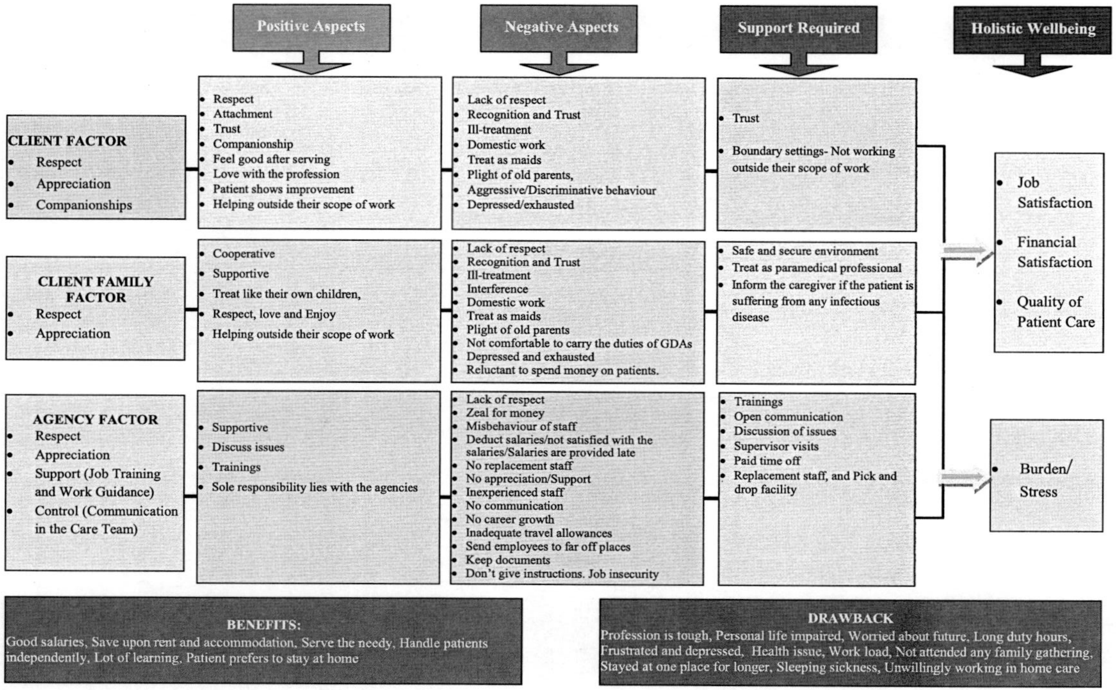

Fig. 8.1: Overall Factors affecting Home Health Care Workers Holistic Well-being.

workers who were complaining of back injuries related to lifting and transferring the patient in various positions. The personal care assistants worked continuously at one place for a period of more than two years as observed in the study undertaken by (Kaye *et al.*, 2006). A majority of the respondents had been with the patient for a period of 6 months to three years. It was found that other low wage occupations had fewer demands and better benefits. Retaining these workers could be difficult, if the conditions did not improve according to the current study.

Through an in-depth information from the respondents, the researcher came with a detailed model where in the overall factors affecting home health care workers holistic well-being was highlighted. The researcher also elaborated on the benefits and drawbacks through the analysis.

8.1.2 Caregivers Burden Scale Findings

- The burden experienced by family caregivers and paid caregivers is the most important caregiver-related variable in care at home in the care of a chronically-ill person. It was found that 7.5 per cent of the nurses, 28 per cent of the family caregivers, and 2.6 per cent of the home aides, BSFC score ranges from 56 to 84, that means 90 per cent of those caregivers have an above-average extent of physical symptoms. The extent of subjective burden (which is borne by the caregivers) has a significant impact on the emotional and physical well-being of the family caregivers and the paid caregivers (nurses and general duty assistants).
- Burden scale was further analyzed for age, gender, marital status, religion, current residence, and socio-economic status of the respondents. Maximum respondents in the age group of 26-28, i.e. 66.7 per cent of the nursing staff were moderately burdened as compared to the other age groups respectively. With regard to the general duty assistants, 50 per cent of the respondents in the age groups of (23-25) were moderately and (17-19, 20-22) were

severely burdened. Further, it was found that 81 per cent of the female nursing staff's BSFC scores ranged from 42 to 55. Thereby, meaning that the female staffs were at an increased risk and a very high risk of psychosomatic symptoms as compared to just 19 per cent of the male staff. However, the burden visualized by the unmarried respondents in the study was much more than the married respondents. Almost all the patients' and their families preferred caregivers speaking the local language and most of the patients' and families' preference was care providers from Hindu and Sikh religions respectively.

- It was examined from the data that whether it was nurses or general duty assistants, the respondents who stayed at the patient-owned residences were moderately to severely burdened. As they sense that their professional value was undermined by family members as they perceived them as housemaids.
- The analysis of the socio-economic status of respondents shows the burden felt by them at the workplace, 33.3 per cent of each of the nursing staff was severely burdened in the upper middle, upper lower and lower segments. When asked about their job challenges, home health workers said that due to financial problems in the family they have to unwillingly work in home care. Moreover, the hospitals no longer provide jobs to ANMs and GNMs, and also the salaries provided in home care to nursing staff are pretty good. Personal duty assistants also faced job challenges and shoulder the bulk of emotional labour while caring for the geriatric population.

8.2 Elderly Population and their Confrontations

Elderly population in India is at a disadvantageous position as compared to other countries in terms of geriatric specialist, health care and insurance benefits. However, it is important for every country to reassess and redesign its health care system to cope with the challenges put forward by demographic and financial variables. As per a study conducted by UN, 62.1 per cent of the elderly are deprived of long term and palliative care. Managing home care for the elderly is a grave challenge as multiple service providers such as agencies, physiotherapists, medical suppliers are small scale and unorganized (Singh, 2017). The state of the elderly in the country is such that they are without any social or health safety nets in the sunset years of their lives. Among this section, the most deprived are the ones who are bedbound or in need of home care round the clock.

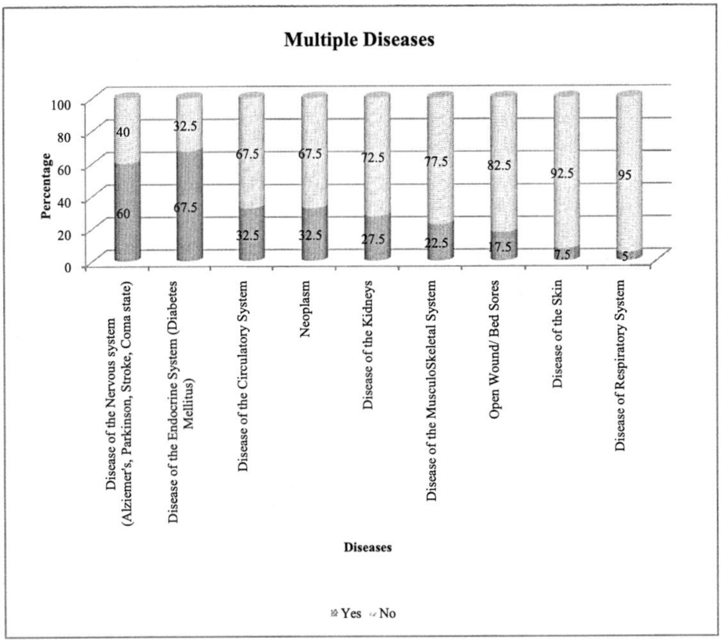

Fig. 8.2: Multiple Diseases Afflicting the Elderly.

In the present study, 67.5 per cent were suffering from the disease of the endocrine system (Diabetes mellitus), 60 per cent were suffering from disease of the nervous system (Alzheimer, Parkinson, paralytic attack), 32.5 per cent of the respondents were living with Neoplastic diseases (means conditions that causes tumor growth), an equal percentage (32.5%) were suffering from disease of the circulatory system (heart disease). The patients were also found to be suffering from cancer of the brain, bones, lungs, breast in females and prostate cancer in case of males. About 22.5 per cent of the respondents were suffering from Musculoskeletal diseases such as injury and fracture. There were 17.5 per cent of the respondents who had open wounds or have developed bedsores as a part of their disease. 7.5 per cent were suffering from the disease of the skin and about 5 per cent were suffering from respiratory diseases such as asthma, lung cancer, chronic obstructive pulmonary disease (COPD). It was also examined that 55 per cent of the respondents were suffering from hypertension in the study. However, majority of the patients were cared by their daughter's and son's (50%), while 27.5 per cent were cared by their spouses. However, 15 per cent were cared by their relatives (such as their sisters, daughter-in-law, brothers). Just meagre percentages (7.5%) of them were cared by their paid help as their immediate families have shifted abroad. However, 52.5 per cent of the patient faced problems with the caregiver work, as it was investigated from in-depth interviews that few of the caregivers used to talk on phone all the time; they were not ready to wash patient's clothes and change diapers while few of the nurses were not ready to even clean their own bed, and were reluctant in changing patient diapers as they believed that changing diapers is the work of home care aides. Even few of the home health care aides were inexperienced and untrained, which has lead to adverse problems in patients.

8.2.1 Zarit Burden Scale Findings

Finding assimilated through the Zarit Burden Scale found that 7.5 per cent of the family caregivers were severely burdened followed by 35 per cent were moderately to severely burdened followed by 32.5 per cent were mildly to moderately burdened. Moreover, 66.7 per cent of the family caregivers followed by 33.3 per cent were severely burdened in the upper middle, and lower middle segments. However, the results were found to be significant as is evident from Chi-square value which is equal to 15.9* showing association of socio-economic class with the burden perceived by the family caregivers. Henceforth, female family caregivers were at an increased risk and at a very high risk of depression as compared to male family caregivers and where the patient is cared by the spouses were severely burdened. The present study also understands the journey of the patients as narrated by their primary caregivers and how this formal caregiving has helped them through the years, as the responsibilities of family caregivers extend beyond personal care and involves sophisticated forms of treatment which are handled by trained nurses and caregivers.

8.3 Important Measures taken by Home Care Agencies

- **Interaction:** The need for interactions and trainings are very crucial for the running of any organisation. Continuous improvement is necessary for the smooth functioning of the organisation.
- **Documentation for the Patients:** Thorough documentation is necessary for clear and consistent information. Agencies maintain client information booklet which carries patient information, their age, gender along with the complete address, even more the document information for the client (Person who is entering the agreement with the agency). Additionally, they take information regarding the scope of service, i.e. professional caregiving/nursing, length of engagement, shift preferred, gender, language and the mode of payment. For the safety of the caregivers, agencies ask additional information such as home setting of the patient, whether lives alone or lives with family, will the client provides personal protective equipment to the caregivers and is the locality safe for the female caregivers to operate. The agencies retain the information by entering the data in electronic form for easy retrieval of information.
- **Documentation for the Caregivers**: The agencies mission in home care is to provide trusted platform enabling

nursing and professional caregiving to chronically ill and bedridden seniors. Agencies maintain caregiver diary, caregiver personal information, caregiver work shift pattern, patient services provided by the caregivers, escalating problems and raising the issues with the agency supervisors, in case they have witnessed any risk that could endanger them and the patients. Additionally, caregiver's code of conduct, recommended behaviour for the caregivers (working with the patients, staying in the hostel, travelling and their financial safety). While working with the clients, the caregivers are required to mark their attendance manually or by calling at the given numbers. Rules are also documented for the termination of the caregivers.

- **Trainings and Supervision:** The care team includes the operation manager, nurse manager, nursing staff and the caregivers. Ongoing trainings with the staff, supervision by the nurse managers helps to analyse the condition of the patient and issues concerning the caregivers. Training the caregivers according to the underlying conditions thus tends to improve the condition of the patient.
- **Clinical Handling Over:** It refers to the transfer of professional responsibility as it's a real time process of passing information between the caregivers, nursing staff to ensure safety and continuity in patient care. It has been examined that 80 per cent of the medical errors occurs due to miscommunication between the medical providers during handling over the process (Solet *et al.*, 2005). A study of 334 patients examined that handing over incidents found that the most common error besides incomplete handling over was reported by (45.2%) and while in 29.3 per cent of cases there was no handling over at all (Pezzolesi *et al.*, 2010). Standardised protocols and checklists are maintained by the home care agencies such as patient condition and illness, patient care plan includes

the services to be provided, name of the medicines, dose of medicine, timing (when medicines to be given after breakfast/after lunch/before lunch/empty stomach/before bed/at bed time) and vitals to be checked such as blood pressure, temperature, heart rate/pulse, respiration rate or random blood sugar. The adherence to these protocols ensures improvements in teamwork and assured continuity of care.

8.4 Policies for the Home Care Staff

The researcher is of the opinion that the certain suggestions may be included at the policy level for the caregivers (Nurses and GDAs) immediately to help them reduce their physical and economic burdens, which negatively impacts upon their quality of life such as:

- No caregiver shall be allowed to work for more than eight hours a day, while maximum weekly hours of work will be 48 hours per week.
- The workers willing in excess of eight hours per day will be entitled to pay overtime. Weekly offs should be made compulsory. Every agency employing caregivers shall constitute a safety committee.
- The workers should be entitled to earn an hour of paid time off for every 40 hours worked.
- The women's who are working between 8pm and 6am shall be provided transport pick and drop facility.
- There should be a provision for health insurance for the caregivers and their dependents.
- The minimum wage rates should be fixed by the government.

8.5 Steps taken by Healthcare Federation of India

In an attempt to **increase inclusivity** and bring together perspectives from **industry stakeholder** and government recommendations, the Healthcare Federation of India has come up with a white paper entitled "Indian Home Healthcare 2.0: Redefining the Modern Care Continuum" in January 2022, which aims to create significant growth opportunities for home health care services in India. The highlights from the plan are discussed under the subheads as follows:

8.5.1 Regulatory and Governance Focus

- For streamlining care delivery there is an urgent need of establishing minimum standards for home care and a transparent process for national licensing standards as part of the clinical establishments act or altogether a separate policy.
- There is a need for integration of medical care being provided outside health care institutions with the primary health care unit. Simultaneously, steps must be taken to mainstream QAI's accreditation standards for home care.
- A transparent care delivery system is the need of the hour which can be efficiently managed by maintaining trust, safety, and privacy by defining the data security regulations.
- Ensuring that data sharing between the health care providers and families through accessibility and visibility.

8.5.2 Capacity Building Focus

- Focus is to be put on establishing a specialised home care workforce by introducing curriculum and training standards for home care personnel.
- Aspirants' interest may be maintained and their schedules can be adapted through the organisation of numerous learning models.
- Periodic renewal processes should be in place for specialised role-based licensing of home care professionals.

8.5.3 Care Financing Focus

- Standard Treatment Guidelines must be implemented immediately based on national and international norms

(STG) and care funding to be ensured for ongoing treatment and a diverse patient ecosystem.
- For new entrants, 10-year tax holiday to be put in place, this could be associated with care delivery in government focus areas or schemes.
- Incentives, such as tax breaks could encourage health care provision in rural and semi-urban regions and GST benefits to be laid out for institutional health care providers.

In India, the market for home health care services is gaining increasing attention with many private insurance providers expanding their coverage to include these services. Max Bupa Health Insurance for senior citizens covers home care services prescribed by doctors. Under domiciliary treatment, the company covers home health care services. Religare Health Insurance also pays about 10 per cent of the sum insured for in home care.[2]

8.6 Conclusion

Regulatory authorities imposing paperwork on HHC nurses and aides, in addition to the shortage and turnover of both certified and unregistered nurses and HHC aides, is an ongoing chronic challenge for the home care industry. There is a lot of demand on HHC institutions, nurses, and aides to offer high-quality care while also keeping costs low. Due to the nature of their work, home care nurses and GDAs sometimes face stressful environments, such as uncleanliness, aggression, and unpredictable client and patient behaviour. At the same time, needle stick injuries among HHC staff raise the risk of contracting life threatening diseases such as the HIV and other blood-borne diseases. Very sick and elderly patients are often seen by HHC nurses and aids at their homes because of the high cost of hospitalization, early discharge, or discharge against medical recommendation. In addition, in order to visit their patients, the nurses and aides who work for HHC have to travel significant distances; hence, the time and money spent on travelling have a negative impact on the quality of care they provide. It has been highlighted that people and patients are still afraid to use home care devices at home, which is a big problem that HHC organizations will have to deal with. The patients and their families have been doubly jeopardized, i.e. on one hand, they want cost-effective care at home, and on the other hand, they are afraid the patient wouldn't live once they are sent home. In addition, patients largely prefer to be treated in a hospital where they get comprehensive care under one roof. Along with, the cost of distributing products and services is a big part of what HHC organizations have to pay for. So, they need to work on making a new, less expensive way to get technology to patients. Needless to mention, big part of the HHC service is not organized, which raises questions of safety and ethicality too.

The findings from the study provide evidence for many current state and national organisations to recognise the needs of direct support workers in home care and long-term care in improving their job conditions. The importance of respect, appreciation and the value of understanding the vital job functions cannot be overlooked if retention of workers is required. Building supportive work environments that allow home care workers to flourish will require recognising, valuing and acknowledging workers full scope of work. The study also pointed towards the role ambiguity that has added to the work stress. Ongoing advocacy and education of the public and policy makers will be necessary in order to assure that direct support workers in home health care are paid livable wages and have access to health care benefits. Without these improvements, recruitment and retention problems will remain impregnable. As the study showed, Home health care workers are facing a host of emotional demands on and off the job. For a high quality work force will require us to build a supportive work environment. In combination with the supportive structural benefits without jeopardising their economic stability, these programmes not only improve their skills but also make them feel valuable and heard at work place. Researchers, policy makers and employers must consider total worker well-being in designing jobs, payment and worker support system that can better satisfy their physical and emotional needs. By valuing the full scope of home care workers labour force, we can improve their well-being and retain and build a committed and skilled work force which our aging population will need.

As home-based care the expectation that family caregivers are always available at home to support patients. The tradition of family caregiving is recognised as fundamental to our society and family caregivers are deeply motivated towards their commitments to the patients. The demographic trends have placed elderly population in double jeopardy, suggesting that there is need for formal caregivers, as the family members are not always available for care when needed. Further the family caregivers expressed that home care team needs more training as the home care staff has the sole responsibility of looking after the patient and they should be well trained according to the underlying condition of the patient and also agencies should identify patient characteristics associated with hospitalization as high-risk patients require specialized intervention beyond the traditional home care services provided. However, in many cases, with the support of caregivers, the families which were earlier not able to carry their activities of daily routine were freed due to the help provided by the home care staff. Thus, such support has resulted in providing the family a breathing space and a break from caregiving stress. It is concluded that to ensure successful and long term care for the elderly, the agencies should understand the demand and value for trained manpower. It is very important to explore the family caregivers, community and health care professionals model where these all should be trained and a detailed training curriculum should be designed to built their capacities to take care of elderly at home.

8.7 The Future of Home Care in India

As we evaluated the impact of COVID-19 pandemic on our health care system in India. Health care facilities faced a dual challenge. Firstly to address the needs of COVID-19 patients and secondly to provide timely care to non-covid patients ensuring no adverse clinical outcomes for these chronic patients amid of ongoing transmission of virus. To address these challenges and reduce the strain on hospital resources, many home care providers, hospitals as well as home care agencies together scaled up the operations of home health care to vulnerable patients.

Home health care provided patients numerous options outside the hospitals creating better quality care at low prices. For the hospitals, home care services have emerged as an essential part of the patient care by extended bed capacity outside the physical hospital. This also implies a much better utilisation of critical care services such as: BiPAP/Mechanical ventilator support for tracheotomised and palliative care patients. The future of home health care services is quite bright as several patients get complex tests, various diagnostic modalities at home with facility of tele-consultations with experts of different specialties. This integrated approach of home health care services will eventually play a critical role in early disease detection, management and treatment thus ensuring service delivery and standardised care at home.

8.8 General Suggestions

The suggestions for the present study have been curated on the completion of the study.

- Worker's stress was most often related to role ambiguity because the families were not given clear instructions about the duties to be carried out.
- Other important areas to be explored are the physical and mental health outcomes, the emotional and financial impact of patient death on the respondents and how workers and families can better negotiate the roles and boundaries with the help of agencies.
- Agencies should incorporate training, care plans, specific job descriptions and payment models.
- Future research can be incorporated on the relationship between the socio-economic status and the financial strain

experienced by family caregivers according to the severity of the disease.

- More research is also needed to determine mechanisms to keep nurses and general duty assistants informed and supported by providing disease specific education material according to the illness of the patient.
- Home health care campaigns should run special training/ educational programmes on fall prevention, safety management, proper medication administration and treatment of various diseases at home.
- A Safe Handling guidebook for the health care providers and patients should be initiated by the health care experts. As these guidelines will altogether improve patients safety, comfort which in return will lead to reduced risk of fall and other injuries. Moreover, home health care staffs will also benefit with less burden at work and improved job satisfaction at the end of their shifts. This will eventually help in achieving more dedication and quality of life outside of work.

Notes

1. India Home Healthcare Market Size, Share & Trends Analysis Report by Equipment (Therapeutic, Diagnostic, Mobility Assist Equipment) by Services (Skilled Home Care, Unskilled Home Care), and Segment Forecasts, 2022-2030 (researchandmarkets.com)
2. https://www.expresshealth care.in/news/nathealth-home-care-forum-launches-white-paper-on-indian-home-health care-2-0-redefining-the-modern-care-continuum/432802/

Bibliography

American Association of Retired Persons (AARP) (2015). *Caregiving in the U.S. research report.* AARP Public Policy Institute. http://www.aarp.org/content/dam/aarp/ppi/2015/caregiving-in-the-united-states-2015-report-revised.pdf. Published June. (accessed February 15, 2019).

Access Community Health (2012). *Job description.* http://www.access.org.nz/content/hr support_worker_jd.pdf (accessed December 17, 2021).

Addington-Hall, J.M., L.D. MacDonald, J. Chamberlain, P. Freeling, J.M. Bland, and J. Raferty (1992). Randomised controlled trial of effects of coordinating care for terminally ill cancer patients. *British Medical Journal Clinical Trial,* 305 (6865): 1317-22.

Adams. E., M. Boulton, and E. Watson (2009). The information needs of partners and family members of cancer patients: a systematic literature review. *Patient Education and Counseling Journal,* 77: 179-86.

Adelman, R.D., L.L.Tmanova, D. Delgado, S. Dion, and M.S. Lachs (2014). Caregiver burden: a clinical review. *The Journal of the American Medical Association, 311*(10):1052-1059.

Alam, M (2000. Ageing in India: a country profile. *Bold 10* (3): 5-22.

Alam, M., and A. Karan (2010). *Elderly Health in India: Dimensions, Differentials, and Over Time Changes.* Building Knowledge Base on Ageing in India: A series of Programmatic and Research Studies. New Delhi: United Nations Population Fund.

Aiyar, S., and S.I. Rajan (2008). *Population Projections for India, 2001-2101.* Thiruvananthapuram: Centre for Development Studies.

Altun, I. (1998). Role in patient care giving difficulty of close states.I. *National Home Health Care Congress* 71-78.

Alzheimer's Society (2009). *Counting the cost: caring for people with Dementia in hospital wards.* AS: London.

Ambady, N., J. Koo, R. Rosenthal, and C.H. Winograd (2002). Physical therapists' nonverbal communication predicts geriatric patients' health outcomes. *Journal of Psychological Aging, 17*(3): 443-452.

American Nurses Association (1999). *Scope and Standards of Home Health Nursing Practice.* Washington, DC: ANA.

American Nurses Association (2006). Nursing-sensitive indicators for community-based non-acute care settings and ANA's safety and quality initiative. http://nursingworld.org/readroom/nurssens.htm. (accessed January 15, 2022).

Andersson, H., M. Lindholm, M. Pettersson, and L.L.Jonasson (2017). Nurses competencies in home health care: an interview study. *BMC Nursing* 16:65.

Angra, S.K., G.V.S Murthy, S.K. Gupta, and V. Angra (1997). Cataract related blindness in India and its social implications. *Indian Journal of Medical Research, 106*: 312-324.

Anthony, A., and P.N. Milone (2005). Factors attracting and keeping nurses in home health care. *Home Health Nurse, 23* (6): 372-377.

Arafa, M.A., M.W. A. Nazel, N.K. Ibrahim, and A. Attia (2003). Predictors of psychological well-being of nurses in Alexandria, Egypt. *International Journal of Nursing Practice, 9*(5): 313-320.

Arts, S.E., A. Kerkstra, J. Van Der Zee, and H. Huyer Abu-Saad. (1999). Workload, capacity for coping and psychological and physical outcomes amongst home helps in the Netherlands. *Health & Social Care in the Community, 7*: 79-90. doi:10.1046/j.1365-2524.1999.00167.x

Ashley, A., S.S. Butler, and N. Fishwick (2010). Home care aides' voices from the field: Job experiences of personal support specialists. *Home Healthcare Nurse, 28*(7): 399-405. doi:10.1097/NHH.0b013e3181e325eb.

Bairwa, M., M.Rajput, and S. Sachdeva (2013). Modified Kuppuswamy's socio-economic scale: social researcher should include updated income criteria, 2012. *Indian Journal of Community Medicine, 38*(3):185-6. doi:10.4103/0970-0218.116358

Banijamali, S., A. Hagopian, and D. Jacoby (2012). *Why they leave: turnover among Washington's home care workers*. Washington: SEIU Healthcare 775NW.

Banijamali, S., A. Hagopian, and D. Jacoby (2014). Characteristics of home care workers who leave their jobs: a cross-sectional study of job satisfaction and turnover in Washington State. *Home Health Care Services Quarterly, 33*(3): 137-158. doi: 10.1080/01621424.2014.929068.

Barsade, S.G., and O.A. O'Neill (2014). What's love got to do with it? A longitudinal study of the culture of companionate love and employee and client outcomes in a long-term care setting. *Administrative Science Quarterly*, *59*: 551-598. doi:10.1177/0001839214538636

Baumgarten, M., R.N. Battista, C. Infante-Rivard, J.A. Hanley, R. Becker, S. Gauthier (1992). The psychological and physical health of family members caring for an elderly person with dementia. *Journal of Clinical Epidemiology*, *45*: 61-70.

Baumgarten, M., J.A. Hanley, C. Infante-Rivard, R.N. Battista, R. Becker, S.Gauthier (1994). Health of family members caring for elderly persons with dementia. A longitudinal study.*Annals of Internal Medicine*, *120*:126-32.

Beer, J.M., S.E. McBride, T.L. Mitzner, and W.A. Rogers (2014). Understanding challenges in the front lines of home health care: a human-systems approach. *Applied Ergonomics 45*:1687-99.

Bektas, H., and N. Akdemir (2006). Kanserli Bireylerde Fonksiyonel Durumlarinin Degerlendirilmesi. Turkiye Klinikleri. *Journal of Medical Sciences*, *26*: 488-99.

Benjamin, A.E., and R.E. Matthias (2004). Work-life differences and outcomes for agency and consumer-directed home-care workers. *Gerontologist, 44*(4): 479-488. [PubMed: 15331805].

Bergquist, S. (2001). Subscales, subscores, or summative score: evaluating the contribution of Braden Scale items for predicting pressure ulcer risk in older adults receiving home health care. *The Journal of Wound, Ostomy and Continence Nursing, 28*(6): 279-89.

Bianchi, M., L.D. Flesch, E.V.S. Alves, S.S.T. Batistoni and A.L. Neri (2016). Zarit burden interview psychometric indicators applied in older people caregivers of other elderly.*Revista Latino-Americana* de *Enfermagem* 24:e2835.

Blais, R., N.A. Sears, D. Doran, G.R. Baker, M. Macdonald, L. Mitchell and S. Thales (2013). Assessing adverse events among home care clients in three Canadian provinces using chart review. *BMJ Quality and Safety, 22*: 972-974.

Blustein, D.L. (2008). The role of work in psychological health and well-being: a conceptual, historical, and public policy perspective. *The American Psychologist* 63: 228–240. doi:10.1037/0003-066X.63.4.228

Blustein, D.L., D.E.P. Schultheiss, and H. Flum (2004). Toward a relational perspective of the psychology of careers and working: a social constructionist analysis. *Journal of Vocational Behaviour 64*: 423-440. doi:10.1016/j.jvb.2003.12.008

Bly, J.L., and P. Kissick (1994). Hospice care for patients living alone: results of a demonstration programme. *Journal of Hospice & Palliative Nursing, 9*: 9-20.

Brannon, D., T. Barry, P. Kemper, A. Schreiner, and J. Vasey (2007). Job perceptions and intent to leave among direct care workers: evidence from the better jobs better care demonstrations. *The Gerontologist, 47*(6): 820-29. doi:10.1093/geront/47.6.820.

Browne, G., J. Roberts, S. Watt, A. Gafni, M. Stockwell, and S. Alcock (1994). Community rehabilitation: strategies, outcomes, expenditures. *Canadian Journal of Rehabilitation, 8*: 9-22.

Butler, S.S., N. Simpson, M. Brennan, and W. Turner (2010). Why do they leave? Factors associated with job termination among personal assistant workers in home care. *Journal of Gerontological Social Work, 53*: 665-681.doi:10.1080/01634372.2010.517236.

Butler, S.S., S. Wardamasky, and M. Brennan-Ing (2012). Older women caring for older women: The rewards and challenges of the home care aide job. *Journal of Women and Aging, 24*: 194-215. doi:10.1080/08952841.2012.639667

Bruera, E., N. Kuehn, B. Emery, K. MacMillan, and J. Hanson. (1990). Social and demographic characteristics of patients admitted to a palliative care unit. *Journal of Palliative Care, 6*: 16-20.

Bullock, R. (2004). The needs of the caregiver in the long term treatment of Alzheimer disease. *Alzheimer Disease and Associated Disorders, 18*(1): S17-23.

Buyck, J.F., S. Bonnaud, A. Boumendil, S. Andrieu, S. Bonenfant, M. Goldberg, M. Zins, and J. Ankri (2011). Informal caregiving and self-reported mental and physical health: results from the Gazel Cohort Study. *American Journal of Public Health, 101*(10): 1971-79.

Canadian Study of Health and Aging Working Group (1994). Patterns of caring for people with dementia in Canada: the Canadian Study of Health and Aging. *Canadian Journal of Aging, 13*: 470-87.

Careers, N.Z. (2014). *Nursing support and care worker.* http://www.careers.govt.nz/jobs/health/nursing-support-and-care-worker/job-opportunities (accessed September 14, 2021).

Carr, K.K., and M.K. Kazanowski (1994). Factors affecting job satisfaction of nurses who work in long-term care. *Journal of Advanced Nursing, 19*: 878-83.

Census of India (2011). *Provisional Population Totals. Rural Urban Distribution.* Chandigarh: Directorate of Census Operations *2*(2).

Centres for Medicare and Medicaid Services (2006). *Home Health Quality Initiative Overview.* http://www.cms.hhs.gov/Home HealthQualityInits. (accessed February 19, 2020).

Centers for Medicare and Medicaid Services (2006). *Quality monitoring using case mix and adverse event outcome reports.* http://www.cum.hhs.gov/HomeHealth QualityInits/Downloads/HHQIOASISOBQMCaseMix.pdf. (accessed August 23, 2021).

Centers for Disease Control and Prevention (2019). *Chronic Kidney Disease in the United States*, Atlanta, GA: US Department of Health and Human Services.

Chang, Y.J., Y.C. Kwon, W.L. Jin, Y.R. Do, L. Keun Seok, H. Tae Kim, S. Ryun Park, Y Seon Hong, I. Chung, and Y. Ho Yun (2013). Burdens, needs and satisfaction of terminal cancer patients and their caregivers. *Asian Pacific Journal of Cancer Prevention, 14*: 209-15.

Chappell, N.L. (1992). *Social Support and Ageing.* Toronto: Butterworths.

Chamber, M, A.A. Ryan, and S.L. Connor (2001). Exploring the emotional support needs and coping strategies of family carees. *Journal of Psychiatric and Mental Health Nursing, 8*: 99-106.

Chappell, N.L., and M. Penning (1996). Behavioural problems and distress among caregivers of people with Dementia. *Ageing & Society, 16*: 57-73.

Chichin, E.R. (1992). Home care is where the heart is: The role of interpersonal relationships in paraprofessional home care. *Home Health Care Services Quarterly, 13*(1-2): 161-77.

Chhugani, M., and J. Mary Merlin (2017). Challenges faced by nurses in India—The major workforce of the health care system. *Nursing & Care Open Access Journal, 22*(4): 112-114. doi: 10.15406/ncoaj.2017.02.00045.

Cieza, A., K. Causey, K. Kamenov, S.W. Hanson, S. Chatterji, and T. Vos (2021). Global estimates of the need for rehabilitation based on the Global Burden of Disease Study 2019: a systematic analysis for the Global Burden of Disease Study 2019. *The Lancet, 396*(10267): 2006-2017.

Clipp, E.D., and L.K. George (1993). Dementia and Cancer: a comparison of spouse caregivers. [Review].*Gerontologist, 33*: 534-41.

Cohen, D. and C. Eisdorfer (1988). Depression in family members caring for a relative with Alzheimer's disease. *Journal of the American Geriatrics Society, 36*: 885-89.

Corbett, C.F. (2003). A randomized pilot study of improving foot care in home health patients with diabetes.*The Science of Diabetes Self-Management and Care, 29*: 273-82.

Covinsky, K.E., and L. Goldman, and E.F. Cook (1994). The impact of serious illness on patients' families. *Journal of the American Medical Association, 272*: 1839-44.

Coyte, P.C., and W. Young (1997). Applied home care research. *International Journal of Health Care Quality Assurance* 10: i–iv.

Craven, C., K. Byrne, J. Sims-Gould, and A. Martin-Matthews (2012). Types and patterns of safety concerns in home care: staff perspectives. *International Journal for Quality in Health Care, 24*(5): 525-31.

Cryer, L., S.B. Shannon, M.V. Amsterdam, and L. Bruce (2012). Costs for hospital at home patients were 19 per cent lower, with equal or better outcomes compared to similar inpatients. *Health Affairs (Millwood), 31*(6):1237-43. doi:10.1377/hlthaff.2011.1132.

Delp, L., S.P. Wallace, J. Geiger-Brown, and C. Muntaner (2010). Job stress and job satisfaction: Home care workers in a consumer directed model of care. *Health Services Research, 45*: 922-40. doi:10.1111/j.1475-6773.2010.01112.x

Denton, M., I.U. Zeytinoglu, S. Davies, and J. Lian (2002). Job stress and job dissatisfaction of home care workers in the context of health care restructuring. *International Journal of Health Services,* 32: 327-57.

Desai, K. (2019). House calls make a comeback. In *Times of India.* Chandigarh (Dance of Democracy). Sunday, 14 April. p. 11.

Dey, S., D. Nambiar, J.K. Lakshmi, K. Sheikh, and K.S. Reddy (2012). Ageing in Asia. In *Health of the elderly in India:*

challenges of access and affordability, James P. Smith and M. Majmundar, eds. pp. 371-86. Washington, D.C: The National Academies Press.

Dias, A., M.E. Dewey, J. D'Souza, R. Dhume, D.D. Motghare, K.S. Shaji, R. Menon, M. Prince, and V. Patel (2008). The effectiveness of a home care programme for supporting caregivers of persons with Dementia in developing countries: a randomised controlled trial from Goa, India. *PLoS ONE, 3*(6): 1-7.

Donaldson, C., and A. Burns (1999). Burden of Alzheimer's disease: helping the patient and caregiver. *Journal of Geriatric Psychiatry and Neurology, 12*: 21-28.

Donovan, R. (1989). Work stress and job satisfaction: A study of home care workers in New York City. *Home Health Care Services Quarterly, 10*(1-2): 97-114. doi:10.1300/J027v10n01_08

Dreze, J. (1990). *Widows in Rural India.* London: Development Economics Research Programme.

Duke, M., and A. Street (2003). Hospital in the home: constructions of the nursing role—a literature review. *Journal of Clinical Nursing, 12*: 852-59.

Dunlop, R.J., R.J. Davies, and J.M. Hockley (1989). Preferred versus actual place of death: a hospital palliative care support team experience. *Palliative Medicine, 3*: 197-201.

Elderly in India (2016). Central Statistics Office. Ministry of Statistics and Programme Implementation, Government of India, www.mospi.gov.in.http://mospi.nic.in/sites/default/files/publication_reports/ElderlyinIndia_2016.pdf.

Ellenbecker, C.H., S.C. Frazier, and S. Verney (2004). Nurses' observations and experiences of problems and adverse effects of medication management in home health care. *Geriatric Nursing Journal, 25*(3): 164-70.

Ellenbecker, C.H., L. Samia, and L. Neal (2006). What nurses are saying about staying and leaving. *Home Healthcare Nurse 24*(5): 315-24.

Ellenbecker, C.H., L. Samia, M.J. Cushman, K. Alster, and Ronda G. Hughes (2008). Patient safety and quality in home health care. In *Patient Safety and Quality: An Evidence-Based Handbook for Nurses.* pp. 1-301-1-340. Rockville (MD): Agency for Healthcare Research and Quality (US): Chapter 13.

Elwer, S., L. Alex, and A. Hammarstrom (2010). Health against the odds: experiences of employees in elder care from a gender perspective. *Qualitative Health Research, 20*(9): 1202-12.

Eustis, N.N., R.A. Kane, and L.R. Fischer (1993). Home care quality and the home care worker: Beyond quality assurance as usual. *Gerontologist, 33*(1): 64-73.doi: 10.1093/geront/33.1.64

Fast, J.E., N.C. Keating, and L. Oakes (2014). *Conceptualizing and operationalizing the costs of informal elder care.* Ottawa: Report to the National Health Research Development Programme.

Fatemi, N.L., H. K. Moonaghi, and A. Heydari (2019). Perceived challenges faced by nurses in home health care setting: a qualitative study.*International Journal of Community Based Nursing and Midwifery,* 7(2): 118-127.7

Federal Register (1997). Department of Health and Human Services. Health Care Financing Administration.42 CFR Part 484, Medicare and Medicaid programme; revisions of conditions of participation for home health agencies and use of outcome assessment information set (OASIS); proposed rule.

Feldman, P.H. (1997). Labor market issues in home care. In *Home-based care for a new century.* D.M. Fox, and C. Raphael eds. pp. 155-83. Malden, MA: Blackwell.

Ferrara, M., E. Langiano, T. Di Brango, E. De Vito, L. Di Cioccio, and C.Bauco (2008). Prevalence of stress, anxiety, and depression in with Alzheimer caregiver. *Health and Quality of Life Outcomes* 6:93. Data from http://www.ncbi.nlm.nih.gov/pmc/articles/PMC2586019/. [PubMed: 18990207]

Ferrell, B.A., K. Josephson, P. Norvid, and H. Alcorn (2000). Pressure ulcers among patients admitted to home health care. *Journal* of the *American Geriatrics Society* 48(9): 1042-47.

Ferri, C.P., M. Prince, C. Brayne, H. Brodaty, L. Fratiglioni *et al.* (2005). Global prevalence of dementia: a Delphi consensus study. *Lancet, 366*(9503): 2112-17.

Flojt J., U.L. Hir, K. Rosengren (2014). Need for preparedness: nurses' experiences of competence in home health care. *Home Health Care of Management and Practice,* 26: 223-29.

Fontaine, K., L. Briggs, and B. Pope-Smith (2001). Designing humanistic critical environments. *Critical Care Nursing Quarterly, 24*(3): 21-34.

Fortinsky, R.H., E.A. Madigan, T. J. Sheehan, S. Tullai-McGuinness, and J.R. Fenster (2006). Risk factors for hospitalization among Medicare home care patients. *WesternJournal of Nursing Research* December (28): 902-17.

Franzosa, E., E.K. Tsui, and S. Baron (2018). Who's caring for us? Understanding and addressing the effects of emotional labour on home health aides' well-being. *The Gerontologist, 59*(6): 1055-1064. doi: 10.1093/geront/gny099

Franzosa, E., E.K. Tsui, and S. Baron (2019). Home health aides' perceptions of quality care: goals, challenges, and implications for a rapidly changing industry. *New Solutions: A Journal of Environmental and Occupational Health Policy,* 27: 629-47. doi:10.1177/1048291117740818

Fuscaldo, D. (2007). *What patients want and expect from health care providers.* Fox Business. https://www.foxbusiness.com/features/what-patients-want-expect-from-health-care-providers (accessed January 21, 2023).

Gallagher, D., J. Rose, P. Rivera, S. Lovett, and L.W. Thompson (1989). Prevalence of depression in family caregivers. *Gerontologist,* 29: 449-56.

George, E., L. Hale and J. Angelo (2017). Valuing the health of the support worker in the aged care sector. *Ageing & Society, 37*: 1006-24.

Gillespie, L.D., W.J. Gillespie, M.C. Robertson, S.E. Lamb, R.G. Cumming, and B.H. Rowe (2003). Interventions for preventing falls in elderly people. *Cochrane Database System Reviews, 4*: CD000340.

Given. B., C. Given, and S. Kozacki (2001. Family support in advanced cancer. CA *Cancer Journal for Clinicians, 51*: 213-31.

Goswami, A., V.P. Reddaiah, S.K. Kapoor, B. Singh, S.N. Dwivedi, and G. Kumar (2005). Tobacco and alcohol use in rural elderly Indian population. *Indian Journal of Psychiatry, 47*(4): 192-97. doi:10.4103/0019-5545.43050.

Government of India (2011). *National Programme for the Health Care of the Elderly (NPHCE). Operational guidelines*. New Delhi: Government of India.

Grafstrom, M., A. Nordberg, and B. Winblad (1993). Abuse is in the eye of the beholde. Report by family members about abuse of demented persons in home care.A total population-based study.*Scandinavian Journal of Social Medicine* 21:147-255.

Granberg, O. (2014). *Learn or learn: about skills and education planning in working life (in Swedish)*. Lund: Studentlitteratur.

Grant, I., K. Adler, T.L. Patterson, J.E. Dimsdale, M.G. Ziegler, and M.R. Irwin (2002). Health consequences of Alzheimer's caregiving transitions: effects of placement and bereavement. *Psychosomatic Medicine, 64*: 477-86. http://www.psychosomaticmedicine.org/content/64/3/477.full. [PubMed: 12021421].

Grasel, E. (1995). Somatic symptoms and caregiving strain among family caregivers of older patient with progressive nursing needs. *Archives* of *Gerontology* and *Geriatrics, 21*: 253-66.

Grasel, E. (1998). Home care of dementia and non-dementia patients (Part II): health and burden of family caregivers. *Journal of Gerontology and Geriatrics, 31*: 57-62.

Grasel, E. (1999). Predictors in maintaining home care. *Journal of Gerontology and Geriatrics, 32* (S2-II): 185.

Gratao, A.C.M., T.R.P. Vendruscolo, L.F.S. Talmelli, L.C. Figueiredo, J.L.F. Santos, and R.A.P. Rodrigues (2012). Burden and the emotional distress in caregivers of elderly individuals. *Texto & Contexto Enfermagem, 21*(2): 304-12.

Gruenberg, E. (1977). The failure of success. *Milbank Memorial Fund Quarterly/Health and Society*, 55: 3-24.

Grunfeld, Eva., R. Glossop, L. McDowell, and C. Danbrook. 1997. Caring for elderly people at home: the consequences to caregivers. *The Canadian Medical Association Journal, 157*(8): 1101-05.

Gupta, Indrani, and D. Sankar (2002). *Health of the elderly in India: A multivariate analysis.* Discussion Paper 46. New Delhi: Institute of Economic Growth. Available: http://iegindia.org/dis_ind_46.pdf.

Gupta, Prakash C., K. Pallab, K. Maulik, Mangesh S. Pednekar, and S. Saxena (2005). Concurrent alcohol and tobacco use among a middle-aged and elderly population in Mumbai. *National Medical Journal of India* 18 (2): 88-91.

Hadley, J., D. Rabin, A. Epstein, S. Stein and C. Rimes (2000). Post hospitalization home health care use and changes in functional status in a Medicare population. *Medical Care, 38*(5): 494-507.

Hahnel, Elisabeth., U. Blume-Peytavi, C. Trojahn, G. Dobos, I. Jahnke, V. Kanti, C. Richter, A. Lichterfeld-Kottner, N. Garcia Bartels, and J. Kottner (2017). Prevalence and associated factors of skin diseases in aged nursing home residents: a multicentre prevalence study. *BMJ Open, 7*(9): e018283. doi: 10.1136/bmjopen-2017-018283

Hakanen, J.J., W.B. Schaufeli, and K. Ahola (2008). The job demands-resources model: A three-year cross-lagged study of burnout, depression, commitment, and work engagement. *Work & Stress, 22*: 224-41. doi:10.1080/02678370802379432

Han, S.J., H.K. Kim, J. Storfjell, and M.J. Kim (2013). Clinical outcomes and quality of life of home health care patients. *Asian Nursing Research (Korean Social Nursing Science),* June *7*(2): 53-60.

Harris, M.D. (1998). The impact of the balanced budget act of 1997 on home health care agencies and nurses. *Home Healthcare Nurse, 16* (7): 199-206.

Hazelwood, D.M., S. Koeck, M. Wallner, K. Hoehn Anderson, and H. Mayer (2012). Patients with cancer and family caregivers: management of symptoms caused by cancer or cancer therapy at home. *Heilberufe Science, 3*: 149-58.

Hendrix, C., and C. Ray (2006). Informal caregiver training on home care and cancer symptom management prior to hospital discharge: a feasibility study. *Oncology Nursing Forum, 33*: 793-98.

Hinds, Cora (1985). The needs of families who care for patients with cancer at home: are we meeting them. *Journal of Advanced Nursing, 10*(6): 575-81.

Hinton, John (1994). Can home care maintain an acceptable quality of life for patients with terminal cancer and their relatives. *Palliative Medicine*, 8(3): 183-96.

Hoffman, M., and B. Nazario (2020). *Lung Diseases Overview.* https://www.webmd.com/lung/lung-diseases-overview. (accessed November 21, 2021).

Hoppe, A., C.A. Heaney, K. Fujishiro, F. Gong, and S. Baron (2015). Psychosocial work characteristics of personal care and service occupations: A process for developing meaningful measures for a multiethnic workforce. *Ethnicity & Health, 20*: 474-92. doi:10.1080/13557858.2014.925095.

Howarth, G., and K.B. Willison (1995). Preventing crises in palliative care in the home. Role of family physicians and nurses. *Canadian Family Physician, 41*: 439-45.

Hsu, H.C., Y.W. Kung, H.C. Huang, P. Y. Ho, Y. Ying Lin, and W. Shin Chen (2007). Work stress among nursing home care attendants in Taiwan: A questionnaire survey. *International Journal of Nursing Studies, 44*: 736-46.

Huppert, F. A., and T.T. So (2013). Flourishing across Europe: application of a new conceptual framework for defining well-being. *Social Indicators Research, 110*: 837-61. doi:10.1007/s11205-011-9966-7

Hughes, L.C., L.A. Robinson, M.E. Cooley, I. Nuamah, S.J. Grobe, and R. McCorkle (2002). Describing an episode of home nursing care for elderly postsurgical cancer patients. *Nursing Research, 51*(2): 110-18.

Ingle, G.K., and A. Nath (2008). Geriatric health in India: concerns and solutions. *Indian Journal of Community Medicine, 33*: 214-18.

Istjanson, L.J. (1989). Quality of terminal care: salient indicators identified by families. *Journal of Palliative Care, 5*: 21-8.

Iyer, M. (2022). Cancer cases in India in 2020. In *Times of India*, Chandigarh (Times Property). Sunday, 25 September, p. 14.

Jerant, A.F., and R. Azari, and C. Martinez (2003). A randomized trial of tele-nursing to reduce hospitalization for heart failure: patient-centred outcomes and nursing indicators. *Home Health Care Services, 22*(1): 1-20.

Jha, Prabhat., V. Gajalakshmi, C. Prakash, C. Gupta, R. Kumar, P. Monty, N. Dhingra, and R. Peto (2006). Prospective study of one million deaths in India: rationale, design, and validation results. *PLoS Medicine,* 3: 18.

Johnson, R.W., D. Toohey, and J.M.Weiner (2007). *Meeting the long-term care needs of the baby boomers: how changing families will affect paid helpers and institutions.* The Urban Institute, May. http://www. urban.org/sites/default/files/alfresco/publication-pdfs/311451-Meeting-the-Long-Term-Care-Needs-of-the-Baby-Boomers.PDF. (accessed August 2, 2016).

Jorgensen, D., M. Parsons, M.G. Reid, K. Weidenbohm, J. Parsons, and S. Jacobs (2009). The providers' profile of the disability support workforce in New Zealand. *Health and Social Care in the Community, 17*(4): 396-405. https://doi.org/10.1111/j.1365-2524.2008.00839.x.

Josefsson, K. (2012). Registered nurses' health in community elderly care in Sweden.*International Nursing Review, 59*: 409-15.

Josefsson, K., and S. Peltonen (2015). District nurses' experience of working in home care in Sweden. *Health Ageing Research, 4*: 37.

Juozapavicius, K.P., and J.A. Weber (2001). A reflective study of Alzheimer's caregivers. *American Journal of Alzheimer's Disease and Other Dementia, 16*(1): 11-20.

Kaiser Family Foundation (2005). *Medicare Chart Book* http://www.kff.org/medicare/7284.cfm. (accessed January 23, 2022).

Kalra, A (2022). Frequent urination in men over 50 years of age should be investigated thoroughly. In *Times of India*. Chandigarh (Chandigarh Times). Sunday, 25 September, p. 8.

Karimi, L., C. Cheng, T. Bartram, S.G. Leggat, and S. Sarkeshik (2015).The effects of emotional intelligence and stress-related presenteeism on nurses' well-being. *Asia Pacific Journal of Human Resources, 53*: 296-310. doi:10.1111/1744–7941.12049

Katz, D., and L. Festinger (1953). *Research methods in the behavioural sciences*. New York: The Dryden Press.

Katz, S., A. Ford, R. Moskowitz, B. Jackson and M. Jafee (1963). Studies of illness in the aged: the index of ADL, a standardized measure of biological and psychosocial functioning. *Journal of the American Medical Association, 185*: 94-101.

Kaye, H.S., S. Chapman, R.J. Newcomer, and C. Harrington (2006). The personal assistance workforce: trends in supply and demand. *Health Affairs (Millwood), 25*(4): 1113-20. doi:10.1377/hlthaff.25.4.1113

Keepnews, D., J. Capitman and R. Rosati (2004). Measuring patient-level clinical outcomes of home health care. *Journal of Nursing Scholarship, 36*(1): 79-85.

Keenan, T.A. (2010). *Home and community preferences of the 45+ Population.* AARP, November, http://www.aarp.org/research/topics/community/info-2014/home-community-services-10.html. (accessed August 12, 2021).

Kemper, P., H. Brigitt, T. Barry, D. Brannon, J. Angelelli, J. Vasey, and M. Anderson-Knott (2008). What do direct care workers say would improve their jobs? Differences across settings. *Gerontologist, 48* (Special Issue 1): 17-25. [PubMed: 18694983]

Kerkstra A, and J.B.F. Hutten (1996). Organization and financing of home nursing in the European Union. *Journal of Advanced Nursing, 24*: 1023-32.

Kosuke, Imai., and S. Soneji (2004). On the estimation of disability-free life expectancy: Sullivan's method and its extension. *Journal of the American Statistical Association, 102* (480): 1199-1211.

Kothari, C.R. (2009). *Research methodology methods and techniques*. New Delhi: Newage International Publishers.

Kroposki, M., and J.W. Alexander (2006). Correlation among client satisfaction, nursing perception of outcomes, and organizational variables. *Home Healthcare Nurse, 24*(2): 87-94.

Kumari, R.S.S (2001). Socio-economic conditions, morbidity pattern and social support among elderly women in a rural area. Medical College, Thiruvananthapuram, Kerala.

Kumari, R.S., and Sarasa (2001). Socio-economic conditions, morbidity pattern and social support among elderly women in a rural area. Medical College, Thiruvananthapuram, Kerala. http://www.cds.ac.in/krpcds/report/sarasakumari. pdf. (accessed on July 17, 2019).

Kumari, B.S. Kaur, M. Dutta, A. Bahl, and P. Barwad (2020). Awareness of patients regarding self-management of heart failure attending a tertiary care hospital of North India. *International Journal of Noncommunicable Diseases, 5*(4): 158-64.

Kumar, V. (2023). Remote training to caregivers cut Punjab's Covid hospitalisations'. In *Times of India*. Monday, 30 January, p. 7.

Kuppuswamy, B. (1981). *Manual of Socio-economic Status Scale (Urban).* Delhi: Manasyan.

Landers, Steven., E. Madigan, B. Leff, R.J. Rosati, A. Barbara A. McCann, R. Hornbake, R. MacMillan, K. Jones, K. Bowles, and D. Dowling, L.Teresa, T. Moorhead, S. Rodriguez, and E. Breese (2016). The Future of home health care: A strategic framework for optimizing value. *Home Health Care Management & Practice, 28*(4): 262-78.

Lena, A., K. Ashok, M. Padma, V. Kamath, and A. Kamath (2009). Health and social problems of the elderly: A cross-sectional study in Udupi Taluk, Karnataka. *Indian Journal of Community Medicine, 34*: 131-34.

Ley, D.C.H. (1989). The elderly and palliative care. *Journal of Palliative Care, 5*: 43-45.

Livingston, G., M. Manela, C. Katona (1996). Depression and other psychiatric morbidity in carers of elderly people living at home. *Biomedical Journal, 312*: 153-56.

Lubin, S. (1992). Palliative care—could your patient have been managed at home? *Journal of Palliative Care, 8*: 18-22.

Lutgendorf, S.K., and M.L. Laundenslager (2009). Care of the caregiver: stress and dysregulation of inflammatory control in cancer caregivers. *Journal of Clinical Oncology, 27*(18): 2894-28. http://jco.ascopubs.org/content/27/18/2894. [PubMed: 19433678].

Lynch, S.M., S. J. Brown, and M.G. Taylor (2009). The demography of disability. In *A International Handbook of Population Ageing*, P. Uhlenberg, eds. London: Springer-Verlag.

Martens, K.H., and S.D. Mellor (1997). A study of the relationship between home care services and hospital readmission of patients with congestive heart failure. *Home Healthcare Nurse, 15*(2): 123-29.

Magnusson, A.B., and K. Lutzen (2002). Nurses' views on situations related to privacy in providing home care for persons with long-term mental illness: an exploratory study. *Issues in Mental Health Nursing, 23*: 61-75.

Miner, L., P. Bolding, J. Hilbe, M. Goldstein, T. Hill, and R. Nisbet, *et al.* (2015). *Socio-economic Status—An overview. Science Direct Topics* [Internet]. https://www.sciencedirect.com/topics/medicine-anddentistry/socioeconomic-status (accessed March 21, 2020).

Malik, R. (2022). Heart of the matter. In *Times of India*. Chandigarh (Times Nation). Thursday, 29 September, p. 11.

Mathur, R (2022). How home health care can help patients with serious kidney ailments keep their condition under check. In *Times of India*. Rajiv Mathur in Voices. India (Lifestyle). Monday, 14 March. 8:25 PM IST. TOI. https://timesofindia.indiatimes.com/blogs/voices/how-home-health care-can-help-patients-with-serious-kidney-ailments-keep-their-condition-under-check/.

McCorkle, Ruth, Neville E. Strumpf, Isaac F. Nuamah, Diane C. Adler, Mary E. Cooley, Christopher Jepson, Edward J. Lusk, and M. Torosian (2000). A Specialized Home Care Intervention improves Survival among Older Post Surgical Cancer Patients. *Journal of the American Geriatrics Society, 48*: 1707-13.

McDowell, B.J., S. Engberg, S. Sereika, N. Donovan, M.E. Jubeck, E. Weber, and R. Engberg (1999). Effectiveness of behavioural therapy to treat incontinence in homebound older adults. *Journal of American Geriatric Society, 47*: 309-18.

McMillan, S.C. (1996). Quality of Life of primary caregivers of hospice patients with cancer. *Cancer Practice. 4*: 191-98.

McWhinney, I.R., M.J. Bass, and V. Orr. (1995). Factors associated with location of death (home or hospital) of patients referred to a palliative care team. *The Canadian Medical Association Journal, 152*: 361-67.

Medicare Payment Advisory Commission (2012). *Report to Congress: Medicare Payment Policy.* Published March.http://medpac.gov/documents/reports/march-2016-report-to-the-congress-medicare-payment- org/data/topic/topic.aspx?cat=18. (accessed July 10, 2019).

Medicare Payment Advisory Commission (2016). *Health Care Spending and the Medicare Programme: A Data Book.* Published March. http://www.medpac.gov/documents/data-book/june-2016-databook- policy.pdf?sfvrsn=2. (accessed July 10, 2019).

Megaritis, C., E. Sakellari, Psychogiou, M.A., Tzenalis V. Krepia, G. Charalambous and D. Sapountzi-Krepia (2018). Exploring home care nurses' perceptions regarding their services in economic crisis: A qualitative approach. *Nursing Forum, 53*: 521-28.

Meeker, M.A., D. Finnell, and A.K. Othman (2011). Family caregivers and cancer pain management: a review. *Journal of Family Nursing, 17*: 29-60.

Michel, J P., D. Zekry, R. Mulligan, E. Giacobini, and G. Gold (2001). Economic considerations of Alzheimer's disease and related disorders aging. *Aging Clinical and Experimental Research, 13*: 255-60.

Modified Kuppuswamy Scale (2021). *PSM Made Easy* [Internet]. http://www.ihatepsm.com/blog/modifiedkuppuswamy-scale (accessed April 15, 2022).

Modin, S., and A.K. Furhoff (2004). The medical care of patients with primary care home nursing is complex and influenced by non-medical factors: a comprehensive retrospective study from a suburban area in Sweden. *BMC Health Services Research, 4*: 22. http://www.biomedcentral.com/1472-6963/4/22 (accessed January 22, 2019).

Montgomery, R.J., L. Holley, J. Deichert, and K. Kosloski (2005). A profile of home care workers from the 2000 census: How it changes what we know. *Gerontologist, 45*(5): 593-600.

Morris, R.G., L.W. Morris, and P.G. Britton (1988). Factors affecting the emotional well-being of caregivers of dementia sufferers. *British Journal of Psychiatry, 153*:147-56.

Morris, L (2009). Quits and job changes among home care workers in Maine: The role of wages, hours, and benefits. *Gerontologist, 49*(5), 635-50. doi:10.1093/geront/gnp071.

Muller-Spahn, F. (2003). Behavioral disturbances in dementia. *Dialogues in Clinical Neuroscience, 5*(1): 49-59.

Mutharayappa, R., and T.N. Bhat (2008). Is lifestyle influencing morbidityamong elderly. *Journal of Health Management, 10*(2): 203-17. doi:10.1177/097206340801000203.

National Center for Injury Control and Prevention (2006). *Falls and hip fractures among older adults.* http://www.cdc.gov/ncipc/factsheets/falls.htm. (accessed on February 25, 2021).

National Clearinghouse on the Direct Care Workforce (2005). *Results of the 2005 national survey of state initiatives on the long-term care direct care workforce.* Raleigh, NC: Direct Care Workers Association of North Carolina.

National Advisory Committee on Rural Health and Human Services (NACRHHS) (2009). The 2009 report to the Secretary: Rural health and human services issues. Retrieved from the Department of Health and Human Services/Health Resources and Services Administration website July 17, 2009 at http://ruralcommittee.hrsa.gov/nacpubs.asp.

National Association for Home Health Care and Hospice (2006). *Basic Statistics about Home Health Care.* http://www.nahc.org/04HC_Stats.pdf. (accessed on April, 2019).

National Institute for Occupational Safety and Health (2010). *NIOSH hazard review: Occupational hazards in home health care*. Washington, DC: Centres for Disease Control and Prevention.

National Sample Survey (2004). Chronic disease profile of elderly in Home health care: The missing link in health delivery system for Indian elderly population—A narrative review. *International Journal of Research Foundation of Hospital & Health Care Administration* July-December, *5*(2): 89-94.

Naylor, M.D., D.A. Brooten, R.L. Campbell, G. Maislin, K.M. McCauley, and J.S. Schwartz (2004). Transitional care of older adults hospitalized with heart failure: a randomized, controlled trial. *Journal of the American Geriatrics Society*, *52*(5): 675-84.

Neff, D.F., E. Madigan. and G. Narsavage (2003). APN-directed transitional home health care model: achieving positive outcomes for patients with COPD. *Home Health Nurse, 21*: 543-50.

Nelson, Robert G.V. Shane Pankratz, Donica M. Ghahate, Jeanette Bobelu, Thomas Faber, and Vallabh O. Shah (2018). Home-based kidney care, patient activation, and risk factors for CKD progression in Zuni Indians. *Clinical Journal of the American Society of Nephrology*, *13*(12): 1801-09. http://www. ncbi.nlm. nih.gov/pmc/articles/PMC6302341.doi: 10.2215/ CJN.06910618

Oberst, M., and R.H. James (1985). Patient and spouse adjustment following cancer surgery. *Journal of Clinical Nursing, 7*(1): 46-57.

Ohaeri, J. (2003). The burden of caregiving in families with a mental illness. *Current Opinion in Psychiatry*, *16*(4): 457-65.

Oresland, S., S. Maatta, A. Norberg, M.W. Jorgensen, K. Lutzen (2008). Nurses as guests or professionals in home health care. *Nursing Ethics, 15*(3): 371-83.

Ortman, J.M., V.A. Velkoff, and H. Hogan (2014). *An Aging Nation: The Older Population in the United States, Current Population Reports*. US Census Bureau. https://www.census. gov/prod/2014pubs/p25-1140.pdf. (accessed July 10, 2019).

O'Toole, G. (2012). *Communication core interpersonal skills for health professionals*. 2nd ed. Chatswood: Elsevier.

Ory, M.G., and D.M. Cox (1994). Forging ahead: linking health and behaviour to improve quality of life in older people. *Social Indicators Research, 33*(1-3): 89-120.

Parth, S. (2022). Cancer medicines may get cheaper: India UICC prez. In *Times of India*. Chandigarh (Times Nation). Monday, 26 September. p. 7.

Patel, V., and M. Prince (2001). Ageing and mental health in a developing country: who cares? Qualitative studies from Goa, India. *Psychological Medicine, 31*(1): 29-38.

Patel, Vikram., A.K. Shiva Kumar, V.K. Paul, K.D. Rao, and K.S. Reddy (2011). Universal health care in India: The Time is Right. *The Lancet, 377*(9764): 448-49.

Pezzolesi, C.F. Schifano, J. Pickles *et al.* (2010). Clinical handover incident reporting in one UK general hospital. *International Journal Quarterly Health Care, 22*(5): 396-401.

Philp, I., K.J. McKee, P. Meldrum, B.R. Ballinger, M.L.N. Gilhooly, D.S. Gordon, W.J. Mutch and J.E. Whittick (1995). Community care for demented and non-demented elderly people: a comparison study of financial burden, service use, and unmet needs in family supporters. *Biomedical Journal, 310*: 1503-06.

Piko, B. (1999). Work related stress among nurses: a challenge for health care institutions. *Journal of Royal Society of Health, 199*: 156-62.

Prinja, S., P. Bahuguna, A. Duseja, M. Kaur, and Y.K. Chawla (2018). Cost of intensive care treatment for liver disorders at tertiary care level in India. *Pharmaco Economics Open, 2*(2): 179-90. doi: 10.1007/s41669-017-0041-4.

Rajan, S.I (2001). Social Assistance for poor elderly: how effective. *Economic and Political Weekly, 36*: 613-17.

Rajan, R.G., and E.S. Prasad (2008). A pragmatic approach to capital account liberalization. *Journal of Economic Perspectives 22*(3): 149-72.

Rajan, S.I., and S. Aiyar (2008). Population ageing in India. In *Institutional Provisions and Care for the Aged: Perspectives from Asia and Europe*. S.I. Rajan, C. Risseeuw, and M. Perera, eds. pp. 39-54. New Delhi: Anthem Press.

Rajan, S.I. and S. Kumar (2003). Living arrangements among Indian elderly: new evidence from National Family Health Survey. *Economic and Political Weekly, 38*(3): 75-80.

Rajan, S.I., and Sreerupa (2008). Disease, disability and health care utilization among the aged. In *Institutional Provisions and Care for the Aged: Perspectives from Asia and Europe*. S.I. Rajan, C. Risseeuw, and M. Perera, eds., pp. 39-54. New Delhi: Anthem Press.

Raju, S. (2000). Ageing in India: An overview. In *Gerontological Social Work in India: Some Issues and Perspectives*. M. Desai and S. Raju, eds. New Delhi: B.R. Publishing.

Raju, S. (2006). *Ageing in India in the 21st Century: A Research Agenda. Mumbai: The Harmony Initiative.* http://harmonyindia.org/hdownloads/Monograph_FINAL. pdf.

Rao, M. (2006). Economic and Financial Aspects of Ageing in India. Paper presented at the UN Regional Workshop on Gender-Responsive Health Security for the Elderly, September 18-19, Seoul, Republic of Korea. Available: http://www.unescap.org/esid/gad/issues/Socialprotection/Report-RegWkshp-HealthSecurity-18-19Sep06-Seoul.pdf.

Rastogi, T., M. Vaz, D. Spiegelman, K.S. Reddy, A.V. Bharathi, M.J. Stampfer, W.C. Willett and A. Ascherio (2004). Physical activity and risk of coronary heart disease in India. *International Journal of Epidemiology, 33*(4): 759-67. doi:10.1093/ije/dyh042.

Robison, J., R. Fortinsky, A. Kleppinger, N. Shugrue, and M. Porter (2009). A broader view of family caregiving: effects of caregiving and caregiver conditions on depressive symptoms, health, work, and social isolation. *Journal of Gerontology: Psychological Sciences & Social Sciences, 64*: 788-98.

Rodrigues, I., and M.F. Megie (2006). Prevalence of chronic wounds in Quebec home care: an exploratory study. *Ostomy Wound Manage, 52*(5): 46-8, 50, 52-57.

Rodat, C. (2014). *Training New York City's home care aides: A landscape survey.* New York: PHI.

Romagnoli, K.M., S.M. Handler, and H. Hochheiser (2013). Home Care: more than just a visiting nurse. *Biomedical Journal of Quality & Safety, 22*(12): 972-74. doi: 10.1136/bmjqs-2013-002339.

Romito.F., G. Goldzweig, C. Cormio, M. Hagedoorn, and B.L. Andersen (2013). Informal caregiving for cancer patients. *Cancer, 119*: 2160-69, doi: 10.1002/cncr.28057.

Roy, G.S. (1994). Morbidity related epidemiological determinants in Indian aged: An overview. In *Public Health Implications of Ageing in India*, C.R. Ramachandran and B. Shah, eds., pp. 114-25. New Delhi: Indian Council of Medical Research.

Russell, D., R.J. Rosati, T.R. Peng, Y. Barron, and E. Andreopoulos (2013). Continuity in the provider of home health aide services and the likelihood of patient improvement in activities of daily living. *Home Health Care Management & Practice, 25*: 6-12. doi:10.1177/1084822312453046.

Sansoni, J., E. Vellone, and P. Giovanni (2004). Anxiety and depression in community-dwelling Italian Alzheimer's disease caregivers. *International Journal of Nursing Practice, 10*: 93-100. [PubMed: 15056348].

Sarkar, S. and K.S. Anand (2013). Assessing the burden on family caregivers. *Asia Pacific Journal of Research, I*(X): 64-74.

Schulte, P.A., R.J. Guerin, A.L. Schill, A. Bhattacharya, T.R. Cunningham, S.P. Pandalai, and C.M. Stephenson (2015). Considerations for incorporating "well-being" in public policy for workers and workplaces. *American Journal of Public Health, 105*: e31–e44. doi:10.2105/AJPH.2015.302616.

Schulz, R., P. Visintainer, and G.M. Williamson (1990). Psychiatric and physical morbidity effects of caregiving. *Journal of Gerontology, 45*(5): 181-91.

Schulz, R., and S.R. Beach (1999). Caregiving as a risk factor for mortality. The caregiver health effect study. *Journal of the American Medical Association, 282*: 2215-19.

Seavey, D. (2010). Caregivers on the front line: building a better direct care workforce. *Generations, 34*(4): 27-35.

Serfelova, R., K. Ziakova, and L. Jezova (2012). Family caregiving at the end of life care. *Journal of Nursing, Social Studies, Public Health and Rehabilitation, 2013*, 62-71.

Selltiz, C., M. Jahoda, M. Deutsch, and S.W. Cook (1962). *Research Methods in Social Relations.* New York: Holt Rinehart and Winston.

Selvaraj, S., A. Karan, and S. Madheswaran (2010). *Elderly workforce in India: labour market participation, wage differentials and contribution to household income.* Unpublished report. New Delhi: Public Health Foundation of India.

Sergi-Swinehart, P. (1985). Hospice Home Care: how to get patients home and help them stay there. *Seminars in Oncology, 12*: 461-65.

Shah, B., and A.K. Prabhakar (1997). Chronic morbidity profile among elderly. *Indian Journal of Medical Research, 106*: 265-72.

Sheikh, M.S., and S. Jan. Shah (2021). Modified Kuppuswamy socio-economic scale updated for the year 2021. *Indian Journal of Forensic and Community Medicine, 8*(1): 1-3.

Sherbourne, C.D., and A.L. Stewart (1991). The MOS Social Support Survey. *Social Science & Medicine, 32*: 705-14.

Shrestha, L.B. (2000). Population aging in developing countries. *Health Affairs, 19*(3): 204-12.

Simon-Rusinowitz, L., D.M. Loughlin, R. Chan, K.J. Mahoney, G. Martinez Garcia, and K. Ruben (2010). Expanding the consumer-directed workforce by attracting and retaining unaffiliated workers. *Care Management Journal, 11*(2): 74-82.

Singh, A. (2017). Home health care: The missing link in health delivery system for Indian elderly population—A narrative review. *International Journal of Research Foundation of Hospital & Health Care Administration*, July-December, *5*(2): 89-94.

Smeds., A.L., C. Tishelman, S. Runesdotter, and R. Lindqvist (2014). Staffing and resource adequacy strongly related to RNs' assessment of patient safety: A national study of RNs working in acute-care hospitals in Sweden. *Biomedical Journal of Quality & Safety, 23*: 242-49.

Sokolovsky, J. (2001). Living Arrangements of Older Persons and Family Support in less Developed Countries. *Population Bulletin of the United Nations*, Spl. Issue (Living arrangements of older persons—Critical issues and policy responses) *42/43*: 162-92.

Solet, D.J. (2005). Lost in translation: challenges-to-physician communication during patient hand-offs. *Academic Medicine Journal, 80*:1094-99.

Sreerupa (2006). Gender, ageing and widowhood: health vulnerability and socio-economic influences. M.Phil. Dissertation. New Delhi: Jawaharlal Nehru University.

Stacey, C.L. (2011). *The caring self: The work experiences of home care aides*. New York: Cornell University Press.

Stone, R.I., and S.L. Dawson (2008). The origins of better jobs better care. *Gerontologist, 48*(Spec No. 1): 5-13.

Stenberg, U., C.M. Ruland and C. Miaskowski (2010). Review of the literature on the effects of caring for a patient with cancer. *Psycho-Oncology, 19*: 1013-25.

Stommel, M., C.W. Given, and B.A. Given (1993). The cost of cancer home care to families. *Cancer, 71*:1867-74.

Stone, R.I., and J.M. Wiener (2001 October). *Who will care for us? Addressing the long-term care workforce crisis*. Princeton, NJ: The Robert Wood Johnson Foundation.

Sudha, S., C. Suchindran, E.J. Mutran, S.I. Rajan, and P.S. Sarma (2006). Marital status, family ties and self-rated health among elders in South India. *Journal of Cross-Cultural Gerontology, 21*(3-4): 103-20.

Suk Jung, H., H.K. Kim, and S. Judith (2013). Clinical outcomes and quality of life of home health care patients. *Asian Nursing Research, 7*: 53-60.

The Dartmouth Atlas of Health Care (2012). Inpatient days per decedent during the last six months of life, by gender and level of care intensity. End of life care. The Dartmouth Institute 278 Home Health Care Management & Practice, *28*(4) for Health

Policy and Clinical Practice. http://www.dartmouthatlas.org/data/topic/topic.aspx?cat=18. (accessed August 12, 2021).

Terence, Ng., C. Harrington, M. Musumeci, and Erica L. Reaves (2012). *Medicaid home and community-based services programmes: Data Update.* Kaiser Family Foundation. http://kff.org/medicaid/report/medicaid-home-and-community-based-services-programs2012-data-update/. Published in November 2015 (accessed August 22, 2022).

Temmink, D., A.L. Francke, J.B.F. Hutten, J. van der Zee and H. Huijer Abu-Saad (2000). Innovation in the nursing care of the chronically ill: a literature review from an international perspective. *Journal of Advanced Nursing, 31*: 1449-58.

Thome, B., A.K. Dykes, and I.R. Hallberg (2003). Home care with regard to definition, care recipients, content and outcomes: systematic literature review. *Journal of Clinical Nursing, 12*: 860-72.

Thomas, A (2017). *Communicate, Care, Cure: A guide to health care communication,* 2nd ed. New Delhi: Wolters Kluwer (India Pvt. Ltd).

Tsigaroppoulos, T., T.E. Mazaris, E. Chatzidarellis, A. Skolarikos, I. Varkarakis, and C. Deliveliotis (2009). Problems faced by relatives caring for cancer patients at home. *International Journal of Nursing Practice, 15*(1): 1-6. doi: 10.1111/j.1440-172X.2008.01725.x.

Todd, K., S. Roberts, and C. Black (2002). The living with cancer education programme I. Development of an Australian education and support programme for cancer patients and their family and friends. *European Journal of Cancer Care, 11*: 271-79.

Townsend, J., A.O. Frank, D. Fermont, S. Dryer, O. Karran, A. Walgrove, and M. Piper (1990). Terminal cancer care and patients' preference for place of death: a prospective study. *British Medical Journal, 301*(6749): 415-17.

U.S. Bureau of Labor Statistics (2009). *State occupational employment and wage estimates: Washington.* Washington, DC: Author.

United Nations Department of Economic and Social Affairs, Population Division (2008). *World Population Prospects (2008 Revision)*. http://esa.un.org/unpp/index.asp? panel=2.

Ugur, O., A. Elcigil, D. Arslan, and A. Sonmez (2014). Responsibilities and difficulties of caregivers of cancer patients in home care. *Asian Pacific Journal of Cancer Prevention, 15*: 725-29.

Van Walraven C., C. Bennett, A. Jennings, P.C. Austin and A.J. Forster (2011). Proportion of hospital readmissions deemed avoidable: a systematic review. *CMAJ: Canadian Medical Association Journal, 183*: E391-402.

Varela, G., L. Varona, K. Anderson, and J. Sansoni (2011). Alzheimer's care at home: a focus on caregivers strain. *Professioni Infermieristiche, 64*(2): 113-17.

Vaz, M. and A.V. Bharathi (2004). Perceptions of the intensity of specific physical activities in Bangalore, South India: Implications for Exercise Prescription. *Journal of the Association of Physicians in India, 52*: 541-44

Vyasamoorthy, P. (2014). Elder abuse by professional care givers in residential setting: some case studies. International Conference on Elder Dignity and Abuse: Trivandrum, Kerala. https://www.researchgate.net/publication/262070344_ Elder_abuse_by_Professional_Care_givers_in_Residential_Setting.

Waite, L.J. (2004). Ageing, health, and public policy: demographic and economic perspectives. *Population and Development Review, 30*(Suppl.): 239-65.

Wang, S.Y., Y. Zhao, and X.Y. Zang (2014). Continuing care for older patients during the transitional period. *Chinese Nursing Research, 1*: 5-13.

Ward-Griffin, C., and P. McKeever (2000). Relationships between nurses and family caregivers: partners in care? *Advances in Nursing Science, 22*(3): 89-103.

Welch, H.G., D.E. Wennberg and W.P. Welch (1996). The use of Medicare home health care services. *The New England Journal of Medicine, 335*(5): 324-29.

Weaver, F.M., S.L. Hughes, O. Almagor, R. Wixson, L. Manheim, B. Fulton, R. Singer (2003). Comparison of two home health care protocols for total joint replacement. *Journal of the American Geriatrics Society, 51*(4): 523-28.

Wen, K.Y. and H.D. Gustafson (2004). Needs assessment for cancer patients and their families. *Health Quality of Life Outcomes, 2*: 1-12.

Wilner, M.A., and A. Wyatt (1999). *Initiative by paraprofessional health care Institute*. Washington, DC: AARP.

Wilkerson, K.B. (2001). *No Place Like Home: A History of Nursing and Home Care in the United States*. Baltimore: Johns Hopkins University Press.

Wilkerson, K.B. (2007). Care of the chronically ill at home: an unresolved dilemma in health policy for the United States. *Milbank Quarterly*, *85*(4): 611-39.

World Health Organization (2002). *Reducing Stigma and Discrimination against Older People with Mental Disorders.* Geneva: World Health Organization and World Psychiatric Association. http://whqlibdoc.who.int/hq/2002/WHO_MSD_MBD_ 02.3.

Xavier, V.K., S. Sarkar, R. Rao, R. Padukone, R. Dorai, U. Maiya, and K.V. Varambally, Jagadeesh (2007). *Research Methodology*. Sikkim Manipal University of Health, Medical and Technological Sciences: Manipal Press Limited.

Yaffe, K., P. Fox, R. Newcomer, L. Sands, K. Lindquist, K. Dane and K.E. Covinsky (2002). Patient and caregiver characteristics and nursing home placement in patients with Dementia *The Journal of the American Medical Association*, *287* (16): 2090-2097.

Zarit, S.H., K.E. Reever, and J.Bach-Peterson (1980). Relatives of the impaired elderly: correlates of feelings of burden. *Gerontologist, 20*: 649-55.

Zarit, S.H., O.N., and J.M. Zarit (1985). *The memory and behaviour problems checklist, in families under stress: caring for the patient with Alzheimer's disease and related disorders*. New York: University Press.

Zimmer, J.G., A. Groth-Juncker, and J. McCusker (1985). A randomized controlled study of a home health care team. *American Journal of Public Health, 75*: 134-41.

Internet Cites

https://www.niddk.nih.gov/health-information/kidney-disease/chronic-kidney-disease-ckd/what-is-chronic-kidney-disease
www.kanomodel.com
https://www.rch.org.au/rchcpg/hospital_clinical_guideline_index/Wound_assessment_and_management/
https://www.peacehealth.org/medical-topics/id/abq1767
https://www.affordablemedical.com/how-to-change-adult-diapers/
https://www.yashodahospitals.com/blog/endocrine-disorders-symptoms-causes-diagnosis-treatments/
http://www.albrightstonebridge.com/health care_india/
http://health care.financialexpress.com/201101/anniversaryspecial09.shtml http://silverinnings.blogspot.ae/2011/05/support-for-our-elders-1298-senior.html
http://www.health-policy-systems.com/content/9/1/42
www.lifecircle.in

Index